14-120-357

ADMINISTRATION
OF
ACTIVITY THERAPY SERVICE

ADMINISTRATION
OF
ACTIVITY THERAPY SERVICE

Compiled and Edited by

GERALD S. O'MORROW, M.Ed.
Coordinator of Activity Therapy
Logansport State Hospital
Logansport, Indiana

With

12 Contributing Authors

And a Foreword by

S. T. Ginsberg, M.D.
Commissioner, Department of Mental Health
Indianapolis, Indiana

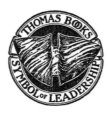

CHARLES C THOMAS · PUBLISHER
Springfield · Illinois · U.S.A.

Published and Distributed Throughout the World by
CHARLES C THOMAS • PUBLISHER
BANNERSTONE HOUSE
301-327 East Lawrence Avenue, Springfield, Illinois, U.S.A.
NATCHEZ PLANTATION HOUSE
735 North Atlantic Boulevard, Fort Lauderdale, Florida, U.S.A.

© *1966 by* CHARLES C THOMAS • PUBLISHER
Library of Congress Catalog Card Number: 65-25744

With THOMAS BOOKS careful attention is given to all details of manufacturing and design. It is the Publisher's desire to present books that are satisfactory as to their physical qualities and artistic possibilities and appropriate for their particular use. THOMAS BOOKS will be true to those laws of quality that assure a good name and good will.

Printed in the United States of America
N-1

THE AUTHORS

Ora R. Ackerman, Ed.D.

Coordinator of Activity Therapy, Department of Mental Health, Indianapolis, Indiana.

Formerly, Coordinator of Activity Therapy, Evansville State Hospital, Evansville, Indiana.

Representative to the Council for the Advancement of Hospital Recreation, Hospital Recreation Section, American Recreation Society.

Geographical Representative, American Recreation Society.

Representative, Great Lakes District Advisory Committee, National Recreation Association.

President-Elect, Indiana Parks and Recreation Association.

Past-Chairman, Ill and Handicapped Section, Indiana Parks and Recreation Association.

Formerly, Member, Executive Committee, Hospital Recreation Section, American Recreation Society.

Daryl B. Adrian, M.A.

Instructor in English, University of Missouri, Columbia, Missouri.

Formerly, Supervisor, Educational Therapy Department, The Menninger Foundation, Topeka, Kansas.

Formerly, Lecturer in English, Evening College, Washburn University, Topeka, Kansas.

Shirley M. Bowing, M.A., O.T.R.

Supervisor, Vocational-Industrial Therapy, Western State Hospital, Fort Steilacoom, Washington.

Formerly, Head, Division of Occupational Therapy, Department of Physical Medicine and Rehabilitation, University of Washington School of Medicine, Seattle, Washington.

Bruce Fessenden, O.T.R.

Industrial Therapy Consultant, Bureau of Mental Health Services, Department of Public Welfare, Harrisburg, Pennsylvania.

Formerly, Industrial Therapy Supervisor, Retreat State Hospital, Pennsylvania.

Formerly, Chairman, Psychiatric Subcommittee, American Occupational Therapy Association.

Herbert Gerjouy, Ph.D.

Research Psychologist, Research Division, Educational Testing Service, Princeton, New Jersey.

Consultant, New Jersey Bureau of Research in Neurology and Psychiatry, Trenton, New Jersey.

Formerly, Chairman, Department of Psychology, University of Toledo, Ohio.

Developer of Industrial Therapy Curriculum, University of Toledo, Ohio.

Robert Goril, R.R.T.

Activity Program Coordinator, Philadelphia State Hospital, Philadelphia, Pennsylvania.

Formerly, Industrial Therapy Supervisor, Norristown State Hospital, Norristown, Pennsylvania.

Formerly, Industrial Therapy Director, Terrell State Hospital, Terrell, Texas.

Past-Chairman, Industrial Therapy Section, American Association for Rehabilitation Therapy.

Formerly, Representative, Industrial Therapy Section, Registry Committee, American Association for Rehabilitation Therapy.

Lucille Kline Leuschner, Certified Librarian

Librarian, Agnews State Hospital, San Jose, California.

Formerly, Librarian, Veterans Administration Hospital, Tomah, Wisconsin, and U. S. Naval Hospital, Portsmouth, Virginia.

Past Chairman, Membership Committee, Wisconsin Library Association.

Albert L. Meuli, M.Ed.

Supervisor of Activity Therapies, Division of Mental Health, Department of Institutions, Olympia, Washington.

Formerly, Coordinator of Activity Therapy, Dr. Norman Beatty Memorial Hospital, Westville, Indiana.

Past-Chairman, Hospital Recreation Section, American Recreation Society.

Past-President, Indiana Parks and Recreation Association.

Vice-President, Washington State Recreation Society.

Gerald O'Morrow, M.Ed.

Coordinator of Activity Therapy, Logansport State Hospital, Logansport, Indiana.

Formerly, Director of Recreation, Dr. Norman Beatty Memorial Hospital, Westville, Indiana.

Past-Chairman, Hospital Recreation Section, American Recreation Society.

Formerly, Member, Executive Committee, Ill and Handicapped Section, Indiana Parks and Recreation Association.

Formerly, Secretary, Ill and Handicapped Section, Indiana Parks and Recreation Association.

Leighton A. Price, M.S.

Research Assistant, Research Division, Educational Research Group, Educational Testing Service, Princeton, New Jersey.

M. Geraldine Shevlin, M.A., O.T.R.

Head, Division of Occupational Therapy, Department of Physical Medicine and Rehabilitation, University of Washington School of Medicine, Seattle, Washington.

Myrtle Fish Thompson, B.A., R.M.T.

Director of Music and Creative Art Therapies, Essex County Overbrook Hospital, Cedar Grove, New Jersey.

Formerly, Music Director, Lyons Veterans Administration Hospital, New Jersey.

Past-President and Honorary Life Member, National Association for Music Therapy.

FOREWORD

THE SCIENCE OF MEDICINE recognizes that man is a complex animal and that the treatment of disease requires full consideration of the individual as a whole person and not just a diseased organ needing special care.

The treatment of the whole person concept has turned hospitals into small communities which must provide, in addition to medicine, bed, and board, programs of work, recreation, and education. In point of fact, a modern mental hospital and many general medical and surgical hospitals are self-contained communities, where life goes on with a full range of activity, the same as one would require when living at home. For many it is home. For others it is preparation for living at home in the mainstream of community life.

This wide range of activities, particularly the programs usually grouped together as Activity Therapy, requires imaginative leadership and coordination to assure harmony in performance and singleness of purpose, which should be helping to get the patient well and back home to family and friends.

Good management principles require the grouping together of similar activities, under expert supervision or coordination, to allow the smallest number of people reporting to the chief executive or his deputy (or deputies). This is particularly true in a hospital where there is an almost endless number of important and necessary people representing a specialized discipline or skill. No hospital administrator, chief of staff, or clinical director can function effectively with twenty or more people reporting directly to him.

This text spells out clearly how sound management principles can be applied to a group of treatment modalities, coordinated for efficiency and harmony in performance, without destroying the uniqueness of each discipline or the traditional doctor-therapist relationship. Each can continue to make its special contribution to the ultimate recovery of the patient.

ix

I am particularly pleased that this first book is being edited by a Coordinator of Activity Therapy in the Indiana Department of Mental Health, where so many pioneering efforts have been undertaken in past years. My gratitude also goes to the many other members of the Department who have contributed their expert knowledge to this text.

S. T. GINSBERG, M. D.
Commissioner
Department of Mental Health
Indianapolis, Indiana

PREFACE

THE IDEA FOR THIS BOOK resulted from the labor and uncertainty that the author has experienced as an administrator of an Activity Therapy Service within a public institution, as well as discussing and listening to mutual problems by other coordinators, directors, and state consultants who are responsible for similar services. During the years as an administrator, the author was and still is confronted with looking to other texts for a philosophy or guide to assist him in administrating such a program. To my knowledge, no book or seres of articles to date has attempted to put forth, within one publication, the philosophy and theory of the various departments that usually constitute the Activity Therapy Service and the administration of them.

This book is concerned primarily with administration as it can be applied to an Activity Therapy Service. Although this publication is slanted toward the administration of the service within federal, state, public, and private mental health institutions, there is no reason why the principles expressed herein cannot be applied within general medical and surgical hospitals having a rehabilitation department. It is realized by the author that the administration of such a service varies in different agencies and institutions, but it is hoped that the book will give a basic foundation and manner of approach to those who are now, or will be in the future, administrators of an activity therapy service. The author also seeks to enlighten those who are directly related, but outside of the activity therapy service, and those indirectly related to the philosophy and functioning of such a service.

The Activity Therapy Service, as defined in this book, is a philosophy of administration as applied to all specialties working within this specific area of service. No attempt is made in this publication to defend or extol any of the specialties discussed since it is the firm conviction of the author that each specialty makes a significant contribution regardless of the setting. At the

same time, although there are similarities and differences, with
more similarities than differences, between the specialties intensified research is needed before an overall theory concerning functional coordination can be developed.

Frequent reference is made to *Project 52: A study in Adjunctive Therapies Coordinator* which was supported by the Office of
Vocational Rehabilitation Administration. This study, although
now nearly seven years old, still contains invaluable information
in the opinion of the author as it relates to administrative and
clinical coordination as well as being the only reliable study to
date involving all of the specialties discussed within this publication.

Part I serves as an introduction and orientation to the specialties that constitute the Activity Therapy Service. Since the author
did not feel complete confidence in the philosophy and techniques
of all the various services, he requested the assistance of others
who are specialists within their profession, or have had a considerable amount of experience in these areas to provide the
material for this section.

Part II deals with the organization aspects of the service, to
include organizational patterns of these services within the various
agencies and institutions, the scope and specific goals of the total
program, programming, principles and practices of administrative management, staff development and in-service education programs, facilities and equipment requirements, records and reports,
budget planning, evaluation, and research.

The appendix is provided for assistance to those who are interested in knowing about schools of training within the specific
disciplines, professional organizations, job descriptions of the
various agencies employing an administrator responsible for such
a service and a selected library reference of books for use in the
Patient's Library. In addition, a very comprehensive bibliography
of reading references in the area of vocational and industrial
therapy is offered. This, I believe, is the first time such a comprehensive bibliography has ever been prepared in this area.

Throughout the book, examples of operation within the Activity Therapy Service of Logansport (Indiana) State Hospital
are used. This, in no way, suggests that this is a superior method

to any other or a substitute for any other, because the author feels there is no correct or wrong way since every agency operates differently. They are used only as examples to show how one specific hospital handles the specific problem or situation.

The author is indebted and fortunate to have the help of many associates, colleagues, and others interested in this general problem of administration. Several have contributed chapters; others have assisted in the preparation of certain chapters. Those contributors who gave of their time and effort under heavy work loads to assist in making this publication a first are listed in the table of contents. In addition to these, various colleagues have aided in the preparation of the book by suggesting additions and revisions; specifically, Albert Meuli, who began as my co-editor but who had to later withdraw because of additional work assignments and further education, Ora Ackerman, Ed. D., Coordinator of Activity Therapy and Martin Meyer, Ed. D., Director of Evaluation and Planning, both of the Department of Mental Health (Indiana) who encouraged the writing of this publication from the start, and James Pratt, Director of Adjunctive Therapy, The Menninger Clinic, who along with Mr. Meuli and Dr. Meyer reviewed the whole book and served as critics.

Generous service was provided by Mrs. Laurine Schawitsch who typed the original draft, Mrs. Marian Bonhomme, who did the complete final typing of the whole book, and Mrs. Susanne Jargstorf, former Medical Librarian, who secured the books and magazines, sometimes on a moment's notice.

The editor also wishes to acknowledge, with thanks, the help of the various individuals and organizations that assisted in providing or gathering materials for this publication. These were from the various state Departments, Divisions, or Bureaus of Mental Health, Hygiene, or Hospital Services, Lee Helsel, former Chief, Rehabilitation Services and his former assistant, Norman Sayen (California) ; Louis E. DeMoll, Supervisor of Rehabilitation and Casework Services (Texas) ; Elizabeth Ridgway, O.T.R., Patient Activities Consultant (Pennsylvania) ; Thomas J. Clark, Chief, Activity Therapy (Illinois), and Patricia Thornton, O.T.R., Chief, Activity Therapy (Wisconsin) ; from public and private psychiatric hospitals, Sidney Acuff, Director, Activity

Therapies, Western (Washington) State Hospital; Margaret Adams, O.T.R., Coordinator of Rehabilitation Therapies, Terrell (Texas) State Hospital; Charlotte L. Cox, Coordinator; Activity Therapy Services, Athens (Ohio) State Hospital; Fred Humphrey, Director of Activity Therapies, Jamestown (North Dakota) State Hospital, and John D. Patton, M. D., Clinical Director, Highland Hospital, Ashville, North Carolina; from general medical and surgical hospitals and rehabilitation centers, Jean Chapman, Supervisor, Department of Physical Medicine, University Hospital, University of Wisconsin; Harry Dando, Coordinator, Rehabilitation Center, Fairview Hospital, Minneapolis; Ralston Bauer, former Director, Activity Therapies, Minneapolis (Minnesota) General Hospital; Shirley Wolf, O.T.R., former Supervisor, Occupational Therapy, Cleveland (Ohio) Clinic; Roy E. Patten, Ll.D., Executive Director, Crossroads Rehabilitation Center, Indianapolis, Indiana, and Frances J. Kane, Jr., M.D., Acting Director, Inpatient Service, North Carolina (Chapel Hill) Memorial Hospital; from federal agencies, C. C. Bream, Jr., former Chief, Recreation Services and Richard Silver, Director, Personnel Services, both from the Veterans Administration, Washington, D. C.; August Hoenack, Chief, Architectural and Engineering Branch, Division of Hospitals and Medical Facilities, Marjorie E. Moore, Research Program Analyst, Division of Research Grants and Demonstrations, both from the Department of Health, Education, and Welfare, Washington, D.C.; and from professional organizations, Mildred Schwagmeyer, O.T.R., Assistant Director of Education, and Marjorie Fish, O.T.R., former Executive Director, both representing the American Occupational Therapy Association; National Association of Music Therapy, Inc., Lawrence, Kansas; Pat Vosburgh, Editor, *Mental Hospitals,* American Psychiatric Association, Washington, D. C., the American Hospital Association, and the Hogg Foundation for Mental Health.

I am also grateful for the editorial assistance from Harry Edgren, Ed. D., on Chapter 12, Mr. James Frohbeiter, M. H. A., for his review of Chapters 9 and 10, Mr. Lawrence C. Olson, architect, for his floor design in Chapter 12, and finally to the staff of Charles C Thomas, Publisher, for their total assistance and undertaking of this publication.

The author welcomes comments, good or bad, from all individuals serving presently as administrators in such a service, and hopes, in addition, that this publication will act as a springboard to others to analyze and develop further what is herein written.

G. S. O'M.

CONTENTS

ADMINISTRATION
OF
ACTIVITY THERAPY SERVICE

Part I
Foundation of the Activity Therapy Service

Chapter I

THE CONCEPT OF ACTIVITY THERAPY

GERALD S. O'MORROW, M. Ed.

IT IS INTERESTING to note that during the past twenty-five years, but especially since World War II, there has been a considerable expansion and a division of labor according to the training of individuals within the professions and/or specialties that make-up the activity therapies. This has primarily been true in the federal and state psychiatric hospitals, although hospitals for the treatment of general medical and surgical patients, emotionally ill and handicapped children, and long-term patients have witnessed a similar expansion.[1][2][3][4][5][6][7]

These professions and/or specialties which have been involved in this expansion and which provide activities to meet the needs and interests of the patients include occupational therapy, medical recreation, music therapy, vocational and/or industrial therapy, educational therapy, volunteer services, and patient library services. Although these specialties usually constitute the basic departments or units of the activity therapies, there may be other specialties which operate as a separate department, service, or sub-section of a specialty within the total framework. These other specialties may be dance therapy, drama therapy, art therapy, horticulture therapy, manual arts therapy, corrective therapy, and in some agencies, physical therapy, audiology and speech therapy, and blind rehabilitation.

This expansion of services has, in turn, brought many new administrative problems to departments or divisions of mental health, superintendents, managers, and administrators of various public and private hospitals. Possibly, the tendency towards specialization within this country has contributed to this situation. Each agency, therefore, has had to face these problems and develop solutions for them, commensurate with the tax dollar or public funds available, staff and facilities presently available, and particular federal, state, and community hospital authorities. As Doniger and Dundon[7] point out, "Each time a hospital became aware of, or interested in the possible contribution of a new kind of activity as therapy, a new department or sub-service was set up in a different section of its organization or physical plant in order to include the new activity. . . . The results of such piecemeal, rather than overall planning, have not always been completely satisfactory." Dunlop[8] has observed that one of the major problems existing today in the rehabilitation process "is the development of methods that will ensure thorough-going integration of all services."

As in any period of change, the major barrier to achievement of progress is creating an awareness of the need to change. Present problems can not be successfully managed with yesterday's solutions. Therefore, one important factor which has developed from the situations mentioned above is the grouping together of similar therapeutic specialties into an activity therapy service or department under the direction and leadership of an administrator.[1 2 3 4 5 6 9] Such grouping takes advantage of the specialized knowledge and skill of each discipline which can be, in turn, fully utilized for the benefit of the patient. Thornton,[10] in discussing the roles of the specialties in Wisconsin, observed that in the past, the different specialties were defined on the basis of the medias each utilized, while, at the present time, "the role of the various specialties are defined on the basis of the objectives and methods rather than the media used."

Project 52: A Study in Adjunctive Therapies Coordination[11] pointed out, "that when (mental) hospitals employ a large number of full-time activity therapy staff, there is a tendency to coordinate more fully activity therapy programs." Key,[6] in conjunction with this same study, found that "there is a need for and a trend toward administrative coordination in hospitals as well as in state departments of mental hygiene." He goes on to say that "there is a . . . trend toward emphasizing the similarities among the activity groups and de-emphasizing their differences based on . . . (their) skills." Further support of this thesis is given by Meyer:[12] "The extent of inclusion of these services within a separate department usually depends upon precedent and the ingenuity of the agency in providing good administrative systems to avoid costly duplication." Cox[13] not only feels that it offers a less complicated assistance to the patient, but is more practical from an economic standpoint.

Another indication of the trend toward the grouping of similar services can be found in the conference held at Allentown, Pennsylvania, which was concerned with the development of a "Core-curriculum" for the training of all activity therapists. A second conference sponsored by the Washburn Project[1] discussed the advantages and disadvantages of coordination and the problems of training coordinators.

Specifically, the literature reveals that the grouping of these specialties, in a vast majority of cases, is done with six basic reasons in mind: (1) that the patient will benefit because all specialties will be working toward one goal; (2) that it protects the patient from competition among the specialties; (3) individual specialties will benefit because of their togetherness, thereby giving greater strength to the total program and enhancing its effectiveness; (4) it improves the communication of interdepartmental contacts; (5) there is equal status with other treatment services, and (6) it reduces the number of personnel reporting to and receiving direction from the clinical director; director of professional services, or chief of rehabilitation services. Moreover, the very multiplicity of all or part of these specialties each reporting to the clinical director can only lead to confusion, departmental jealousy, and extreme independence, not to say anything about the resulting fragmentary life for the patients. A situation in point was that in 1960, the Veterans Administration incorporated the recreation section within the Department of Physical Medicine and Rehabilitation Services, thereby bringing about better program planning, unity, and coordination.

To coordinate the grouping of these specialties, some state agencies, the Veterans Administration, general medical and surgical hospitals, have appointed or promoted from within one of the specific specialties, the service of a "coordinator," "director," or "chief," although the Washburn Study[1] did indicate that the coordinator may be from a work experience or academic specialization other than those previously mentioned. Briefly, the coordinator is primarily an administrator responsible for the total coordination of the other specialties as they relate to the administrative and clinical philosophy of the hospital. The Veterans Administration defines the role of the coordinator as being "responsible for administrative supervision of the functions of these various therapies (occupational therapy, recreation, etc.) and with other medical services and rehabilitation functions within the agency."[14] In some agencies, as will be discussed later, the administrator or director may be a physician.

The department or service for which the coordinator is responsible, within the various public and private mental health or hygiene agencies, is called, as an example, "Activity Therapy" in Indiana, Ohio, Washington, and Wisconsin; in California and Maryland, "Rehabilitation Services;" Minnesota uses "Rehabilitative Services;" in Pennsylvania, "Patient Activities," while Kansas, Michigan, and Tennessee use "Adjunctive Therapies;" and others use "Ancillary Services." It should be noted here that various private and public agencies utilize these same terms, at times, to denote a particular philosophy of treatment.* The Veterans Administration hospitals group their specialties within the

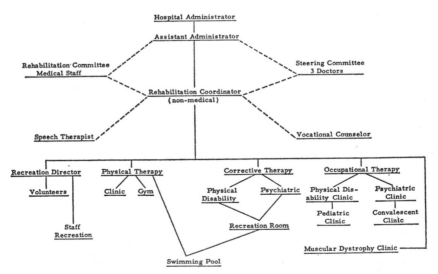

Figure 1. Organizational Chart, Fairview Hospital, Minneapolis, Minnesota (courtesy of Fairview Hospital).

*In this publication, the terms for the grouping of these specialized departments will be used only as a collective term.

department of "Physical Medicine and Rehabilitation Service" which had its beginning as a major service in the Department of Medicine and Surgery as early as 1946. General medical and surgical hospitals, specialty hospitals or homes, and homes for the long-term or aged use similar names of titles that have been previously mentioned. Regardless of name, the department services includes those programs which are of an activity nature, general or specific, performed directly with and for the benefit of patients.

Since the structure of the activity therapies or similar services vary so much in their lines of formal authority and organizational patterns within public and private hospitals, they will be fully explored in Chapter IX. However, two basic organizational charts (Figs. 1 and 2) are hereby inserted at this point to illustrate the relationship that one might find in a typical large institution employing a full activity therapies staff.*

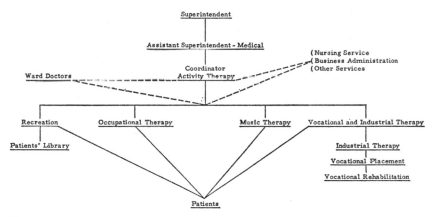

Figure 2. Organizational Chart, Department of Mental Health, Hospitals for the Mentally Ill, Indianapolis, Indiana (courtesy of Department of Mental Health).

GOALS OF ACTIVITY THERAPY

Although this book is primarily concerned with the concept and administrative aspects of an activity therapy service, it would be well to briefly review the goals of this service in both a neuropsychiatric setting and in a general medical and surgical hospital

*See Chapter IX for other organizational charts.

having a physical medicine and rehabilitation unit which serves the physically handicapped. It should be kept in mind that in many large general hospitals the physical medicine unit serves both the physically and mentally handicapped.

Relatively little has been written about the goals common to an activity therapy service in a public or private neuropsychiatric hospital. This is partly due to the newness of the concept as well as the continuing concern of each department in the development of their own particular goals. What has been written has revolved from within particular public and private hospitals and departments of mental health who have developed and are utilizing an activity therapy concept. Four goals most frequently mentioned in a neuropsychiatric setting are as follows:[15 16 17 18 19 20 21]

1. Opportunities are Provided for Structured Normal Activities of Daily Living. The activities are fashioned to help the patient deal with his basic problems and motivate him toward participation in less protected activities in a healthy way. The therapist uses the activity as a tool to bring about desired changes in behavior. In addition, the activity permits the healthy part of the patient's personality to continue to function.

2. Assist in Diagnostic and Personality Evaluation. The trained therapist assists with diagnostic and personality evaluation through observation of the patient while he is participating in the activity. The choice of the activity by the patient, the manner in which he participates, the interaction with other patients and therapist all assist in understanding the personality structure.

3. Augment Psychotherapy and Other Therapeutic Efforts. Opportunities for the expression of emotional needs and drives is available through the interpersonal relationship between activity therapist and patient, and the activity.

4. Assist the Patient to Bridge the Gap Between the Hospital and the Community. Opportunities are provided for work experience and utilization of community resources.

Specifically, the goals of a physical medicine and rehabilitation unit in a general medical and surgical hospital are designed to restore function to a maximum level to which the patient is capable, to evaluate the degree of impairment and the extent of residual capacity for social and economic activities and to furnish practical and effective motivation for rehabilitation.

While the total activity therapy service and the physical medicine and rehabilitation services have common goals, each of the services make different, though often overlapping contributions and they have different professional roots with different approaches and techniques.

SERVICES RENDERED IN DIFFERENT MEDICAL SETTINGS

The services rendered in different medical settings are many and varied and should not be looked upon as diversional activity, but according to Kahn,[22] "viewed and used as primary forces for therapy-functioning in an integrated total program." Since the tools used by the various specialties to assist physical and mental restoration will be thoroughly covered in the following chapters, we will only summarize here the services rendered in the various agencies.

Naturally, a balanced program of all types of activities within the aims and objectives of the particular agency should be provided. However, the type of program depends upon the agency size, services provided, and the staff personnel available, especially qualified personnel who have been trained to utilize their tools in the particular setting and facilities available. The therapist has two responsibilities; first to provide certain activities, and secondly, to see that these activities contribute toward returning the patient to society or to his maximum level of functioning. Judgment is always necessary in planning the type of program most needed for the handicapped since all patients do not necessarily benefit from the same type of program. Moreover, it is assumed that a certain amount of overlapping will occur when occupational therapist, medical recreators, physical therapist, and many others work together on any program. But with cooperative and coordinated action on the part of each service, a practicable plan, with allowance, can be worked out.

In order for activities to be used more successfully in any agency setting, medical prescription, referral, clearance or approval will be received from the clinical director or ward physician. In turn, the therapist will be responsible for recording the progress of the patient in the activity. The importance of the trend toward "team conference" communications, both as to referrals and discussion of observed behavior should not be overlooked compared to the more formal method of communication represented by the written prescription and "progress note." Frequency of the "progress note" will be determined by the request of the physician and by changes in the patient worthy of explanation. Some departments, because of the modality that they use and the particular handicap involved, require more medical direction. Reference here is made primarily to general medical and surgical and specialty hospitals which work with the physically handicapped and neuropsychiatric patient. State hospitals, hospitals for long-term patients, and homes for the aged usually only give clearance or approval for activities although some patients in these settings will receive specific prescriptions.

State hospitals for the mentally ill and retarded, like the Veterans Administration and some private psychiatric hospitals, provide the greatest variety in programming. This is due to the fact that all types of specialists are employed and, in addition, newer professional specialties have been more readily accepted in these hospitals.

Programming within general medical and surgical hospitals with or without a psychiatric unit will be restricted to those departments usually found in a rehabilitation unit—physical and occupational therapy and recreation. The program itself is usually prescribed within the limits of the facilities by the patient's physician. Some hospitals will utilize a "rehabilitation steering committee" to assist in the treatment of the patient as well as discuss matters of mutual concern or interest. When services are provided for both physical disabilities and psychiatric patients in a general hospital, two separate programs, which may or may not be administered separately, are usually in operation for each group or type of patients with some overlapping in areas, although facilities to some degree are usually shared by the various departments.

A comment should be made here, before continuing, about the number of activities conducted for patients on a daily basis.

In the sampling of public and non-public psychiatric hospitals by the Washburn University research group, it was found that forty-one hospitals of the seventy-nine sampled "had six or more activity programs (arts and crafts, music, athletics, special interest groups, etc.) available for patients; twenty-six hospitals program three to five activities; and twelve hospitals utilized less than three programs."[1] Although public psychiatric hospitals provide a variety of activities because of the large patient population, it should be noted, "that not all patients in public hospitals receive a full program of activities"[1] because they require full-time custodial care or are so regressed that they are only able to make minimal use of the activities. The Washburn study also indicated that "occupational and recreational therapies are used proportionately more than any of the other activity therapies in both public and non-public (psychiatric) hospitals."[1] Music therapy was used in over half of the hospitals reporting with manual arts and industrial therapy close behind.

Taking the more extensively used specialties to discuss, we find that occupational therapy concerns itself with a combination of remedial programs and therapeutic work and play experiences regardless of the setting. Spackman[23] states that "the unique contribution of occupational therapy is that it uses a program of normal activity to aid in the psychosocial adjustment of the patient, as specific treatment or as simulated work situation." The scope of the treatment program does not tend to conform itself to a particular hospital setting; rather, here is overlapping of programs between hospital settings. However, the program may be limited by the personnel available, type of facilities, diagnostic groups to be treated, and patient needs and interest. The range of programs utilized is quite broad and include arts and craft activities, educational and academic services, recreation activities, prevocational and industrial activities and vocational counseling. In addition, the occupational therapist may be called upon to adapt or devise equipment, such as splints and other self-help items to assist the patient in achieving a greater degree of independence. As we will see later, some of these aforementioned programs are also planned and conducted by other disciplines within particular settings.

In the general-medical and specialty hospitals, large or small, occupational therapy is a part of the department of physical medicine and/or rehabilitation. Activities provided in this setting are usually of a short-term nature unless there is a particular physical or mental handicap needing additional attention. Basically, rehabilitation of these patients may be psychological or physical or, in some cases, a combination of the two. Moreover, the general hospital may also provide an outpatient clinic in occupational therapy for those patients who are continuing a treatment program after discharge from the hospital. The suggested daily load per therapist, as discussed in the *Manual on the Organization and Administration of Occupational Therapy Departments*,[24] is twenty to thirty patients, but this varies according to the type of patients being treated and the disability involved. In this setting, there should be frequent conferences between the therapist and the patient's physician to discuss the progress of the patient and the adequacy of the treatment program.

The occupational therapist in hospitals for the mentally ill, as in general hospitals, is concerned with total personality. But, in addition, more emphasis is put upon the development or redevelopment of establishing satisfactory interpersonal relationships which lead to a better social adjustment for the patient and prepare him for involvement in the work and play experiences of the hospital. The particular medias, whether chosen by the therapist or patient, allow the patient to express his emotional feeling. Moreover, as with other therapies within this type of setting, occupational therapy assists in environmental adjustment, adjunct to other therapies (psychotherapy, electro or insulin shock, etc.) as an aid in diagnosis, and as a supportive form of therapy in the prevention of deterioration of patients with chronic disorders.[25]

Occupational therapy in children's hospitals and schools, and departments of pediatrics in general hospitals serves primarily as a tool in the psychological adjustment as well as assisting in the physical and social re-adjustment of the child. As Schad[26] points out," . . . the occupational therapist on the pediatric service assists the ill or handicapped child to recover from illness or injury. It is the whole child who is of central concern."

The application of occupational therapy is also utilized in the treatment of tuberculosis, visually handicapped, amputees, and for disabilities and handicaps resulting from multiple sclerosis, poliomyelitis, arthritis, cerebral palsy, and nerve injuries. In addition, we find therapists working in sheltered workshops and vocational rehabilitation centers.

Medical recreation in any setting allows the patient the opportunity to enjoy a satisfying experience as well as contributing to the patient's rehabilitation. Whether the activity should be called therapy or not is not clearly understood because of the semantic interpretation given by various authorities. Regardless of what it is called, recreation provides activities with therapeutic results to aid in the development of inter-personal relationship in addition to providing an education in the use of leisure-time.

The selection of recreation activities depends upon the type of patients the therapist is serving. Activities can not always be based upon the particular needs of the patient since the patient's activity may be limited for a period of time because of an injury or disease; therefore, it is often necessary, as commented upon by Knudson,[27] "to modify and interpret recreation to meet peculiar needs and limitations." Hence, the therapist must provide a wide variety of activities to assist the physician in getting his patient well. The program content of recreation for the ill and handicapped, according to Chapman,[28] includes (1) arts and crafts; (2) audio-visual activities; (3) dance activities; (4) dramatic activities; (5) hobbies and special interest programs; (6) musical activities; (7) nature and outing activities; (8) social recreation activities; (9) special events, and (10) sports and games. Undoubtedly, the reader realizes these activities overlap other specialties but the author feels that the distinction can be made as to when and how they are used.

In the general medical and surgical hospitals, the recreator works closely with the other members of the rehabilitation team by providing activities which fill the leisure time of the patient while he is convalescing. In addition, the therapist may be asked, through medical prescription, to provide an activity which will develop coordination or strengthen particular muscles while providing enjoyment or amusement at the same time. It is well worth mentioning the importance of developing activities which can assist in the social readjustment of the physically handicapped individual when he leaves the hospital. Recreation for children in special hospitals provides an atmosphere of warmth and understanding. Not only are activities used for functional and psychological purposes but as an educational tool in developing the whole child.

Recreation in hospitals for the mentally ill and mentally retarded provides purposeful and absorbing leisure-time activities which are designed to assist the patients achieve general, as well as specific treatment goals. It focuses on the general, developmental and social needs of the individual which are so essential to establishing a therapeutic environment and an atmosphere desirable for recovery. In addition, the program is medically approved and guided.

Hunt's[29] *Recreation for the Handicapped,* Chapman's[30] *Recreation Activities for the Handicapped,* and Rathbone and Lucas's[31] *Recreation in Total Rehabilitation* provide excellent examples of what type of recreation activities are best suited for ill and handicapped persons.

A survey of the literature in the specialty of music therapy renders a wide range of use for music as both a therapeutic agent and as an adjunctive to other therapies in all kinds of hospitals. The wide use of music therapy today is partially due to the results of its use in military hospitals during the war. At the present time, there remain some misconceptions of its use, but this can be partially explained by the fact that it is a new profession, organized professionally in 1950, and hospitals have not yet realized its scope and purpose. In general, music has been used in the hospitals for the mentally ill and retarded, with the physically handicapped, in institutions for emotional and behavioral problems of children, as an adjunct to surgery, in tubercular hospitals, and in dentistry. Also, a considerable amount of research has been done in the area of physiological effects of music (muscles, skin, pupillary reflexes, blood pressure, pain threshold, heart rate, respiration, vascular changes, gastric reaction), affective responses, projection techniques, personality testing, and the development of various musical tests. The National Association for Music Therapy is one specific organization leanding dynamic impetus to this field of endeavor.

What is here referred to as vocational and industrial therapy is variously termed work therapy, occupational therapy, vocational retraining, vocational therapy, industrial therapy, and a number of other officious titles as opposed to the sheltered workshop or community rehabilitation clinic. Although recently a newly re-organized profession with new methods and techniques of opera-tion, it has been used as a therapeutic agent, for many years, gain-ing its precedence primarily in state institutions and the Veterans Administration.

The place of the vocational and industrial therapy program in the hospital organization differs from one institution to the next. Often it is placed under the auspices of the occupational therapy department. A vocational and industrial therapy department is sometimes regarded as an independent clinical unit directly re-sponsible to the clinical director. Some hospitals utilize a very unstructured procedure whereby the hospital industries make their requests for workers directly to the ward personnel or the ward physician. Other hospitals designate the department as an adjunct or activity therapy and is a part of the activity therapy service. This latter approach is becoming the most accepted in in-stitutions.

In many institutions, industrial therapy, vocational placement or counseling and vocational rehabilitation may all exist in one department. In others, there may be in name only one of these therapies operating within the institution, but doing the work of all three. Some states have worked out arrangements whereby the Vocational Rehabilitation Division of a state agency has developed programs within and outside the hospital.

Industrial therapy is usually concerned with the assignment and management by medical prescription of a patient in any activity in which the hospital, or some department of the hospital, derives a service from the efforts of the assignee, and from which the patient receives some benefit. In short, it involves the produc-tivity of the patient in the hospital industries and the solution of interpersonal problems as they relate to productivity as well as providing the opportunity for vocational evaluation in a "reality" oriented work situation.

A distinction is made between Industrial Therapy and Vocational Training because the latter denotes the actual instruction and training of patients in specific vocational skills. Some large psychiatric hospitals, but especially the Veterans Administration, have a section comparable to the vocational training program called manual arts therapy which is concerned with providing actual or simulated work situations of "an industrial and agricultural nature which have vocational significance."[32] In addition, it provides an activity which yields tangible results.

A third area, which in the past was a service found only outside the hospital but is now beginning to operate on a small scale within the hospital, is vocational placement. Its primary purpose is the counseling of patients for job placement within the community. The work of the therapist in this area may also involve the surveying of local industry needs for patient placement in addition to determining the factors involved in successful or unsuccessful employment behavior of the patient.

In any given case, vocational and industrial therapy can provide therapeutic benefits to the patient definitely prescribed for the individual consistent with treatment goals as determined by the physician or medical staff.

Volunteer services, which may or may not be a part of activity therapies, is used in all hospitals. The service is concerned with providing a service to the patients and to the hospital. Their activity may range from directly leading or assisting in activities to escorting patients to activities, shopping, providing parties and transportation to and from clinics or writing letters for the mentally ill, physically handicapped or short term patient. Most of all, they provide a link between the hospital and the social and cultural life of the community.

Educational therapy programs within all types of hospitals are becoming more prevalent every day, although the Veterans Administration has had such a program for a considerable number of years. The program implies not only a formal education process, but a concern for the psychodynamics of the patient under treatment. In addition, many patients, because of their handicap which prevents them from participating in activities, need the gratification and stimulus which education activities provide.

Some educational programs, within various hospitals, are accredited by the particular state's department of education, the local board of education, or the Commission on Accreditation of Service Experience of the American Council on Education. On the other hand, some schools have only attempted to maintain the student at the level in which the student was before leaving the community school.

Daily sessions are usually established for the adolescent consisting of basic studies on both the elementary and secondary level. In many instances, the home schools of patients are consulted so as to insure continuity of studies. In other situations, students are permitted to enter the local high school and return to the hospital following the school day. Adult education programs which may or may not be conducted during the daytime and on a voluntary basis provide not only courses based upon known patient interest, but regular classroom instruction or correspondence courses in which the patient receives credit or attains a diploma.

Approximately 40 per cent of the hospitalized sick receive some form of library service.[33] This service is influenced by the particular type of hospital it is, the illness treated, length of hospitalization, census, and the ratio of ambulatory patients.

The place of the patient's library within the hospital structure varies from hospital to hospital. In some, it is a part of the medical library, in others, it may be a part of either the recreation or occuptional therapy department, and in others, it may be a department of its own, directly responsible to the superintendent. Regardless of where it is placed within the hospital structure, its objective is to ". . . furnish reading material for all patients, for the purpose of contributing to their recovery and welfare."[33]

The patient library service has three purposes, according to Tews,[33] (1) recreational, in that it provides a means of relaxation, a change of activity, and a source of gratification; (2) educational, whereby it assists in developing new interest and keeping the patient in contact with reality, and (3) it is inspirational and therapeutic.

Other services which may be provided with the assistance of

the librarian include special reading programs, book reviews, planning radio programs, story hours for children, hospital newspaper publication, group discussion clubs, audiovisual-aids material including talking books and books in Braille. The librarian may also be called upon to assist other departments in working with patients such as providing books which deal with particular hobbies or assisting in the academic and vocational training of patients. At times, the librarian may be asked to provide specific books which will assist the doctor in the treatment of his patients. This latter form of assistance is usually referred to as "Bibliotherapy."

GENERAL ORGANIZING PRINCIPLES FOR ACTIVITY THERAPY

The major objective of any hospital is getting the patient well so that he can leave the hospital or, if this is impossible, to assist the patient in becoming as independent as possible within the hospital setting. Good organizing, consistent with the treatment objectives, assists the hospital and doctor to achieve these objectives. However, the organization is only a means to the treatment end and should not be considered of primary importance, lest the patient be lost within its framework. Nevertheless, without good organization, treatment objectives lack strength and vigor.

How to organize and integrate various departments within a hospital to provide maximum therapy with a minimum amount of wasted energy, effort, or money has always been a challenge to administrators. Consideration must be given to many factors which influence the organization's effectiveness with the solution being within reality limits. Among the most noteworthy trends during recent years, as discussed earlier in this chapter, has been the grouping of various activity therapists into a single coordinated department. Such a grouping takes into consideration the inherent nature of the activities which are conducted by these therapists. This type of organizational grouping provides the best programming available so as to insure accomplishment of the objectives — enhancing the total hospital treatment program. Furthermore, saving of energy and a minimum of friction and frustration can be avoided in addition to a decrease in duplication of effort. In too many hospitals, department obstacles are not recognized but are indifferently accepted as fixed difficulties of that particular department. But the grouping of these specialties does away with many of these obstacles thereby bringing a proper balance among work effort.

The concept of activity therapies, as observed by Meuli,[34] "is not intended to 'blur' professional roles or to bring about a 'loss of identification' of the various professions involved. To the contrary, experience has proven that well-coordinated activity therapy services result in strengthened professional identity and clarification of professional roles."

In organizing for an activity therapy service, difficulty may be encountered due to the educational training and experience that is required within each specialty. At times, there is a tendency to disperse the efforts of each specialty rather than unify them. This is primarily due to the fact that over the years there has been a prescribed area of work which has been determined on a functional and physical basis by the particular specialty. Within the specialization, each department head may tend to exaggerate the importance of his particular work as compared with other departments. In addition, the department head may be so concerned with his own department accomplishing their goals that in many instances he will purposely avoid involvement in other areas. It is not uncommon to observe specialties becoming so engrossed in their program and goals that the specialty becomes the entire activity therapy program. Dunlop[8] observes that this type of situation has developed, "as much as a result of the functionalized nature of many institutions and agencies, as from any lack of sympathetic understanding of the resources and limitations of other services and skills." Since each specialty can be viewed as a specialized team within the hospital, with their particular invested goals, education, and training, the conditions emphasize the need for organization and coordination in order to better synchronize the efforts of all departments. The advantages of this include the fuller use of specific abilities of individuals and departments. Each department has strong and weak points, and by developing and assigning activities based upon their different abilities greater efficiency and broader programming is secured.

The first step toward effective organization must begin in the individual departments of the the activity therapy service whereby each department has an understanding or acceptance of the general purpose of activity therapy within the hospital. It is important that all common goals of the activity therapies be spelled out as well as the unique goals of each service. The next step is one of integration of these specialties into a whole and finding the effective balance between them to meet the specific aims and objectives of the hospital. The contribution of one department toward the objectives must be balanced against the contribution of another department. Objectives give rise to the program, where each department has some contribution to make to the achievement of the objectives. Each department must be helped to understand and respect the contribution made by other departments. Thirdly, is the development of the proper lines of communication between departments and to the administrator who is responsible for the total program. This final point does not only include inter-action between individuals and departments, but implies authority invested in the administrator to accomplish objectives.

If the predetermined objectives are to be obtained through the organizing of the activity therapies, it logically follows that there is a need for coordination. Coordination deals with the blending of efforts of people to attain a stated objective. By what means, then, we may ask ourselves, can effective coordination be obtained. Briefly, we can say that a knowledge and acceptance of the various tools used by all departments is basic to coordination as well as an understanding of the objectives of the particular hospital. This involves making sure adequate personnel and facilities are available and that the departments are capable of obtaining the objectives. Encouraging members and department heads to discuss and exchange suggestions and ideas, participation in formative stages dealing with program content (planning) of all the specialties affords the better coordination. In turn, each department knows what the other departments are programming and good relationships between departments are attained. Direction, supervision, and leadership is needed to insure effective total collaborative staff participation as well as proper evaluation of work progress so that goals are achieved.

Again, referring to *"Project 52,"* the following aspects were found to be desirable for coordination.

"1. It could lessen confusion on the part of the patient. He would be protected from feelings of competition among disciplines.

2. It would encourage a sense of security among workers. Security could result from a lack of competition among disciplines resulting from knowledge gained in a training program. Therapists could then work in a relaxed manner with a patient.

3. It could retard regression. The coordinator could promote prescriptions for specific treatment needs of the patient and utilize them in treatment planning, thus preventing regression.

4. It could improve communication between doctor, staff, and patient.

5. It could result in more economical use of staff and save the time of the psychiatrist.

6. It could centralize interdepartmental contacts. The social workers felt that outside departments would find it easier to work with a coordinated department.

7. It could control patient contacts. Patients would be protected from having too many interpersonal relationships at a time when this might be difficult for them.

8. It could encourage intradepartmental cooperative efforts. Staff members could serve as consultants or co-workers in other areas than one's specialty, e.g., an adjunctive therapist worker could be consulted by a recreational worker faced with preparing decorations for parties."[35]

In conclusion, we can say that effective organization and coordination results in the best use made of departments, personnel, and facilities.

THE ACTIVITY THERAPY ADMINISTRATOR

Regardless of the title used for the administrator of an activity therapy service, his function is primarily that of administration.

This administration of the activity therapy service involves the synchronization of efforts of others to attain specific objectives.

As an administrator, he is concerned with two specific roles; one, clinical coordination, seeing that the objectives of the hospital as they relate to the activity therapies and as determined by the clinical director are met, and secondly, administrative coordination, whereby administrative functions common to all of the activity therapies are combined and centralized. However, clinical and administrative coordination should not interfere with the lateral communication between the therapist and the physician. This is a professional relationship which supersedes the administrator's authority. Likewise, the administrator does not impose treatment practices on the various activity therapy specialties.

These two functions of coordination are interwoven, interrelated and sometimes overlapping; one function does not stop before the next one begins. However, some procedures tend to come before others and greater emphasis is placed on others.

Before proceeding further, some comments are needed concerning the shift from a department head to an administrator. How successful this shift is made determines the success of the program. As sometimes happens, the administrator continues to remain as a specialist. It is important that the specialist recognizes the distinction. The special skills of the therapist are important in conducting activities but the administrator does not require this special skill. Many administrators are specialists before advancing to this new role, and although the special skill may be helpful, another skill is now required — administrating effectively. As Barton[36] points out, "Exceptional ability to manage people is of greater value than technical ability. Also important is the intellectual ability to reason through a problem that is essential to the selection of the best plan from the alternates." It is unfortunate, but in so many situations, the administrator of the activity therapy unit has had little formal training in administration.

The administrator, for effective administration, must have a basic understanding of the over-all hospital purpose and goals. The purpose and goals will determine the program content of the activity therapies. As Finer[37] comments, "The aims or goals of an institution are reflected in the policies set up to govern its activities; it inspires the whole and its parts and gives them coherence and direction. That goal can be achieved only to the degree that all sub-divisions of the institution accept it as their own."

No administrator can function successfully without knowledge about the elements involved in the over-all objectives, and the immediate objectives and broad concepts of the various specialties. It is also necessary that each specialty understand its contribution to the accomplishment of the goals regardless of how direct or indirect this may be. Although each specialty will have its own specific goals, set to some degree by professional standards, these goals will be contained within the overall objectives of the whole hospital. If the administrator understands the purpose and goals; the organization and integration of the specialties into a whole flows clearly therefrom.

The administrator must be concerned with the planning and coordination of the specialties. Effective planning is deciding in advance what is to be done and how it is to be done to achieve the goals. It is a fundamental function. Two prerequisites, in order to accomplish the goals, will be the surveying of staff potential to determine the treatment load which each of the specialties are capable of handling and the amount of equipment and facilities. With this information, the administrator is prepared to present to the clinical director the type and extent of services available in all of his service areas. The final results of this planning will be the development of a master schedule of activities which is distributed among the clinical services. This not only is a means of communication, but is a method of evaluation and examination of the distribution of services.

As many times happens, the extensiveness of planning is overlooked. Planning not only includes the development of the activity program, but policies which provide and give meaning to the goals; procedures, which deal with a specific course of action such as scheduling; decision-making, in the sense that one decision must not conflict with other decisions, else coordination will be made most difficult; and creativity, whereby the administrator and his department heads exercise some degree of imagination and resourcefulness. Competent planing draws heavily upon creativeness and the ability to put together a format of required activities to meet the treatment needs. In the final analysis of the planning process, the administrator must be concerned with the education of his staff through staff-development or in-service training programs. Concepts are always changing in the health sciences. Such a program increases the competency and confidence of the staff.

The administrator must be aware of controlling. Direction, supervision, and leadership are of primary importance in helping to achieve coordination. Communication in controlling can not be ignored. The wise administrator is easily accessible and ready to the problems confronting any of the department heads. Much is gained through regularly scheduled conferences. It is important to remember that the conditions for effective total collaborative staff participation can exist only in a setting that has competent administrator and professional leadership.

Budgetary control is another area which is an integral part of the administrative process. It aids the administrator in several ways, the most obvious of which is the balancing of activities. It assists also in making the administrator think in advance, to project future program and facilities, personnel, supplies and equipment. These parts must be in harmony with the treatment goals.

Finally, the administrator must have the means of evaluating how effective the activity program is in achieving its goals of treatment, learning how to utilize past experience in order to achieve that goal more effectively. For this purpose the question of how successful treatment is must be answerable at any time: how the treatment is being done; at what cost in terms of personnel, facilities, and money. Records are essential; records that will explain things by analysis and comparison and serve as a guide in the making of plans.

In summary, the qualities of a top administrator, according to Finer,[38] must include the four C's: consciousness, constancy, coherence, conscientiousness.*

---

*For further information concerning the role of a lay-administrator in a physical medicine and rehabilitation service under the direction of a physician or psychiatrist, see Pattison, Harry A., ed.: *The Handicapped and Their Rehabilitation,* Springfield, Illinois, Charles C Thomas, 1957, Ch. 18.

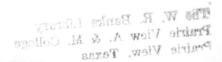

QUALIFICATION OF AN ACTIVITY THERAPY ADMINISTRATOR

Before bringing this chapter to a close, it would be wise to discuss briefly the qualifications for an administrator of an activity therapy service (sample specification and qualifications for an "Activity Therapy Coordinator, Director, or Chief" can be found in the Appendix).

Owing to widely different public and private hospitals, there is no uniformity in the titles and qualifications for activity therapy administrator positions throughout the United States, although hospitals are increasingly tending to adopt some type of a standard nomenclature. This is due in no small measure to the increase of activity therapy administrators in all types of hospitals.

The selection of a competent administrator is a most important function performed by the hospital authorities. His duties are comparable in many respects to those of the business administrator and the clinical director combined. Most of his time is spent in planning, organizing, directing, clinical and business conferences and promoting the work and interest of the activity therapy department.

The administrator must have a fundamental knowledge of the philosophy of the activity therapies. He must be capable of looking at the entire scope of the hospital program rather than at isolated phases. In addition to having administrative ability, he must possess the qualification of a good clinician in his particular profession. Likewise, a familiarity of the various specialties that comprise the activity therapies is essential: knowledge of facilities and equipment used by each specialty; knowledge of the principles and methods involved in development of a budget and records; knowledge in conducting research; and knowledge in building up cooperative relationships within the hospital and in the community.

The administrator should be a graduate from an approved school in one of the professions that make-up the activity therapies. In addition, he should have not less than three years' experience of which one year or more has been in a responsible position involving administrative duties. It is highly recommended that the administrator also possess a graduate degree.

Project 52[1] revealed that of the seventy-nine (mental) hospitals surveyed, nearly all of the coordinators were from a "work experience and academic specialization" other than medicine. The non-medical administrator usually has a bachelor's degree in one of the activity therapy specialties with an internship or field work experience in that specialty from six to twelve months in length. Approximately half of the administrators in the sample were from the specialization of either recreation or occupational therapy. In addition, 50 per cent of the coordinators had graduate study.

The Veterans Administration, like larger general and medical hospitals, require their chiefs of physical medicine and rehabilitation service to have a degree in medicine or physiatrics in addition to a working knowledge or experience in the specialties that make up the department. The coordinator in a Veterans Administration[14] hospital has the "responsibility for administrative supervision of the functions of the various specialties and with other medical services and rehabilitation functions within the agency" that do not require the services of the physician. Although the requirements for a coordinator are somewhat flexible, in essence, they require training and education in one or more of the specialties found in a physical medicine and rehabilitation service.

There is a trend in public and private psychiatric hospitals and schools for the retarded in the larger and more progressive states to require a graduate degree in one of the more established specialization to obtain the position as an activity therapy administrator. This trend is also seen in some general medical and surgical hospitals.

In conclusion, it has been suggested that a graduate program be established to train administrators beyond their particular specialization; however, this does not seem feasible at the present time because of various unsolved questions between clinical personnel and educators. It has also been suggested that all the specialties combine into one parent organization, in much the same way as the American Medical Association, whereby each specialty would retain their identity while at the same time, gain secured status.

REFERENCES

1. *Project 52: A Study in Adjunctive Therapies Coordination.* Washburn University, Topeka, Kansas, June, 1958.
2. Meyer, Martin W.: Recreation in a state mental hospital system. In *A Report of the Fourth Southern Regional Institute on Recreation in Hospitals.* North Carolina Recreation Commission, Raleigh, North Carolina, No. 27, 1959, p. 39.
3. Gaston, Thayer E.: The adjunctive therapies. *Music Therapy, 1956.* National Association for Music Therapy, Inc., (Ed) Gaston, Thayer E., Lawrence, Kansas, 1957, p. 222.
4. Meuli, Albert L.: Coordinated activity therapies program. *Ment. Health Res. Inst. Bull., IV* (3) :38, 1961.
5. Clark, Thomas J.: Activity therapies and voluntary services. *Recreation for the Ill and Handicapped, V* (2) :10, 1961.
6. Key, William H.: *Coordination of the Ancillary Therapies.* Convention Address, Sheraton-Lincoln Hotel, Indianapolis, Indiana, December, 1960.
7. Doniger, Joan M., and Dundon, Dwyer H.: Administrative planning of patient activity programs in mental hospitals. *Amer. J. Occupational Ther., XIV* (5) , 1960.
8. Dunlop, Edward: The integration of services in the rehabilitation process. *Occupational Therapy and Rehabilitation,* 1949.
9. Ackerman, Ora: Coordination of activity therapy. *Recreation for the Ill and Handicapped, V* (2) :6, 1961.
10. Thornton, Patricia, Chief, Activity Therapy, Division of Mental Hygiene, Madison, Wisconsin; Personal letter, February, 1963.
11. Project 52, *op. cit.,* p. 90.
12. Meyer, Martin W., *op. cit.,* p. 39.
13. Cox, Charlotte, Coordinator, Activity Therapy Service, Athens State Hospital, Athens, Ohio: Personal letter, January, 1963.
14. Silver, Richard A., Director, Personnel Services, Veterans Administration, Washington, D. C.: Personal letter, December, 1962.
15. Meuli, Albert: Report on activity therapies service. *Annual Report,* Department of Institutions, Division of Mental Health, Olympia, Washington, August, 1962.
16. Owen, Carolyn: An activities group charts its own course. *Ment. Hosp.,* December, 1960, p. 38-40.
17. O'Morrow, Gerald: Activity therapy services. *Annual Report,* Logansport State Hospital, Logansport, Indiana, June, 1962.
18. Acuff, Sidney, Director, Adjunctive Therapy, Eastern State Hospital, Knoxville, Tennessee, Personal letter, March, 1963.
19. Cox, *op. cit.*
20. Humphrey, Fred, Director, Activity Therapies, State Hospital, Jamestown, North Dakota, Personal letter, April, 1963.
21. Ridgway, Elizabeth, Patient Activities Consultant, Bureau of Mental Hospital Services, Department of Public Welfare, Harrisburg, Pennsylvania, Personal letter, March, 1963.
22. Kahn, J. P.: The role of ancillary personnel in the total treatment of psychiatric patients. *Ment. Hosp.,* June, 1959, p. 27.

23. Spackman, Clare S.: Coordination of occupational therapy with other allied medical and related services. In *Occupational Therapy*. 3rd Ed., (eds.) Willard, Helen S., and Spackman, Clare S., Philadelphia, J. B. Lippencott Company, 1963, p. 1.

24. *Manual On The Organization and Administration of Occupational Therapy Department*. American Occupational Therapy Association, Dubuque, Iowa, William C. Brown Company, 1951.

25. Dundon, H. Dwyer: Psychiatric occupational therapy. In *Occupational Therapy*. 3rd Ed., (eds.) Willard, Helen S., and Spackman, Clare S., Philadelphia, J. B. Lippincott Company, 1963, p. 55-74.

26. Schad, Carol J.: Occupational therapy in pediatrics. *Ibid*, p. 75-76.

27. Knudson, A. B. C. and Gibson, James W.: Concepts of recreation in rehabilitation. In *A Report of the Fifth Southern Regional Institute on Recreation in Hospitals*. North Carolina Recreation Commission, Raleigh, North Carolina, No. 29, 1961, p. 20.

28. Chapman, Frederick M.: *Recreation Activities for the Handicapped*. New York, Ronald Press Company, 1960.

29. Hunt, Valerie V.: *Recreation for the Handicapped*. Englewood Cliffs, New York, Prentice-Hall, Inc., 1955.

30. Rathbone, Josephine L., and Lucas, Carol: *Recreation and Total Rehabilitation*. Springfield, Illinois, Charles C Thomas, Publisher, 1959.

31. Rose, A. E., and Brawn, C. E.: Music therapy at Westminster Hospital. *Ment. Hyg.*, January, 1959, p. 93-104.

32. *Orientation Manual*. Department of Medicine and Surgery, Physical Medicine and Rehabilitation, Veterans Administration, Washington, D. C., May, 1959.

33. Tews, Ruth: The patients' library. In *Applied Medical Library Practice*, Keys, T. E., Charles C Thomas, Publisher, 1958.

34. Meuli, Albert L.: On Organizational Complex. In *Recreation in Treatment Center* Washington, D. C., Hospital Recreation Section, American Recreation Society, Vol. II, September, 1963.

35. Project 52. *op. cit.*, p. 106.

36. Barton, Walter: The hospital administrator, *Mental Hospitals*, May, 1962, p. 261.

37. Finer, Herman: *Administration and the Nursing Service*. New York, MacMillan Company, 1952, p. 157.

38. *Ibid.*, p. 222.

Chapter II

OCCUPATIONAL THERAPY

SHIRLEY M. BOWING, M.A., O.T.R., AND
M. GERALDINE SHEVLIN, M. A., O. T. R.

ORIGIN AND DEVELOPMENT OF OCCUPATIONAL THERAPY

OCCUPATIONAL THERAPY, as a profession, is less than a half-century old; and usually classifies itself as a "young and growing" member of the allied medical professions. When considering, however, the youth of many newer specialties in today's burgeoning programs for rehabilitation of the mentally and physically disabled, it might be more appropriate to think of occupational therapy as a small but relatively seasoned veteran.

Self-organization and Self-definition

The use of "occupations" as a treatment tool came into prominence in the hospitals for the mentally ill in the 19th century. By the time of the first world war, the term "occupational therapy" had come into use and, in 1917, a group of persons who were interested in promoting the use of activities for treatment formed The National Society for Promotion of Occupational Therapy. During World War I, "occupations" were used as part of the total medical treatment program in the military services, and their use not only had a positive effect on mental health, but also contributed significantly to the speed of recovery from physical disability. This broadened interest in the potential of occupations for treatment undoubtedly accounted for the breadth of responsibilities inferred in the 1921 definition of occupational therapy: "Occupational therapy may be defined as any activity, mental or physical, definitely prescribed and guided for the distinct purpose of contributing to and hastening recovery from disease or injury."[1] In the years since 1921, this definition remains basically unchanged. Occupational therapy continues to reaffirm its concern for the use of "any activity, physical or mental" in

31

furthering the patients' physical, psychological and social well-being.

The charter membership in the budding profession apparently were a dedicated group with respect for strong organization. In 1921, they changed the name of their association to the present one: The American Occupational Therapy Association, and emerged with a highly centralized organization which has actively governed the development of the profession. Some of the areas of development with which they were concerned are also of significance here and include:

Certification of qualified occupational therapists. The association published the first registry of qualified occupational therapists ("O.T.R.'s") in 1934 and has maintained and published a registry continuously since then. Since 1943, registration has been based on a national qualifying examination as well as on graduation from an approved school of occupational therapy.

Literature. The literature of the profession is largely confined to the publications which have served as the official organ of the profession during these years: 1917-1922 *Maryland Psychiatric Quarterly;* 1922-1924, *Archives of Occupational Therapy;* 1924-1947, *Occupational Therapy and Rehabilitation;* and 1947 to the present; *The American Journal of Occupational Therapy.*

Books on the subject are few and those in common use are listed at the close of this chapter. The single book of most universal influence in the profession is undoubtedly the one edited by Willard and Spackman and currently available in a considerably-revised third edition.[2,3]

Various manuals and institute proceedings have been published by the American Occupational Therapy Association and are essential for the thorough student of occupational therapy.* Some are referred to in this writing; complete lists are available from the association's office.

Training programs. Establishment of training programs for workers in "occupations" came even before the organized profession of occupational therapy existed, with the first one credited to a head nurse who offered a course for her nursing staff in 1906.

---

*A.O.T.A., 250 W. 57th Street, New York, New York.

Other training programs followed and were offered by hospitals for nurses and other personnel, but the first college-centered course was inaugurated at Milwaukee-Downer College, in 1913, and continued uninterrupted to 1964 to become the first school of occupational therapy. Significantly, even these earliest training programs recognized that workers must have a basic medical orientation and the earliest programs emphasized anatomy, physiology and psychology.

From 1923 to 1935, the American Occupational Therapy Association provided direction for training programs and encouraged the establishment of these in colleges and universities rather than in hospitals, as it was early recognized that a liberal education was essential for adequate performance of responsibilities such as those the profession had undertaken. During the past two decades, educational requirements for the bachelor's degree is part of basic preparation for occupational therapy in all of the American schools. A majority of the schools require substantially more than four academic years in order to complete the combined academic and clinical program and still retain a core of general education.

In 1935, the American Medical Association accepted the association's request to assume responsibility for setting up and maintaining official standards for and inspection and accreditation of schools of occupational therapy. Under this continuing program, five schools were accredited by 1939, eighteen by 1945, and thirty-one by 1963.

The American Occupational Therapy Association and the Council on Hospitals and Medical Education of the American Medical Association publishes the *Essentials of an Acceptable School of Occupational Therapy* which outlines minimum requirements. The *Essentials* emphasizes that occupational therapists are trained to work under the direction of qualified physicians and not as independent practitioners and requires that the schools be established only in approved medical schools or in accredited colleges or universities which maintain affiliation with acceptable hospitals. The last revision of these essentials was in 1949 and the revision which is now in process will undoubtedly reflect considerable change in curriculum content. The present *Essentials* establish minimum course content as follows: Out of four years of study, at least 59 per cent (two years) of course credits must be divided approximately thus:

24 per cent . . . . Biologic science; social science; clinical subjects (anatomy, physiology, kinesiology, neuroanatomy, psychology, sociology, psychiatry, neurology, orthopedics, etc.) .

6 per cent . . . . Professional theory (application of occupational therapy in various disability areas) .

20 per cent . . . . Technical training (fine and applied arts, education, recreation) .

The requirements for clinical training are in addition to the above and specify at least three months in psychiatry, two in physical disabilities and four in electives from pediatrics, general medical and other medical services.

Although the *Essentials* form the cornerstone for basic occupational therapy education programs, substantial influence on growth and refinement of existing curriculums has been wielded by an active communication system which involves several committees of the professional association (Curriculum Committee, Student Affiliations Committee, Graduate Education Committee) , its Council on Education, its national Board of Management, plus its Medical Advisory Council.

Graduate Education. The preceding discussion relates to the basic preparation for occupational therapy registration which is on an undergraduate level. With increased specialization and other demands on the profession, graduate programs in occupational therapy have developed in recent years. Five universities now offer programs of graduate study leading to the Master of Arts or Master of Science degree with a major in occupational therapy. The American Occupational Therapy Association does not take the same responsibility for maintaining standards for these curriculums as it has for the undergraduate programs, but does provide consultancy on request. The emphasis in existing programs varies, with some programs established for advanced study in clinical subjects (physical disabilities, psychiatry) and some established particularly for training educators with course work in principles of education, student counseling, administration and supervision, advanced professional theory, and advanced course work in basic sciences particularly pertinent to occupational therapy.

Increased numbers of therapists are now enrolled in predoctoral studies in fields such as psychology, education, social sciences and biologic sciences.

CLINICAL OBJECTIVES AND METHODS OF OCCUPATIONAL THERAPY

Occupational therapy for any patient is appropriately multiobjective. For clarity, however, the writers present an orientation to clinical practice in terms of the following objectives: (1) to assist recovery from mental illness; (2) to promote physical restoration; (3) to assist in training for independent living; (4) to contribute to psycho-social development; (5) to stimulate normal development of the ill and disabled child and (6) to aid in vocational rehabilitation.

Occupational Therapy in Psychiatry

The occupational therapist uses activities with the mentally and emotionally disturbed to further the general goals of psychiatric treatment; that is, to assist the patient to (1) gain self-understanding or insight into his problems; (2) relate successfully and comfortably to other people, and (3) develop his assets and use them constructively toward optimal independence. It is not within the scope of this chapter to go into the complex and controversial theories of psychiatric treatment, although every occupational therapy program reflects the philosophy of its medical setting, depending upon the amount and nature of medical guidance received. Ratio of patients to staff is of equal importance in determining the quality of the occupational therapy program.

Further it should be emphasized that the approach in occupational therapy for children differs distinctly from that for adults. The adult is helped to regain an equilibrium which he has lost, whereas the disturbed child has not yet developed his ego and does not have the background of experiences on which to build his adjustment.

On the basis of their limited training in psychology and human physiological function, the nurses and craft teachers who first called their work "occupational therapy" in the early 1900's were beginning to select activities which appeared to be appropriate for particular types of psychiatric patients. The rationale for the use of occupations as treatment still issues from relatively elementary observations of human behavior as well as from more complex analyses made through psychology and psychiatry. The education of today's occupational therapist should provide an understanding of the dynamics of development of human personality, an appreciation of the fine line between normal and abnormal behavior, a knowledge of the difference between organic and functional causes of mental illness, and an understanding of self. The therapist must see the significance of symptoms, understand the basic needs of patients and appreciate how certain activities can help to meet these needs. The required three months minimum of clinical training in a psychiatric setting provides the student with the opportunity to apply this knowledge under supervision.

The experience and depth of understanding of the therapist is one determinant of the extent to which he is able to take advantage of important aspects of the patient's participation in activity. Another determinant of the therapist's ability to guide the patient effectively is the total information available on the case. Although treatment may start with only a minimum of data from the referring physician, such as symptoms of illness, apparent needs, and precautions to be observed, all those working with the patient can move ahead with more assurance when there is adequate and timely exchange of information. The psychologist, social worker, vocational counselor, and others may supply vital information on a patient's pre-morbid personality, intellectual capacity, educational level, economic status, social aspirations and family life. In turn, the occupational therapist initially can contribute diagnostic information, such as observations of bizarre behavior, of visual-motor incoordination, signs of petit mal seizures, evidence of concrete versus abstract thinking, or other evidences of organic disturbance. Later on, information may be supplied to assist in vocational rehabilitation as described in another section of this chapter.

The usual occupational therapy setting provides a normal atmosphere, reality-oriented although relatively protective, and designed to meet the special needs of the regressed, the depressed, the hostile, the anxious, the withdrawn, the dependent, and otherwise disturbed. Within general climate, some physicians or treatment teams set fairly specific guide lines by prescribing attitudes such as "firmness" or "permissiveness" in approach to certain patients.

Although recognizing that the same activity can mean different things to different people, the occupational therapist has traditionally used certain types of activities to elicit certain behavior. If it is simply a matter of a patient "letting off steam," the therapist channels the hyperactivity by providing vigorous work or play. The patient who has a tendency to withdraw must be tempted with something that will attract rather than threaten him. The guilty, depressed patient may respond best initially to some unimaginative and repetitive chore.

Frequently, in the normal course of activity, the occupational therapist is able to demonstrate to a patient how he responds to certain situations and how others accept or reject him on the basis of his behavior. For example, the occupational therapist may deliberately structure an activity to elicit frustration, so that the patient may be confronted with his own behavioral response. There are varying philosophies among occupational therapists and their co-workers as to the appropriate extent of their participation in psychotherapy beyond the role of observer and reporter; however, the great majority of occupational therapists feel that their function should be limited unless they have had advanced special training, either formal or informal.

In addition to following the psychodynamics of each case, the occupational therapist also plans around the effects of drugs, electroshock therapy and surgery. Side effects of some drugs cause sensitivity to sunlight or temporarily curtail the patient's visual acuity, coordination, or ability to concentrate. Adaptations in occupational therapy are made accordingly. For example, some patients must be discouraged from initiating numerous efforts without following anything to completion, while it may be important for others to have several projects underway when medical treatment causes periodic fluctuations in ability to perform. Very confused or distractible patients are guided in simple procedures appropriate to their attention span. Some patients benefit from projects they can work on at home or on the ward, while others require the presence of the therapists for any successful accomplishment.

In discussing "successful projects," it must be re-emphasized that the activity is not important in itself, but should be recognized as an important natural means through which relationships occur and feelings may be expressed. However, because society places value on things of beauty and usefulness which are made with the hands, or on physical and mental skills which may be learned, and because an individual's progress in this kind of achievement can be an indication of the level of his physical and emotional health, the successful accomplishment of an occupational therapy activity is a realistic secondary goal. The projects created, games played, work done, are all symbols of occupational therapy. Less apparent are the decisions and planning, the sharing of equipment and materials, the give and take that are involved in getting things accomplished. These are intangible tools of the occupational therapist not only in psychiatry but also in other areas of disability.

Aid in Physical Restoration

Increased strength, endurance and coordination of individual muscles or small or large groups of muscles or of the total neuromuscular system is the focus of treatment here. This is the most exact, the most measurable, and probably the most easily understood use of occupational therapy. It is the area of occupational therapy which particularly necessitates study of general anatomy and physiology, neuroanatomy, neurophysiology, kinesiology, neurology, and orthopedics. It is the area of occupational therapy where the medical specialties of neurology, orthopedics and physical medicine are most appropriately looked to for medical guidance of the profession. It is also the area where maximum quality of treatment is particularly affected by good communication and close teamwork with physical therapy, so that each profession makes its particular contribution and the areas of natural overlapping of function are mutually planned and coordinated to assure comprehensive treatment without wasteful duplication of effort.

Occupational therapy's importance in physical restoration is recognition of the complicated interdependence between emotions, intellect and physical functioning. The earliest users of occupational therapy noted that a patient would work longer and more vigorously at a therapeutic exercise if it were part of a purposeful activity which was pleasurable or meaningful to him. Further—repetitive performance of consciously-initiated acts has been generally accepted as essential to the development of those automatic, coordinated neuromuscular performances essential to normal human function. In other words, occupational therapy is important in physical restoration because it emphasizes coordinated performance of the entire psycho-motor system.

The activity program planned to meet these treatment objectives must have these characteristics: (1) It must provide adequate frequency of repetition of the specific motion (s) necessary to exercise the specific muscle (s) ; (2) it must provide the needed amount of resistance to muscle pull; (3) it must require sufficient simplicity or complexity of consciously-initiated movement to meet the requirements for development of coordination; (4) it must be flexible enough to permit increase or decrease in frequency of repetition, amount of resistance and coordination according to the changing needs of the patient; and, finally (5) it should be of interest or pleasurable to the patient to provoke his maximum voluntary participation.

It is understandably difficult, particularly in a medical setting, to provide an array of activities which meet all of the above requirements. Traditionally, the various handcrafts (i.e., woodworking, weaving, printing, ceramics) have provided maximal flexibility within limited space and continue to be emphasized. Ingenious adaptations of looms, printing presses, hand tools, and other equipment have been developed by occupational therapists in order to provide specific exercise and simultaneously offer the patient some choice of activity.

During the early stages of treatment in physical restoration, close supervision by a medically-oriented therapist is essential, as dosage is exact and methods of performance must be closely guided. As the patient progresses and the exercise requirements become more general, direct supervision by the patient's program of "treatment-through-selected-activity" may be by participation in planned work and recreation activities in his own home or in general activity programs in the hospital.

To Assist in Training for Independent Living

This objective of occupational therapy relates to comprehensive rehabilitation (or habilitation) where the total staff's concern is for provision of training and practice for the patient in those functions which are essential to independent living and which he, because of his disability, needs special help to perform. The following functions are typically included: (1) self care (dressing, feeding, bathroom and personal grooming requirements) ; (2) communication (speech, handwriting or typing, use of telephone) ; (3) transportation (walking, use of crutches, use of prosthesis, use of wheelchair, getting in and out of chairs, getting up and down stairs, getting in and out of an automobile); (4) general home responsibilities (use of kitchen equipment, use of cleaning equipment) , and (5) miscellaneous (special demands of school, home or job environment) .

In programs for the physically disabled child or adult, the job of providing necessary training is usually shared in various ways by the rehabilitation nurse, the speech therapist, the physical therapist and the occupational therapist. A division of labor is realistic because of the specialization necessary if the patient is to benefit from the advances in knowledge made in all aspects. The occupational therapist usually has special responsibility for numbers 1 and 2 above (with the exception of speech if a speech therapist is available), and shares responsibility in other areas, according to need and special abilities. The particular contributions of occupational therapy in the total program are those which utilize the following skills of occupational therapy: a knowledge of human anatomy and kinesiology with special emphasis on the upper extremity; knowledge and concern for the importance of human emotions in motivation for independence; a knowledge of a wide variety of manual skills useful in design and construction of special adaptations of equipment.

In programs for the mentally disabled patient, where training in independent living rarely involves physical disability and the concern is entirely with social and psychological disability, the composition of the rehabilitation team will differ from the above. The occupational therapist may share responsibility with the special teacher, with the social worker, and with other members of the staff who have special skills important in helping the patient to function independently in his home and community.

Aid in Psycho-social Development

This is a particularly complex area of occupational therapy and bears a close and frequently overlapping relationship to treatment for the mentally ill patient. It is considered as a separate category, however, because it refers to treatment frequently prescribed for the physically ill or disabled person who is not "mentally ill" in the usual sense, but who is coping with personal-adjustment problems which have been precipitated or accentuated by his illness. Frequently, these are problems of such magnitude that they are interfering with his recovery from a physical ailment. On the other hand, a patient may seem to be currently well-adjusted but this type of treatment is requested as a preventive measure when recurrent emotional stress is anticipated.

This is an area of occupational therapy which requires the therapist to integrate and apply all of the knowledge he has gained about the human being as a physical-psychological and social creature. It requires not only a thorough understanding and appreciation of the patient, but also a sophisticated understanding of the medical setting and its complexity of inter and intra-professional relationships which are affecting the patient and a knowledge of his family and work situation and the supports and stresses he will face there.

The therapist's aim is to help the patient make the best possible adjustment to his immediate institutional life and to his post-institutional life in terms of his psychological and social adjustment to his family, his co-workers, and his community. The aspired level of adjustment needs to be set in terms of the reality of his disability as well as his basic physical, emotional, intellectual, cultural, and social assets.

It would be an unusual occupational therapist who could, with maximum effectiveness, carry out this responsibility unaided. However, occupational therapists are oriented to seeking the guidance of specialists from all other fields (medicine, nursing, psychology, social service, etc.) to gain the best possible understanding of the patient. They can then use this knowledge and their unique "tools" to structure a situation which can be of therapeutic benefit to the patient. The "unique tools" of occupational therapy to which we refer are those various traditions of the profession which can be so advantageous. For example: (1) The occupational therapists typically approach the patient with an emphasis on *that which is well* about him. Their emphasis is properly on what the patient can do, despite his illness or disability. (2) Their traditional orientation to patient-approach is to seek to motivate the patient to voluntary participation. Rarely must they assume an authoritarian role and demand the patient's compliance. (3) They traditionally have enviable freedom in the tools they use, with any activity from manual labor to an extravagantly-conceived entertainment serving as a therapeutic tool. (4) They have traditional freedom to make the occupational therapy department truly a "laboratory for living." It can be business-like and formal or casual and informal; it can be highly directive or very permissive; it can be work-oriented or play-oriented—and all of these in accordance with the needs of the patients who are currently using the clinic. (5) Finally, the occupational therapists can adjust the work setting to regulate the quantity and quality of interpersonal relationships. They can start the patient on an activity where he works alone in an isolated part of the clinic and has no reason to talk with anyone except the therapist; or they can start him on a project which draws him immediately and naturally into a small or large group of patients. They can afford the opportunity for him to learn to accept help from a special type of person, or they can create the opportunity for him to gain quick acceptance from others by constructing a situation where his skills are immediately valuable.

Occupational Therapy in Pediatrics

Certain general goals, based on the common needs of all children, are superimposed upon the immediate need for treatment occasioned by the mental or physical disability of the individual. The primary consideration which makes treatment of children different from that of adults is the fact that their normal growth and development, their potential for adulthood, is threatened by the occasion of illness. Consideration of the role of parents is also a built-in feature of the child's management, since reactions of parents to the disease or disability have a marked effect on the response of the child.

In addition to a background of medical sciences, psychology, and psychiatry, the occupational therapist should have thorough grounding in the processes of normal growth—physical, social, and mental, as well as in speech and personality. Working cooperatively with the doctor, psychologist, social worker, nurse, teachers or others sharing in the care of the child, the therapist can then plan play activities that will provide the child with opportunity to develop his resources to the optimal degree. This may mean structured or unstructured leisure time; it may mean providing stimulation or protecting the child from too much stimulation; it may mean encouraging his participation in group play or teaching him new work or play skills which he may enjoy alone. By guided play, the child practices social as well as physical skills in which his illness has caused him to lag behind. An appropriate activity normally holds a child's interest longer than the average toy and permits him to attempt problem-solving, to learn work habits, cooperation with others, manual skills and standards of achievement.

Although all children tend to regress to some extent when they do not feel well, the therapist trained in child development and knowing the individual problems of the patient can select, adapt, and grade activity at an appropriate level to encourage growth, while at the same time provide pleasurable experiences.

Ideally, the therapist has the opportunity to work cooperatively with the child's parents in order to assist them in understanding and carrying out procedures which have been recommended. On the medical ward, children who are absorbed in an activity program are more cooperative in accepting medical procedures and less preoccupied with illness. They tolerate readmission more readily when it is necessary.

Physical goals may be the same with children as with adults— increased muscle strength, self-care, writing, or other such skills, but the media most frequently used are toys and some form of play.

In work with children, occupational therapy provides a secure and natural milieu where the child under treatment will play and perform with a freedom of expression and with a relaxation that enhances his receptivity and ability to learn. As a constant fixture in this setting, the therapist can make trained observation of the child's abilities as well as his disabilities and can serve as liaison between the medical staff, the parents, and the child.

Aid in Vocational Rehabilitation

In this area of occupational therapy, the therapists' aims are directed toward utilization of their laboratory situation to contribute to assessment of the patient's vocationally-related assets and liabilities and to aid in the development of vocationally-related abilities. The occupational therapist is particularly qualified to make a limited but significant contribution here because his basic medical and psychological orientation and training in manual skills is coupled with training and practice in observing physical and psychological responses of patients in their performance of both creative and manual skills. Because occupational therapists lack an intensive orientation to vocations and industrial work demands, their most effective contribution to the patient's vocational rehabilitation depends upon a close working relationship with, and appropriate guidance from, the vocational rehabilitation department, as well as from the responsible physician.

The methods of reaching the above objectives vary according to the space, equipment and supplies available to occupational therapy and according to the interests and abilities of the individual occupational therapist. The patient may work with unstructured and highly-creative activities (i.e., sculpture, painting) or he may work with highly-structured and industrially-related activities (i.e., assembly-line production of quantity items in the metal shop). Observations of vocationally-related characteristics will necessarily vary in objectivity according to the type and variety of activities used; but, in either instance mentioned above, the therapist can make valuable observations to answer questions such as these: Is he a steady and conscientious worker or is he sporadic and careless? Does he like to go ahead and develop his own ideas or does he prefer to have the therapist plan and detail his work? Does he prefer meticulous detailed work or does he consistently choose vigorous activity which is gross in work demands? Does he accept constructive criticism well and seek to improve the quality of his work or does he resist any suggestions and seem unconcerned if the result is poor in quality? Does he demonstrate a concern for the rights of others and willingness to share? Does he demonstrate any leadership abilities as he works as part of the group? Is he neat and careful with tools and equipment?

The vocational information requested of the occupational therapist also may be centered on the patient's disability, and work projects and observation methods must be modified to discern the answers to questions such as these: Has he recovered sufficient fine finger dexterity to go back to his old job at small-machine assembly? Can he get to and from the employees' lunchroom and restroom independently and in a reasonable time? Can he physically tolerate standing in one position for periods up to two hours? Are his needs for hyperactivity still too great for him to tolerate a sedentary desk job? Does he have sufficient facility with his prosthesis to handle specific machine controls?

The above illustrations emphasize evaluation as it can be

carried out in any occupational therapy department with either physically disabled or mentally ill patients. Frequently, this process can be concurrent with treatment if the patient's disability does not invalidate observations of his vocational aptitudes. This has the advantage of starting the patient and the staff in early planning for the patient's vocational future. More objective evaluation is usually obtained after the patient has received maximum treatment benefit and some occupational therapists are now specializing in what is commonly called "prevocational evaluation" whereby the patient's full time is devoted to either "work sample tests" or actually working in a selected job. As industrial norms can be used in the latter type of situation, both the patient and the vocational counselor can have greater faith in the reliability of the assessment of the patient's abilities.

The aforegoing paragraphs emphasized evaluation as the first division of occupational therapy's responsibility in vocational rehabilitation.

The development of vocationally-related abilities is the second division of this area of occupational therapy and is closely related to everything that is done for the patient under the name of "treatment." However, there are certain habits and abilities which may have particular vocational significance which can be developed through the provision of a training and graded—work program. Some of these are as follows: general work tolerance (to an eight-hour day), special strengths (i.e., ability to lift a 20 lb. object above shoulder height), standing tolerance, tolerance for working in distracting surroundings, habits of punctuality, and neatness in maintenance of work area.

As in all other areas of occupational therapy, economy of effort and success in making a real contribution to the patient's welfare depends on early planning and cooperative effort by all members of the rehabilitation staff who are properly involved. Leadership of the planning team is usually held by the physician if the patient is still undergoing treatment; it is appropriately held by the staff member in charge of vocational rehabilitation services if the patient is discharged from active medical treatment.

CONSIDERATION OF SOME ADDITIONAL ASPECTS

The "Tools" of Occupational Therapy

The "tools" of occupational therapy are these: (1) purposeful activities which are selected and (if necessary) modified to meet treatment requirements; (2) the therapist as a therapeutic personality; (3) the prevailing "climate" created within the occupational therapy department and (4) the person or persons (other patients, other staff, volunteers) who are used to affect therapeutic relationships in the clinic setting. No attempt will be made to describe the direct use of therapeutic relationships as this is a tool shared by all trained members of the rehabilitation team and better described in the writings of experts in the science of human behavior. The creation of a special climate has been presented earlier on page 35, with examples, which it is hoped, will be meaningful to the reader.

It is important, however, to discuss the use of selected and modified purposeful activities in occupational therapy. As was mentioned earlier, occupational therapy, in its earliest self-definition, emphasized that the profession was built on the philosophy that treatment may be given through the use of "any activity, physical or mental." This is a philosophy which occupational therapists have continued to maintain with absolute sincerity, as the therapist is well oriented to individual differences and the truth of the adage that "one man's meat is another man's poison." However, in actual practice, and through tradition, the occupational therapist has usually been limited to the use of the various arts and crafts. The present occupational therapist graduates have less proficiency in most of the skills than therapists of a decade or more ago. There appears to be two principle reasons: (1) The total length of the curriculum has not been increased enough to allow for the constantly increasing number of credit hours required for the biologic, social, and medical sciences. The number of hours devoted to training in technical skills has consequently had to be reduced. (2) The college students of today do not have the background in many usable skills which were taught in the home in earlier years (i.e., many women students have no knowledge of sewing, kitchen activities or basic home management skills).

There is disagreement among occupational therapist as to whether this is an unfortunate trend or not. Some leaders in the profession believe that occupational therapists can make a greater contribution to the patient if they have only a general orientation to a wide variety of skills (creative and manual arts, recreational, industrial, educational) and have a strong academic background which qualifies them to direct activity programs where specialists in skills do the actual teaching and supervision of the patients.

Other leaders in the profession feel that the unique value which occupational therapy has had to the patient lies in the unusual (in our culture) combination of intellectual, personal and manual skills. It is not the prerogative of the writers to predict the final decision of occupational therapy. Worth noting, however, is the increasing trend toward graduate education, and the serious discussions about putting the basic occupational therapy preparation on a graduate level. It is also important to emphasize that the young occupational therapists graduating today must be judged on the basis of their knowledge of human physiological and psychological function and not on the basis of whether they can "sew a fine seam" or "plane a square block."

Specialization in Occupational Therapy

This subject merits special attention in this chapter, if the reader is to have a realistic understanding of occupational therapy's assets and its limitations.

There is, at present, no formal recognition of specialization within occupational therapy. There is no specialization possible in the basic undergraduate curriculum and although graduate curricula offer specialization, there is no method of certification to give official recognition. In actual practice, however, there are many avenues of specialization. Examples of typical specialization are these: (1) Psychiatric occupational therapy: the therapist who works in a dynamic treatment-oriented hospital where team conferences on patients serve as staff training devices, and where the medical library is readily available becomes a specialist in that he has knowledge of the dynamics of mental illness and principles of psychiatric treatment which are far superior in depth and scope to the knowledge held by the therapist who has not had such experience. (2) Treatment of the cerebral palsied: the therapist who works in this complex area in one of the research-oriented programs develops, of necessity, advanced knowledge of neurophysiological principles and theories. (3) Rehabilitation of the severely disabled: therapists who work in these programs develop amazing facility with gadgets and adaptations of equipment, knowledge of kinesiology far beyond the undergraduate preparation, and a more thorough understanding of severe disabilities such as spinal cord injuries and amputations.

Many avenues of specialization are possible, and it may occur in disability areas as in the above, or it may occur in types of treatment as in pre-vocational evaluation. It would seem advantageous for the patient, the therapist, and the administrator if such specialization were more formally recognized.

The Work Setting for Occupational Therapy

The registered occupational therapists who are presently employed are working with acute or convalescent patients in a wide variety of settings. Typical places of employment include the following:

Hospitals, day-care centers and clinics for treatment and rehabilitation of the mentally ill.
General orthopedic, pediatric, and tuberculosis hospitals.
Rehabilitation centers.
Nursing homes.
Schools for handicapped children.
Institutions for mentally retarded.
Sheltered workshops and work programs for homebound adults.

Occupational therapy, since its inception as an organized profession, has emphasized its medical origin and alliance. The profession has always stressed that the use of activities for influencing the physical, psychological and social changes in a patient should not be termed "occupational therapy" unless the program is under the guidance or direction of, or in consultation with, a qualified physician. As a consequence, in most of the above work settings, the occupational therapy department will be placed administratively under medical direction. In many hospitals, the occupational therapy department is a separate service directly responsible to the medical director or a physician designated by him for all matters of patient treatment, and directly responsible to the hospital administrator for purely administrative matters.

In some hospitals (i.e., state psychiatric hospitals) occupational therapy is one of several "activity therapy" or "rehabilitation therapy" groups administered by a coordinator who is usually selected from one of the therapy specialties. Where basic differences, as well as similarities of the various specialties are considered, this organizational structure can promote an effective occupational therapy services.

In other hospitals (i.e., Veterans Administration hospitals), occupational therapy is a section in the department of physical medicine and rehabilitation and is responsible to the physician in charge of the department. The administrative practicality of having the occupational therapy service under the general direction of a single member of the medical staff is accepted by the profession as realistic. Occupational therapists, as members of an organized profession, however, strive for maintenance of a direct line of communication between the occupational therapist and the patient's personal physician. This has particular significance if the profession is to maintain its "general practice" approach to patient care and its breadth of concern for the patient as a physiological, psychological and social being.

The principle of medical "direction" of occupational therapy has, until recent years, emphasized the importance of a written prescription in which the referring physician spelled out exactly what he expected the occupational therapist to do for the patient. After years of attempting to procure this type of prescription, many occupational therapists now recognize that the physician may have enough general appreciation of occupational therapy's function to know that the patient can be helped by its services, but he may not know enough about the details of its service to write a specific prescription. Consequently, in practice, numerous occupational therapists now feel ethical and secure in accepting patients for treatment solely on the basis of a general medical referral, and are willing to assume responsibility for planning a treatment program based on medical information which they obtain through conference with the physician and other members of the medical team and from medical records. It remains essential that the therapist report to the referring physician as to the plan and course of treatment, and that the therapist be well trained in medical science so as to recognize danger areas and seek medical counsel before proceeding with treatment which might be detrimental to the patient.

In some places of employment (schools for handicapped children, sheltered workshops, institutions for mentally retarded), the primary emphasis of the institution's total program is not medical. The occupational therapist may function as part of a small, medically-oriented unit within the program and receive medical guidance from a part-time consultant who assumes responsibility for the total medical care of the persons seen by the occupational therapist and other medically-oriented personnel. In other programs (vocationally-oriented rehabilitation centers, sheltered workshops) the skills of the occupational therapist have been sought to contribute in areas that logically cannot be considered occupational therapy as they are not "treatment" (i.e., adaptation of work equipment and work methods to fit physical or mental limitations of employees).

REFERENCES

1. Dunton, Jr., William R., and Licht, Sidney: *Occupational Therapy - Principles and Practice.* 1st Ed., Springfield, Illinois, Charles C Thomas, Publisher, 1950.
2. Willard, Helen S., and Spackman, Clare S. (Eds.): *Principles of Occupational Therapy.* 2nd Ed., Philadelphia, Pennsylvania, J. B. Lippencott Co., 1954.
3. *Ibid.* 3rd Ed., 1963.

Chapter III

MEDICAL RECREATION

ORA R. ACKERMAN, Ed.D.*

INTRODUCTION

Recreation in a medical setting is relatively new, but recreation for medical purposes is not new. The activities that are now thought of, when one hears the word recreation, have been used through the ages to relieve illness and restore health. The literature reveals that as early as 2,000 B.C., the Egyptians saw the need for games, songs, and dances to provide cures for those suffering from melancholia. The Egyptians and those to follow received recreation as a diversion or an amusement. They did not have the scientific knowledge that is now available and applied to the practice of medicine. With the advent of scientific medicine also came new methods for the treatment of the mentally ill. Physicians were beginning to prescribe physical exercise, handicrafts, reading, and music for their patients. This advancement in medicine took place toward the end of the 18th and the beginning of the 19th centuries. Recreational activities continued to be utilized in the treatment of the mentally ill on a somewhat sporadic basis until World War I. Even though recreation activities were found in the mental hospitals they were still viewed pretty much as diversional. One doctor, at a Massachusetts hospital, in 1822, states that such activities as chess, backgammon, reading, writing, and singing, "were therapeutic in the diversion they afforded from unpleasant subjects of thought, in the mental and physical exercise involved; and in the tranquilizing effect upon the mind, resulting not only in breaking up wrong associations of ideas, but also in inducing correct habits of thinking as well as acting."[1]

Florence Nightingale, as part of her nursing crusade, introduced recreation services to those soldiers hospitalized for reasons other than mental illness. As she introduced and provided

---

*The author wishes to thank Miss A. Margaret Seymour, O.T.R. for her editorial assistance.

recreation opportunities, she came to realize that significant therapeutic values could be attached to recreational activities. She recommended pets for the invalid, after noticing that through the feeding and caring of the animal, the patient would gain a sense of self worth and the feeling of being needed.

World War I provided the opportunity for the recreation movement to expand into the hospital setting. The American Red Cross, through providing incidental recreation services to World War I patients, alerted the hospital administration as to the value of hospital recreation. The Red Cross continued to employ recreation leaders and provide recreation services to military and veterans hospitals until 1931. At this time, the recreation programs in the veterans hospital were made the responsibility of the United States Veterans Bureau.

During the 1920's and 1930's, recreation programs were appearing in some state operated mental hospitals and schools for the retarded. The programs were still diversional in nature and were conducted by untrained personnel, but nevertheless contributed to the hospital's treatment program.

World War II helped recreation to make the transition from recreation in a medical setting to medical recreation. It was during this era that recreation services for the physically and mentally ill were not only suggested - they were demanded. The military and veterans hospitals greatly expanded their recreation service to provide programs and activities to all the patients regardless of their illness or disability.

Recreation in the veterans hospitals was under special services and was not supervised by the Department of Physical Medicine and Rehabilitation Services until 1960. This administrative setup technically prevented recreation from becoming a clinical program. However, recreation programs were available to patients on the general medical and surgery unit, tubercular ward, orthopedic ward, and the neuropsychiatric unit. The type and purpose of the activity or program differed as did the medical services to the patient. A patient with a psychiatric disorder was assigned to a neuropsychiatric ward, and a patient with tuberculosis was placed on a T.B. unit. The treatment program in each case was different because the needs of the patient were different, but it was still a medical treatment. The same principle was true of recreation. The type of activities programmed for the psychiatric ward might have been completely different from the activities programmed for the general medical and surgery ward, but the programs were still called recreation. When the recreation activities were developed and programmed to meet the needs of a specific individual or group of individuals, then the concept of recreation in a medical setting began changing form and began to take on the pattern of medical recreation.

The recreator can plan and schedule various activities for hospitalized patients, but until the program is developed to meet specific medical needs, goals, and objectives, it should not be called medical recreation.

The difference between recreation in a community or in a medical setting and medical recreation is the fact that the goals, needs, and objectives are clearly determined by a physician and not by the professional recreator.

OBJECTIVES

Medical recreation has the responsibility to fulfill three objectives:

1. To help the medical staff meet specific emotional, psychiatric, and physical needs of the patient.
2. To help the patient develop a proper attitude toward the use of leisure time, and then to help him develop commensurate skills that will allow him to pursue an activity or activities of interest to him upon returning to his home community.
3. To help the patient adjust to hospitalization and to make life as enjoyable as possible.

These three objectives are inherent, but not always easily identifiable in the medical recreation program. In some instances, the professional recreator may have in mind all three of the objectives while he is working with a patient. In other instances, he may be focusing on only one objective as he involves a patient in a particular activity. To the competent recreator, this versatility is an asset which allows him flexibility to utilize a great number of activities to meet a variety of needs. To the lay person, all the activities appear to be the same or very similar and seemingly, all meeting only one objective. Too often the recreation program is seen as meeting only the third objective; that of making hospitalization more enjoyable. This is a vital and most necessary function of every recreation program; for every individual, regardless of his place of residency, has the need and right to meet and talk with others, to belong to a group, to be creative, to work off excess energy, to read and relax, and to have vicarious experiences. The physically and emotionally ill also have these same needs and therefore should be provided with opportunities to have them satisfied.

There is no one specific activity or program that can be prescribed to meet any one of these needs; yet nearly any of the needs may be satisfied by different individuals in the same activity. People go to the bowling lanes for various reasons; some to work off excess energy by throwing the ball, others to be with their friends - the actual bowling is incidental, and still others go to watch. Each individual is different. His interests and skills may be different from those of his neighbor. Therefore, the recreation program must be broad in scope and varied in specific activities.

A quality recreation program will provide opportuity for participation in games, sports, music, picnics, reading, trips, dance, dramatics, crafts, and discussion groups. Each of these program areas may also be varied and structured according to the needs and interests of the participants. The athletic activity may be a team dual or individual event; or the dance may be social or folk. With this magnitude of variety and scope the recreator is mandated to provide a full program that will be of interest and therapeutic benefit to the majority of the patients in the institution at any given time. The needs and interests may vary with changing populations and the recreation program must be adapted to meet the present needs.

It is becoming more evident each day that the American public must be educated toward the worthwhile use of leisure time. This educative process includes the development of positive attitudes toward the use of leisure, the acquisition of skills, and a knowledge of available facilities and programs available in which to pursue these leisure time interests. To the experienced medical recreator it is evident that most patients need to be involved in the same educative process. Most patients' histories reveal that the individual does not have a good pattern of leisure time use; nor does he have skills that will allow him to participate if he were so inclined.

The reasons for such a void in this area of total living may be many, as it is with the so-called normal. The physically ill individual may be under the impression that his disability prevents him from taking part in this aspect of life. He does not realize that recreation activities can be modified and adapted to allow for his participation. Too often this individual has the feeling that he "can't do it." Perhaps he tried once and failed. He fails to realize that through proper instruction and continued effort he can participate. More importantly he fails to realize that the participation is not an end in itself, but only a means to the end. The involvement in the activity allows him the opportunity to belong to a group, to be accepted by one's peers, and to have day-by-day interpersonal experiences that strengthens the character and personality, all of which leads toward healthful and meaningful living.*

The mentally ill patient may have also tried and failed. Failure is not unusual in this particular pattern of life. For the most part he has been a failure in all endeavors of life; his family, his work, and his leisure. The primary defense to ward off further failure is to withdraw. If I don't attempt to do anything, I can't fail; if I don't make friends, I can't be hurt. Consequently, life becomes a constant battle of avoiding possible unpleasantries.

There are many other factors or circumstances that may have prevented the mentally or physically handicapped individual from developing a pattern for the worthwhile use of leisure time. The specific reasons are not important at this point. What is important is the fact that the patient, like every other human, has the right to opportunities for healthful use of leisure time. The patient will not remain a patient forever. Upon recovery from his illness, he will return to his community as a useful and contributing citi-

---

*For additional information see Pomeroy, Janet: *Recreation for the Physically Handicapped*. New York, MacMillan Co., 1964, p. 382.

zen. It is the responsibility of the medical recreator to provide the educative process by which the patient may develop the necessary attitudes, skills, and confidence so as to use his leisure time in a healthful manner.

In planning for this phase of the recreation program the recreator must be cognizant of the recreation facilities and programs that are available in the surrounding communities. To have this knowledge of only the community adjacent to the hospital is not adequate. He must know, or have available to him, such information from each and every community that is represented by the hospital's population. If the purpose of this phase of the program is to develop the patient's interest and commensurate skills in recreation pursuits to be used in the home community, then it seems only natural to counsel the patient toward activities that will be available to him. The professional recreator must also be aware of family, religious, cultural, or any other restrictions and limitations that may be placed on specific activities by various communities or groups of people. Without this knowledge, the patient may be encouraged to pursue an interest that would cause conflict and frustration rather than peace, harmony, and adjustment. One young female patient was encouraged to take ballroom dance lessons. After some hesitation, she accepted and proved to be a most acceptable dancer. She enjoyed this activity and attempted to follow through when she returned home. The only problem was that the family did not approve of social dancing; nor was it commonly accepted in the community. This situation was frustrating to the girl and immediately caused a problem within the family. If the recreator had made use of knowledge that may have been available to him, this situation could have been avoided.

The first listed, but last discussed, objective or purpose of the medical recreation program is to help the medical staff meet the patient's specific emotional, psychiatric, and physical needs. These needs are not always self-evident and are usually defined following a complete diagnostic evaluation. In chart rounds or staff meetings, it may be determined that this patient has a need for such things as: release of hostility; socialization; ability to foster independence; strengthening of defenses; help to act out and accept aggressive impulses; socially acceptable means of self-punishment other than self-mutilation; palliatives for expression of anxiety and hostility rather than the rigid control now present; interpersonal exchange in situations where the control can be external as much as possible rather than internal; fostering of responsibilities; a firmer feminine identification; help in relating to both sexes; the ability to express hostility; and many other definitive needs.

Up to the present, the task of meeting these types of needs have been directed toward the psychiatrist, psychologist, social worker, and perhaps the psychiatric nurse or occupational therapist. What do these needs mean to the medical recreator and what can he do to help meet them? In too few instances has the medical recreator been assigned the challenge of meeting these needs. This is partially the fault of the psychiatrist for not using, to the maximum, the ability of the professional recreator and the activity or tools with which he works. The primary responsibility, however, lies with the recreator. He must first have the necessary training to function as a therapist. Secondly, he must accept the responsibility for helping to educate the entire medical service as to recreation's potential as a form of treatment.

PROGRAM ACTIVITIES

If we can think of activities as treatment tools, the medical recreator has a great variety from which to choose. The activity he selects for the patient will depend upon the treatment goals outlined in the psychiatrist's or physician's referral. The recreation therapist has a thorough knowledge of recreation activities. He knows the requirements and prerequisites for participation. He has analyzed each activity and considered participation in terms of functional abilities, physical requirements, degree of coordination, the degree of social involvement and interaction, and the degree of complexity or difficulty. The medical recreator cannot think of an activity only in terms of the whole. He must consider it in terms of its component parts. Consider such well-known recreation activities as bowling, physical conditioning, dancing, reading, and parties. What exactly is required of a patient to participate in one of these activities? Will this activity allow him to meet casually with others, or is the structure such that close contact and participation is demanded? Bowling would allow for a more casual relationship than would dancing. The focus in bowling is placed more on the individual and the personal interaction may vary according to the needs and capabilities of the participants. In ballroom dancing, however, participation necessitates a one-to-one relationship. No matter how much the patient might like to participate, if he is unable to bring himself to this one to one relationship, he will not dance and the treatment objective may not be reached.

Some activities require a certain level of body and/or hand coordination to achieve any degree of satisfaction. If the patient is unable to meet this minimum requirement, then similar or other activities should be scheduled. This might simply involve changing from ballroom dancing to folk or square dance - or from badminton to volleyball.

Many patients are functioning at a level much lower than their potential. The activity planned for this individual must be started at a level which allows the patient to perform at the maximum of his present capability and then progress from there. This does not mean that the adult patient should be expected to participate in childrens' games. The professional must adapt and modify an adult activity to a level of complexity that is comparable to the functioning level of the patient. In the case of the physically disabled, the level of mental complexity may be kept high, but the degree of body involvement may have to be modified.

The effective medical recreator knows the needs of patient, and has analyzed the activities in all program areas so that he knows explicitly the necessary prerequisites necessary for participation in any one activity. The prerequisites must be taken into consideration when a specific activity is selected to help the patient meet a specific mental, physical, or emotional need.

An example of this process is found in the case study of a single white girl from a small town who was admitted to a midwestern state hospital. The girl, in her early twenties, was the youngest of three siblings. She had completed two years of college, but her prime responsibility was to keep house for the family, as the mother was semi-invalid. The patient indicated upon admission to the hospital that she had been interested in church activities, civic clubs, softball, and bowling. Her principle occupations were a college student and housekeeping. Her history also revealed superficial suicide attempts. There were no physical disabilities.

The patient was diagnosed schizophrenic reaction, undifferentiated type, chronic. The general treatment objectives were: opportunity be provided for patient to express her feelings of intense hostility. It is also important that she learn more sublimated (hence, more socially acceptable) means of self-punishment other than self-mutilation. If this can be achieved, then it will be possible to discover and attack the sources of hostility much more directly. The treatment schedule for this individual, based on the general treatment objectives included: individual therapy three times per week, leather class twice per week, ceramics once per week, general occupational therapy once per week, physical conditioning and bowling, each meeting twice per week, a weekly social dance class, and an industrial therapy assignment involving sixteen hours per week. In addition to this schedule, the patient was allowed to participate in the religious services of her choice and in the diversional recreation programs scheduled in the evening. The ceramics and leather classes were supervised by occupational therapy and were selected to help meet the treatment objectives. The question at point is how can the recreation activities, namely physical conditioning, bowling class, and social dance, help meet these treatment objectives?

Bowling provides an excellent opportunity to express the intense hostility. This release is possible through the throwing of the ball. The delivery may be soft or hard as desired and no one really cares. In this particular case, the recreation therapist kept encouraging the patient to throw the ball harder and harder, thus actually fostering the expression of hostility. Release of hostility and self-punishment can also come through the setting of pins. Bowling, to the medical recreator, is more than throwing the ball. It is also the setting of pins, the score keeping, the handing out of balls and shoes, the assigning of the patient to an alley; thus controlling social interaction - and the actual instruction in the technique of bowling.

Physical conditioning allows an excellent outlet for socially acceptable self-punishment. If the individual seems to over-exert the body, the observer distinguishes it as an attempt to attain and keep the body healthy. The various components of physical conditioning such as jumping rope, riding a stationary bike, striking a punching bag, and throwing a medicine ball, all provide an outlet for the expression of hostility.

The dance class, through the rhythmical expression of the body, does provide an opportunity for expression of hostility. The type of music and form of dance utilized is the secret of success. Music with a fast, clear beat that would suggest whole body movement would be selected in place of quiet, slow moving mood music.

This is only a sample of the activities which might be suggested for a particular patient. What must be stressed is that there is no one answer or activity for any given situation. The recreator must know the treatment objectives, the patient, his physical disabilities, any precautionary measures, and have a thorough knowledge of all aspects of recreation activities.

Recreation programs will vary from medical setting to medical setting. The activity or program that is prominent in one institution may not even exist in another. No outsider can accurately say that this is good or bad. Only the medical staff and the professional recreator can determine what should be included in the recreation program at any given institution.

The focus in this chapter has been primarily on medical recreation with the neuropsychiatric patient. This is due partially to the author's experience in this area and, secondly, to the fact that the majority of the medical recreators are employed by state, federal, and private neuropsychiatric hospitals. Medical recreation can be an effective part of the treatment program in schools for the retarded, general hospitals, rehabilitation centers, childrens' hospitals, nursing homes, out-patient clinics, and the comprehensive treatment centers now being developed. The actual medical setting, the physical facilities, the type of patient, and the composition of the treatment team will affect the type of recreation activities offered. It will not, however, affect the objectives of the total recreation program nor the process effected by the professional recreator in utilizing the recreation activity as a therapeutic media. The medical recreator who has a basic understanding of the illnesses and disabilities normally treated in a medical setting and has analyzed into component parts all types of recreation activities can be an effective member of the treatment team regardless of the setting or the type of patients being treated.

Recreation, as a treatment media, has an advantage over many other forms of treatment. This advantage is couched in the concept of fun and play. The patient is oftentimes involved in the activity before he realizes what is really happening. He is having fun and enjoying himself; he does not think of himself as being in a treatment setting. This sense of freedom and naturalness allows for the complete giving of one's self without the conscious awareness of being on guard. The subsequent relationship between the patient and the medical recreator can be most therapeutic. In order to involve a patient in any activity, it is first necessary to know something about the patient. In addition to his physical and mental condition, the recreator must find out the patient's interests. What he did for recreation prior to hospitalization? What are the things he would like to learn to do - does he have any secret ambitions? The list is endless, but the answers to such questions enable the competent recreator to choose an activity that is likely to be of interest to the patient and which will still be adaptable and flexible for use as a treatment tool. There have been many cases reported of patients who have been on the ward for a length of time and seemed to have no interests and no skills, but given the right opportunity, sat down to the piano and started to play. This action amazes everyone and somebody always comments, "I didn't know so and so could play," or "so and so could do anything."

Communication is not always possible, but in too many instances the patient was never given the opportunity to tell anyone that she plays the piano. The recreator should draw from as many resources as possible to obtain all the information of this nature known about the patient. This knowledge, along with his own personality, helps to develop the patient-therapist rapport that is so vital in all forms of treatment.

STANDARDS

The relative newness of medical recreation, as with all new professions, leaves many problems unresolved. The actual labeling of the profession is primary to many. Some use the term of this chapter medical recreation; others prefer therapeutic recreation. Once these semantics are agreed upon, the title given the individual professional should follow. The individuals are now known as medical recreators, recreation therapists, rehabilitation therapists, etc. The titles are numerous, but their duties and responsibilities appear to be similar. In addition to defining and exemplifying the term and function of medical recreation, the profession is concerned with standards for academic preparation and internship training. Many colleges and universities offer courses and degrees in recreation, recreation leadership, recreation administration, etc. These curriculums have been developed primarily to train the student to be employed in community recreation, private and social agencies, youth work, and other agencies or programs housed in the community setting. For the most part, the curriculums have not been designed to provide the student with information that would make him more effective in a medical setting, and certainly do not prepare him to be a professional medical recreator. The graduate of such curriculum has the basic knowledge and skills of recreation; its philosophy; its scope; leadership technique; competent skills to lead and instruct; and some understanding of man as a social being.

The medical recreator must also have this same knowledge, but he must, in addition, have specific training and preparation that will give him the essential common denominators needed to treat patients and to work with the physician, nurse, social worker, physical therapist, psychologist, and occupational therapist. These common denominators are the behavioral sciences and a clinical affiliation.

Some colleges and universities have developed specialized curriculums to give the student this common denominator but, to date, a standardized curriculum of this nature has not been developed. A Therepeutic Recreation Curriculum Development Conference held in February 1961, in New York City, was a beginning attempt in this direction. The participants of this conference, educators, clinicians, and consultants, identified these competencies of a recreation therapist: an understanding of human growth and development of man as an individual and as a special social being; including his needs, desires, and capabilities at all age levels, and in varying degrees of mental, emotional and physical capabilities; an understanding of the learning process and how to expedite it, including skill in the use of appropriate leadership techniques with due regard for the differing needs of individuals; ability to stimulate maximum participation in participant leadership; and proficiency in evaluating outcomes of learning experiences; a fundamental knowledge of the structure in functions of the human body; knowledge of and skill in the use of group processes and other methods of informal education; an understanding of psychological reactions to disability or illness and an awareness of the implications of basic psychological principles for the rehabilitation process; ability to give guidance to ill and handicapped individuals in relation to personal and social lesisure concerns, in order to make possible optional use of available personnel and community resources and facilities; understanding of how impairment of the various organic systems limits activity and how activity affects the function of the various systems; ability to relate the effects of impairment to the patient's relaionship to others, his utilization of his environment (both material and personal) , and his potential participation in activity; understanding of program activity as a means to promote individual expression, to improve inter-personal relationships, or to provide a means of interaction for the ill and handicapped; knowledge of implementation and adaptation of programming for the ill and handicapped; knowledge, understanding in appreciation of such program areas as: arts, acquatics, camping, outdoor recreation, crafts, dance, drama, hobby or special interest groups, mental and linguistic activities, music, physical activities—gymnastics, sports, games—social recreation, and special recreation.

Now that the competencies of a recreation therapist have been spelled out, it is possible to develop curriculums that will more adequately prepare the student for employment in this specialized area of recreation. As the therapeutic use of recreation continues to expand, in both quantity and quality, the employers will insist upon employing professionally qualified medical recreators. The recreation profession will demand that individuals wishing to become a member of the profession be trained and educated at a college or university having an approved curriculum in recreation and some type of option in therapeutic, medical, or hospital recreation, or preferably a graduate degree with a major in this specialized area. In order to be fully trained, it is recognized that the medical recreator will ultimately have to be trained at the master's level or beyond.

The Council for the Advancement of Hospital Recreation has developed professional standards and has established a national registration procedure for two levels of professional hospital recreators. These levels are the hospital recreation director and the hospital recreation leader.

The minimum educational requirements and experience for registration at the director's level is:

1. Master's degree from an accredited college or university with a major in hospital recreation, recreation in rehabilitation, or recreational therapy, and one year of successful full-time, paid experience in recreation for the handicapped in a medical setting. (The required clinical experience for the master's degree may be substituted for an equal portion of successful full-time paid experience.)

2. Master's degree from an accredited college or university with a major in recreation, and two years of successful full-time, paid experience in recreation for the handicapped, in a medical setting.

3. Master's degree from an accredited college or university with a major in a professional field closely allied to recreation and applicable to recreation for the handicapped in a medical setting, an undergraduate degree from an accredited college or university with a major in recreation, or its equivalent (24 college credits in professional courses in recreation), and two years of successful full-time, paid experience in recreation for the handicapped in a medical setting.

The minimum educational requirements and experience for registration at the leaders level is:

Bachelor's degree from an accredited college or university with a major in recreation or in a field of study appropriate to a specialized recreation function within the hospital recreation program (e.g., music, sports, drama, dance).

The Council for the Advancement of Hospital Recreation was organized in *1953* by three professional organizations interested in the specialized field of hospital recreation. These three organizations are (1) The American Recreation Society, Hospital Recreation Section formed in 1948; (2) The National Association of Recreation Therapists, formed in 1952, and (3) The Recreation Therapy Section, Recreation Division of the American Association for Health, Physical Education and Recreation, formed in 1952.

The purpose of the Council is to effect a closer working relationship toward the accomplishment of mutual purposes and to explore the possibilities of eventual amalgamation into one strong professional organization dedicated to the promotion of recreation for the ill and handicapped. The latter purpose is not yet a reality, but the National Registration is. This registration has had its effect upon the hiring practices of many private and governmental agencies. These agencies may not require registration, but they have adopted the majority of the requirements for academic preparation and full-time experience.

It is estimated that there are 2,800 persons employed full-time in recreation programs in a medical setting. As of July 1st, 1964, there were 273 individuals registered at the Directors level with the Council for Advancement of Hospital Recreation, and 105 registered at the Leaders level. In addition, 38 were registered as Recreation Aides. These figures are significant when one thinks of the philosophy of recreation therapy or medical recreation as developed in this chapter and the existing programs that may be termed medical or hospital recreation. The discrepancies in these figures suggest that there may be many untrained recreators and many more untrained recreators conducting and supervising recreation programs in medical settings. These individuals may or may not be conducting a medical recreation program, but it would be unfair to judge now, and in the future, a young profession with a tremendous potential on the basis of existing programs conducted by individuals who are not fully qualified by professional standards.

HOSPITAL-COMMUNITY RELATIONS

The second objective of a medical recreation program assumes that the patient will return to the community to live as a useful citizen. In focusing on this objective, the recreation therapist is concerned with developing the patients' skills and attitudes for his leisure time use. But is this adequate? It is now realized that the patient must be helped in bridging the gap from the hospital to the community. He must be helped to find outlets for his recreational interests. To accomplish this transition it is imperative that the local community be aware of the needs of these individuals. It is not the responsibility of the medical recreator to develop and conduct recreation programs in the community - this is the community's responsibility; it is, however, his responsibility to develop a relationship with individuals or agencies in the community providing recreation programs, and promote an exchange of ideas, that creates a pattern of communication. To help facilitate this action, the Indiana University Department of Recreation in cooperation with the Indiana School of Medicine and the Indiana Department of Mental Health sponsored an Institute on Therapeutic Recreation in the Community. Dr. Janet MacLean[22] in the foreword states, "The basic democratic principle of the right to 'life, liberty, and the pursuit of happiness' makes mandatory an increasing awareness of our obligations to groups with special problems. The ill and the handicapped who live in our communities constitute such a minority. If the recreation profession is to maintain the ideal of 'recreation opportunity for all,' then the recreation needs of this segment of our population present an ever increasing challenge to community recreation personnel, since these groups with extended free time most need satisfying experiences in that leisure."

Recreation professionals have often discussed their responsibility for helping the non-institutionalized mentally ill or mentally retarded in their communities; they have also shown concern for those mental patients who return from the hospital to continue their lives in the local community. All too frequently, the patient released from the hospital must return to the same environment which originally sparked his mental difficulties. Though aware of the need to improve existing conditions, the recreation professionals have often been reluctant to serve these patients or have found difficulty in opening channels for better understanding of the needs of this population. Better communication is needed with other individuals and disciplines which are concerned with the same individuals.

The Institute was aimed at effecting, among those whose responsibility it is to serve recreation needs in local communities, a better understanding of the needs of: (1) patients returning to their communities from the state mental hospitals, and (2) those non-institutionalized individuals who are suffering from mental illness or mental retardation.

The Institute participation was restricted, so that better group interaction might take place among those in attendance. Delegates were invited from: (1) municipal recreation departments with full-time administrative staff and year round community center programs, (2) YMCAs and YWCAs sponsoring community recreation programs, and (3) recreation personnel from the state mental hospitals and schools for the mentally retarded.

Expected outcomes of the Institute included:

1. Closer cooperation and better communication between recreation personnel and other professionals who are serving the needs of the ill and handicapped.
2. For the community recreation personnel:
   a. Increased responsiblity for, and involvement with the non-institutionalized mentally handicapped now living in Indiana communities.
   b. Better understanding of the problems of patients returning to their communities to decrease the reluctance to accept former patient in the present community recreation offerings.
   c. Knowledge of sources of deferral and information concerning problems in mental health.
   d. Development of the optimum therapeutic milieu in existing programs in which returning patients will participate.

3. For the hospital personnel:
    a. Better understanding of the total community offering in recreation and the scope and limitations of that offering.
    b. Up-to-date information or sources of information concerning program offerings in the communities to which patients are returning.
    c. More effective counseling of patients returning home with regard to opportunities for recreation in their local communities."

When the results of institutes such as this and individual contact between community and medical recreators bear fruit, the gap between hospital and community will disappear — thus enabling the patient to be easily assimilated into leisure time activities of his choice.

SUMMARY

Medical recreation has made significant strides in a relatively short period of time. In the early 1930's and the mid 1940's recreation in a medical setting was primarily available only in military, governmental, and a few state hospitals; and the programs were viewed primarily as diversional. The personnel conducting these programs were untrained by today's professional standards, but nevertheless their contribution was significant. The recreation leaders had the necessary skills to teach and conduct recreation programs, but lacked the training and medical direction to program recreation activities for direct therapeutic values. The patients' participation in the various recreation activities was indirectly therapeutic. It provided them an opportunity to belong to a group, to express themselves, to release excess energy, and to have something to do during many otherwise seemingly empty hours.

This objective, a diversional program, is still a vital part of the medical recreation program. However, it is only a part. The professional medical recreator now has the academic training and program skills that enable him to utilize the various recreation activities to meet the patients' specific physical, emotional and psychiatric needs as defined by the physician. This aspect of the recreation program can now be evaluated for its direct therapeutic values. The medical setting, type of patient, etc., will not affect this objective. The medical recreator can be an effective member of the treatment team regardless of the setting or the type of patient.

The medical recreator is now concerned with the carry-over values inherent in the recreation program. The patients, like most "normal" citizens, have not learned or developed adequate leisure time pursuits. They are lacking positive attitudes toward the use of leisure time and have not developed skills that will permit them to actively pursue activities of interest to them. The medical recreator is concerned with the leisure time habits of the patient returning to the community and has assumed this educative process to be a part of his total recreation program.

Professional preparation of the medical recreator is not yet standardized with approved curricula, but the confidences of a recreation therapist have been identified and a national registration has been effected through the Council for the Advancement of Hospital Recreation. The American Recreation Society, Hospital Section, has published the second report entitled, *Basic Concepts of Hospital Recreation*.[3] These basic Concepts further define medical recreation; its function, its purpose, its potential, and the qualifications of its professional personnel. It does not limit its scope of operation. The boundary will be defined only by the professional recreator and his ability to interpret, to conduct, and to evaluate medical recreation.

REFERENCES

1. Frye, Virginia: Historical sketch of recreation in the medical setting. In *Recreation in Treatment Centers*. Washington, D. C., Hospital Recreation Section, American Recreation Society, 1404 New York Avenue, N. W., September, 1962, Vol. I, p. 41.
2. MacLean, Janet R., ed.: *Therapeutic Recreation in the Community*. Bloomington, Indiana, Department of Recreation School of Health, Physical Education, and Recreation, Indiana University, 1962.
3. *Basic Concepts of Hospital Recreation*. Hospital Recreation Section, American Recreation Society, Washington, D. C., 1962.

Chapter IV

MUSIC THERAPY

MYRTLE FISH THOMPSON, B. A., R.M.T.

INTRODUCTION

What and Why

SPECIFICALLY, music therapy is the purposeful use of music in participation or listening experience in the treatment of patients toward better health. More broadly, as one of the arts most universally practiced, it serves toward better functioning of individuals and groups, well or sick. The former use, with patients, and within the framework of a psychotherapeutic situation is our chief concern in this writing, although the discussion cannot be divorced completely from broad sociological concepts of the importance of art and aesthetics to all humans.

Music is the science or art of assembling or performing intelligible combinations of tones in organized structured form, with infinite varieties of expression possible, depending on the relation of its several component factors of rhythm, melody, volume, and tonal quality. *Therapy* has to do with how it may be used to bring about changes in people listening to it, or performing it. The responses will be neurophysiological, endocrinological, psychological and sociological. The latter will differ in different cultures, but more specifically, each person will respond in his own unique way to the wordless meaning of music which stems from its aesthetic quality and emotional content, as colored by his own cultural conditioning, by his environmental background, and perhaps by inherent tendencies. We react through our own interpretations, integrated through our own experiences, augmented by our own emotional feedback system which makes it even more forceful and meaningful.[1]

To influence attitudes and moods by non-verbal communication between music and people (and people and people) ; to create an atmosphere in which tensions may be more easily released and positive transference encouraged; to provide an experience which encourages free sharing of feelings and an added sense of security in being able to relate to others and to dissipate "aloneness;" this is the Gestalt of the whole music response potential.

In music therapy practices, Farnsworth[2] questions whether the emotional character of music is a subjective quality within the listener or an objective quality in the music itself. He finds it impossible to keep these formally apart. Doctor Dillenger[3] cites as potentials: feelings of integration transferred to the listener due to the orderliness of the music, catharsis of repressed aggressive impulses, and sublimation of sensual and sexual components. Doctor Gaston[4] sees in music opportunity for healthy expression of otherwise inexpressible emotions: "From lullaby to dirge, music has spoken for man when words could not." Van de Wall[5] cites systematic procedures and medical guidance as factors of importance. How the therapist functions as a therapeutic person, and how far he is able to accept sick behavior in others are stressed as contributing factors to success. Max Schoen[6] feels that music's healing virtues are derived partly from the physical and expressive aspects of sounds, and partly from the medicinal influence of art forms in general as they provide stimuli pleasurable to experience and recall.

Rudolph Dreikurs, famous Adlerian psychologist,[7] considers results gained in healthier interpersonal relationships to be of equal, if not greater, importance in music therapy practices than beneficial emotional responses, *per se,* from the music. He feels that social maladjustments directed "against the world" can be led, through the nonverbal sharing of the music experience, to relaxed and more friendly social adjustments in which patients find they can now reach "toward" the world, and "toward" each other.

Two or more listening to or making music together have a natural, comfortable situation in which to relax and expand and forget for awhile pressures from without and brooding from within. This is a situation approximating conditions outside a hospital. The music is a ground to meet on, a bridge for making contact; but it is the total milieu that treats the patient, not only the medium. No matter how helpful the music, it is how the music therapist relates to the patients in the situation, how well he understands the psychodynamics, and how effectively he makes pertinent material available to the psychotherapist that count more. In this sense, music is the adjective and therapy the noun, with positive attitudes the goal.[8]

Diserens,[9] many years ago, found that music experiences caused influential physiological reactions in the areas of bodily metabolism, tonus, muscular energy, speed of response and quantity of change in pulse, blood pressure, breathing and pupillary dilation. Depending upon specific qualities of the music, it calmed or stimulated activity. He went on to conclude, in later writing,[10] that music was not merely an aesthetic luxury but an adjunct to economic well-being, as seen in industry, and a tool for therapy through bodily changes of influencing mood, affect, and attitudes.

James Mann[11] stresses positive transference as the heart of any therapy, seeing distortions of faith in others as coloring faith in self. We need someone or something we can trust. We want closeness, but fear it. Music is then a therapy useful for engendering feelings of closeness to people through sharing an agreeable experience. Threat and danger are averted by the pleasant emotional overtones.

Dr. Gaston[12] cites Masserman's first Principle of Biodynamics[13] in describing man's response to music as stemming from one of three basic needs: survival, procreation, and aesthetic creativity — the latter significant and necessary but "indescribable" in words; and stresses Masserman's second Principle by his own theory that each man reflects his cultural and environmental conditioning, plus his personal idiosyncrasies, in responding to music. While exteroceptive pathways bring stimuli from the outside world, proprioceptive add stimuli from reactions within various parts of the body in a constant two-way flow, so that we receive and respond emotionally and intellectually as well as physiologically, exaggerating our feelings with the personal feedback systems determined by our own histories and by "all that in the present makes each himself."

A different interpretation represents the psychoanalytical thinking of Heinz Kohut.[14] He sees the ego as the acting center of the personality, enjoying mastery of the world of sounds, and using musical experiences as catharsis to counteract the tensions and overanxiousness of malfunction and disease. The superego calls on us for "submission to rules of the aesthetic code," accepting our guilt, accepting discipline, and seeking to find in music a restful, socially permissible substitute for regression and defeat.

Finally, Howard Hanson,[15] the eminent conductor and composer, feels that the first importance of music for therapy lies in its use as an art form for the sake of people, — not art for art's sake, nor art for the artist's sake, but to serve all men through inspiration, comfort, and pleasurable experiences.

Before leaving the introductory section on "What Is Music Therapy?" some comment should be made on what it is *not*. Nontherapeutic or antitherapeutic uses of music may occur in many ways through too-great permissiveness, or through carelessness in planning or supervision. Hospital audiences should not be affronted by poorly screened performers, or badly performed programs. Satisfaction to the performer should not be put before enjoyment of patients in the audience. Constant intensity or badly chosen content can inflict a punitive experience on listeners. Too-repetitious rhythm or style may become boring, or it may lead toward an unhealthy mesmerism of performers or listeners, or encourage narcissistic feelings and recapitulation of libidinal expression. Too-great license in exhibitionism by performers, or by an audience drawn into participation that becomes orgiastic, are dangers of certain current popular styles. Dr. Meyer[16] calls attention to the fact that sensuous music is not necessarily beautiful but may savor of "hedonism." He also warns against separation of sounds as "atomism," and against assumption that there can be one, and one reaction only, to any given composition as "absolutism."

Again, if music is used too often as escape from reality or to encourage unhealthy reliance on fantasy it can be a detrimental influence. Too-great preoccupation with any music experience, to the exclusion of other interests, can result in lack of balance and warped, obsessive behavior; or it may fortify a malady or an asocial trait or egocentric concern. Also, with psychotics, it can be dangerous to probe too deeply and too emotionally. Safer music should be chosen rather than to permit a breaking point to be reached, unless this is intentional and under close supervision of a doctor.

Individual dislike of certain kinds of music, or of any music at all at an unwelcome moment should be accepted. If there is indication of pathology in the aversion, the music therapist will want to consult the physician as to pursuing or dropping it. But in addition to respecting valid physiological reasons he should explore psychological ones due to unhappy association with certain music, or to personality factors of performer or therapist, or to any of a number of idiosyncrasies and vagaries which people occasionally must be permitted.

HISTORY

Rhythm is a basic phenomenon of nature and of man. Many of earth's functions — solar system, tides, and seasons, and many human functions — pulse, breathing and motor coordination follow orderly rhythmic patterns. Superimposed on regular rhythmic stresses an infinite variety of movements, an intricate detail, join with melody and harmony to make the sounds of wind and waves.

So with the human race, feeling and expressing rhythms, and making and responding to sounds are instinctive. Out of the steady rhythmic sway of primitive woman comforting her young came the crooning tune of the earliest lullaby. As man herded into communal groups his grunts and tonal sounds, by accent, inflection, and changes of pitch and volume became his language, conveying message and emotion. In time, he combined these with his innate feel for rhythm to create the beginnings of music, tied up almost universally to personal and tribal needs. As he experienced the group's reaction toward flight, or fight, in response to changes in volume and speed, and to rhythmic complexities he came to use these more and more meaningfully. To them he added fierce gesticulations and bodily movements as representations of attack and conquest of his physical enemies, man and beast. Again, in his fear of the unknown — the punishing gods of storm and natural disasters and of disease and death — he sought to placate or drive out evil spirits by the use of this powerful force men could generate when their incantations were used in particular ways.

By 4000 B. C. chants were accepted guarantees of fertility, as well as defense, and on through the ages music played a prominent role in mythology, folklore, sorcery, and conquest, as well as in religion and health.[17] From the early linking of Apollo as both god of music and patron of medicine, through the era of the great philosophers, Homer, Pythagoras, Hippocrates, Plato, all recommended that music be listened to and performed to help prevent negative passions, and to build positive health through elevating and vitalizing experiences.[18] Disease was considered a disharmony between the physical man and his psyche, and fundamentals of the tonal systems wisely used to be palliative measures for changing disharmony to harmony. Later, in Rome, the psychosomatic aspects of health were stressed by Aesculapius, Cicero, and later, Galen, and music used not only in temple rites but in health resorts, along with potions and surgery, in a constant theme of "musico-therapeutics."[18] While early Christianity referred primarily to the joy and efficacy of song and instrumental music in worship (a belief which has continued into the Anno Domini years in the concept of music as the "handmaiden of religion"), the Church in the Middle Ages often considered disease to be punishment for sins, with medicine strongly linked to religious cults and with musicians supposed to be able to supply specific music to heal.

Not until the Renaissance of the 17th and 18th centuries[19] when physicians were also learned men in all the arts, did medicine become a science with a humanistic approach, in the merging of many divergent fields. Diseases were now considered to be temporary disruptions of a natural harmonic state, and medicine increasingly concerned itself with the "whole man," body and mind, with the health of each part intimately involved with the other. Music and physiology came together in manipulation of instruments and in the scientific use of voice production and virtuosity. Communication and associative meanings were also explored by music and medicine in joint effort, and many philosophical works on the effect of music on disease and on man's attitudes and behavior in general, and as related to music, followed.[20]

In the late 19th and early 20th centuries, a measurable increase can be noted in the scientific and critical quality of writing as it moved away from a strongly philosophical emphasis. As psychology became a separate science concerning itself with specific responses to experience, among them artistic and aesthetic ones, legendary data were avoided, and more plausible reasoning and verification required in reporting uses of music in such nervous disorders as hysterias, phobias, conversions, and hypochondria. Physical properties of sound, vibrations, aspects of perception, and psychological factors involved in music enjoyment were beginning to be explored, and writers were already lamenting the absence of prolonged observation and careful note-taking on effects of music in treatment. However, despite these trends and the rich heritage of interest in the functional uses of music, scientists and musicians do not seem to have continued as consistent a pursuit of knowledge in this area as might have been expected. Except for a few researchers in psychological foundations, such as Helmholtz,[21] this period was low in recognition of music as a tool in therapy compared with the classical days of the Greek philosophers and Roman conquerors, or with the high cultural development of the Renaissance period.

In the first decade of the 20th century, although the arts had been growing by leaps and bounds in the performance areas, and in recognition by educators, it took two World Wars to bring the use of cultural activities back into focus for rehabilitation purposes. The need for absorbing interests for service men, particularly when long-term care was indicated, and the eagerness of volunteers to "do" for them—many of these people of professional skill as entertainers and teachers—brought all the arts into use as adjunctive tools of therapy. In the field of movement, Dalcroze[22] was concerning himself with cause and effect of rhythm as involved in individual deficiencies. Eva Vescelius[23] was preaching that health is rhythm, and disease unrhythmical, and that music, by co-ordinating impulses of body and mind, can assuage tensions and distress. Widespread investigation was growing of numerous specific aspects of body and mood responses to music, and studies with varying levels of scientific validity were appearing with growing frequency in professional and lay publications.[24]

More important, built on Helmholz' earlier efforts, an experimental psychology of music had been developed by the 1940's which was founded on pure psychology, musical aesthetics, physics, acoustics, and the anatomy of the auditory and cerebral centers.[25]

Physical properties of sound were as carefully explored and interpreted as physiological and psychological functions of the body; and perception, imagination, and ideation factors were treated exhaustively. Out of this effort came several textbooks on the psychology of music and the influences of music on behavior.[26-31] These are in equal demand by departments of psychology, music, and education. Other books of more general nature have stimulated widespread interest.[32-34]

While music had been used in varying degrees, in private and public institutions for years, the first move toward development of a professional status for hospital musicians began in 1920 with the formation of a Committee for the Study of Music in Institutions operating from the Russell Sage Foundation offices in New York City. This committee enlisted the services of Willem van de Wall, Ph. D., a professional musician with broad academic background and keen sociological interest, to investigate the potential uses of music at Central Islip State Hospital on Long Island. Later, he initiated and supervised music activities in several Pennsylvania institutions in cooperation with that state's Department of Welfare and wrote a comprehensive textbook on the subject of Music in Institutions.[35] Works Progress Administration projects under the leadership of Dr. Ira M. Altschuler[36] gave further impetus to developing institutional music programs.

In 1944, the services of Dr. van de Wall and of Dr. Samuel W. Hamilton of the United States Public Health Service were enlisted by the National Music Council in New York City, to do a survey on uses of music for the mentally ill.[37] Of 341 institutions questioned, 209 responded and of these, 192 indicated they were using music in some form. Almost fifty reported programs embracing several activities, and one was cited as outstanding in scope. Of 187 institutions answering a question on therapy, thirty considered music to be primarily recreation, twenty-three therapy, 134 recreation and therapy. Many stressed the greater value of active participation over passive listening.

By late 1940's, a few midwestern Schools had initiated music therapy degree courses, and two large national music organizations, the National Educator's Music Conference (NEMC) and the Music Teachers National Association (MTNA) had special committees studying uses of music in illness, handicap, and re-habilitation. An "overall" supervisory National Music Council with representation from all branches of music performance, education, and industry had an active Hospital Music Committee which was publishing a widely disseminated "Hospital News-letter."

All this activity culminated in 1950, in the organization of the National Association for Music Therapy.* This is an association of musicians working in rehabilitation areas, doctors, educators, psychologists, students preparing for the profession, and persons interested in supporting its work. Its aims are the progressive development of the uses of music in medicine, the advancement of research, the distribution of helpful information, the establishment of high standards of qualification and training for therapists, and the perfecting of techniques of music programming which will aid medical treatment most effectively. Annual conferences, and publication of a yearly book and of a professional magazine[38] cover all phases of the uses of music in therapy. Its membership of some 700 in 1963 included over 400 Registered Music Therapists.

In 1954, as a followup of the 1944 Russell Sage Survey, this association sponsored a study of the uses of music in 800 institutions of all kinds, first, on aspects of music as therapy; second, on scope of programs; third, on character and training of personnel; and fourth, on factors of facilities and management.[39] In contrast to the one outstanding comprehensive program described in 1944, 77 broadscoped music programs were reported; 52 in mental hospitals covering various uses of music for diversion, stimulus, mood control, as an ancillary tool in evaluation of tolerance and needs, and for the development of good work habits. As in 1944, the value of active participation was stressed — "the more participation, the more therapy." Several institutions indicated that their interest in music therapy was one of long standing.

ORGANIZATIONAL STRUCTURE

Many professional musicians respond best to the stimulus of career goals. Countless gifted amateurs know the joys of per-

*See Appendix A.

formance. While both value the need and satisfaction of study and practice, there are thousands of other devotees who prefer to enjoy their music as listeners and "appreciators." The extent of the use of music and of its impact on our society are reflected not only in the mass use of records, radio, and television, but in the astonishing growth of concerts by touring or locally trained units which permeate not only urban but rural areas throughout the country. Community choruses and large school bands are only matched in size and number by the ubiquitous city-sponsored symphony and opera groups in what is known as the "grass roots" development of American music.

In the field of education, music has also become a major activity not only in conservatories but in separate departments of many general colleges and universities. Course content covers all aspects of pedagogy, performance, composition, conducting, music history, and general musicology including sociological and psychological implications.

Such a growth both in mass uses and in professional training was bound to be directed to exploration of the specific uses for therapy of an activity used so universally for its general therapeutic affect, and with values for patients approximating so closely values for people in general. From out of these concepts grew the professional field of music therapy now recognized by a dozen academic degree courses in the country, and by extensive psycho-dynamically oriented applications in hospitals and institutions for rehabilitation.

The potential uses of music for hospitals run the gamut as to kind, amount, and degree of therapeutic content. In many places, there is music programming which might be considered minimal. For example, any one or two of the following activities might be available regularly, or perhaps all, occasionally: records (usually owned by patients); "day room" radio and television; music with religious services (often volunteer); dances once in a while with records or local talent combos; spontaneous "jam sessions," or more formally planned and conducted community singing; and, in most places, music performance at various levels of acceptability brought into the institution by "well-wishers" from outside. Such a list sounds more impressive than an analysis of actual substance reveals. Not only are events more occasional than routine, but the program must depend for any virility on the initiative and interest of some one patient or employee or volunteer who has leadership qualities as well as interest in the patient's emotional and social needs. Other more formally conceived and developed music programs are of all sizes and varieties depending not only on needs dictated by the specific kinds of illness but on administrative support as to rooms, equipment, and number and degree of special skills of the personnel who implement the program.

Music programs *per se* did not appear until after occupational therapy and recreational therapy were well established as professional activity fields, so that in many parts of the country music was and is still conducted as one of several activities of either occupational or recreational therapy departments. In some private mental hospitals and in many institutions for crippled children and the mentally retarded, it is under the aegis of education. In a few large hospitals, it is a separate department, or one of several coordinated activity therapies of equal status.

There is rationale for each placement. As to recreation, music *is* diversional, — among several potential approaches, and outside of hospitals is a major leisure-time activity. So is it therapeutic occupation for many. It is also a major field of education among the arts. One cannot draw clear-cut lines between what in an art form is recreational, what is uniquely educational, and what is good occupational therapy. While music study belongs in the area of education, it often is also absorbingly healthy occupation, and certainly it is diversion to many. The three approaches have similar goals which each of the arts in therapy shares: They stimulate interest and imagination, encourage application, and use energy productively.

Efficiency of administrative structure is based not solely on practicability but also on advantage to patients. What works best? In the case of music, is it possible by being a separate department of skilled technicians, to more fully explore potential uses of this activity for therapeutic affect? It may be argued so because intensive training in the specialty allows the worker to function at all levels with ease. Occupational therapy and recreational therapy cannot add to already-full academic curricula the level of skill training which a highly specialized art form demands if the activity is to be applied effectively for rehabilitation purposes, with concentration on psycho-dynamic factors. Further, a separate unit usually has freer rein in to initiate and experiment with all aspects of the medium — educational, occupational, and diversional. This seems to have been proven by the amount of activity and spread of uses found in a few large autonomous music or music-and-arts departments of the country.

Whatever the channeling, the activity therapist in the arts who has high skill in his specialty and freedom to use it brings unique stimulus to patients through creative aspects of his art form as well as technical "know-how." For the patient who is to work with him, it is often the driving force of the therapist's special talent, and the obvious satisfaction the latter has found in it, which will capture his own interest, and perhaps touch off a kindred spark. At least he gains a glimpse of the emotional and spiritual satisfactions he too may hope to find in the activity and grows in appreciation as feelings are communicated and shared.

Structural divisions of music programming are concerned with type of service as indicated in the two tables following. Table I covers music service to the total hospital, and Table II the more concentrated and highly specialized uses carried on in the music therapy clinic.

The area of music service to the total hospital, besides assisting in the general climate and functioning of the institution, reaches

TABLE I
PROGRAM BREAKDOWN — TOTAL HOSPITAL SERVICE

(A) Diversional Coverage Outside Music Rooms (Patient Audiences)	(B) Services to General Hospital-Program (Performance)	Activities Outside the Hospital
Ward entertainment Music for ball games picnics, dances, patient parties Concert by guests Concerts/shows by patients	Religious music Large Community sings Music with treatment (EST/Physiotherapy) Background music for hospital functions and professional meetings	Programs by patients Patients to concerts Community talks on MT Articles Information by correspondence Conferences attended Reports to schools on music therapy trainees

not only those patients who receive medical referrals to attend the clinic but the many more patients in public institutions who for reasons of age, health, or behavior are not suited or ready for more-concentrated effort but who have need for enjoyable, though less demanding, occupation, and recreation.

TABLE II.

PROGRAM BREAKDOWN — MUSIC THERAPY CLINIC

A. Participation Activities

Individual Work (patient alone)	Smaller Groups (performance)	Larger Groups (regular coaching)	Performance Opportunities
A pastime	String ensemble	Secular chorus	Ward entertainment
As practice	Wind group	Religious choirs	Community sings
	Fretted group	Men's glee club	Performance Clubs
Individual Work (with the therapists)	2-Piano ensembles	Women's glee club	Formal recitals
	Novelty instr.	Orchestra	Special seasonal
	Rhythm band	Senior band	music
Lessons	Vocal (2-3-4 pts)	Beginner band	Demonstrations of MT
Duets	Popular combos.	Bugle & drum	personnel
Supervised		corps	community
Practice			Skits for holidays
Accompaniment		Special-skill Groups (allied fields)	Large patient shows
Coaching	Smaller Groups (classes)		
Musicology		Dramatics	
		Folk dancing	
Pilot Studies	Theory	Social dance	
	Harmony	Creative dance	
Experimental	Composition	Marching drills	
small/large	History	Baton twirling	

B. Passive Listening

Small Sessions	Group Record Programs
One to three patients	Classical
playing records of	Semi-classical
own choice	Popular

It is in the music therapy clinic, that the real applications of music as therapy are centered. All patients here are directly referred by doctors, or, if suggested by other sources, are approved by followup medical referral. An initial interview and two or three days of getting acquainted and of visiting different activities usually make the patient feel at ease. There should be an early reading of the case history with notes taken for later reference. From these several sources come indications of the patient's capacities, interests, and special needs, so that he may be assigned to suitable activities in a conference of director and therapists.

Records should be kept of the patient's attitudes and behavior, including comments on his progress in the activity as related to his health, and his reactions to the therapist and to other patients. An informal report within two or three weeks either acquaints the doctor with the fact that of several approaches tried none seemed to be suitable for the patient at the time; or, hopefully, that his program is successfully underway. A month or two later, a full formal report should be sent to the referring doctor, with copies to the clinical director for the hospital case history, to the ward personnel, and to any other professional staff particularly concerned. A copy of each report should be kept in the permanent music rooms records.

In the "on-going" period the department must be concerned with what is happening to the patient, as a person, through the activity. Musical progress is of importance only as it is a factor in the working out of his problems and in his personal growth in insight, sense of security, and feelings of self-worth. In this process, as time goes on, frequent change of the patient's music schedule may be advisable. He may be ready to be thrown with more people, or he may depend on people less. He may be ready to face bigger challenges and more-concentrated efforts, or need to do relatively little for a time. He may need stricter group discipline, or more freedom. He may be stimulated by all the music around him to want to try new instruments or groups, or to leave others.

Through branching-out, he is weaned away from leaning on one person or activity too heavily, and he develops independence to accept the reality of the complex world outside in which many things of interest go on simultaneously. Therapists must face the importance of this move toward independence without feelings of rejection. Even when it seems likely music may be a major interest later for certain patients they should be encouraged to think of it avocationally rather than vocationally and should be encouraged to do other things, as well, as part of a reality pattern of living.

When patients request it, and doctors approve, there should be some spot in the total structure of department activity for outpatient return. This may be for lessons or for congenial group performance. It may be better for the music therapist or social service to help him find a suitable outlet in the community.

PROGRAM CONTENT

Rationale

Any planned systematic use of time in work or play contributes to the better functioning of members of a community whether in or out of a hospital. Within the hospital, it is particularly valuable for fighting the lethargy which drives many patients into the nonchallenging acceptance of long hospitalization. Activity programs are no longer considered to be "icing-on-the-cake" extras, but essential tools for building health. The patient must have something to think about, and to do with time, rather than dwelling too much on personal problems; something to get up for in the inevitable new day rather than mark time in inactivity, in indulgence of hostility toward the hospital or other patients, and in feelings of rejection by family or of exclusion from what is going on in the world outside.

Values

Music activities share certain general values with all kinds of activity programs; (1) *stimulation of interest,* so that "positivism" rather than negativism results; (2) *organization of faculties,* which comes from directed effort as opposed to indiscriminate and ineffectual use of energy and time, and (3) *socialization,* the reaching back toward people, as opposed to the isolation of illness with its tensions and hostilities. Added to these general values of all fields of activity are special aspects of art forms involving skill: (1) *creativity,* the urge to do something original, to express artistic ideas in an individual way: (2) *aesthetic enjoyment,* the age-old satisfaction which philosophers described as the "balm" or "peace" found in contemplating beauty or making it ourselves, and (3) *communication of feelings,* sharing with others what we are thinking and feeling and learning to receive this from others without embarrassment. Dr. Gaston[40] describes the specific assets of music for therapy as persuasive, nonpunitive activity in which learning brings the satisfactions of achievement in situations encouraging comfortably controlled behavior. It affords fulfillment of aesthetic needs, allows freedom in performance to dare to express any emotion, and helps establish patterns of sensory and motor reactions which have desirable emotional and social components.

Evaluating the Patient and Activity

In *evaluating the patient* for placement in the music program, kind and degree of illness are weighed, as well as character, temperament, and his capacity at the moment. Does he need the support of individual work, or the discipline of an organized, goal-demanding group? What are his musical associations, good or bad, and his training? Are his bodily movements inhibited and tight, or expansive and euphoric? His personality traits, and his way with people are matters of concern in deciding what activities to try first.

Care must be taken in evaluating the kinds of music activities available. These are potentials only. What is true for one person is not necessarily true for the next. What is true for one person at a certain time, is not necessarily true at another. Rarely is any quality exclusively the value of one activity. However, a general breakdown is often possible as between individual one-to-one work, and group; between small and large groups; study and diversional activities; and certainly between passive listening and participation, for most patients, with the latter heavily weighted for dynamic content.

Caution should be taken not to assign activities which may fortify unhealthy characteristics. Escapism, aloofness, seclusiveness, will not be discouraged, but encouraged, by hours of playing alone. Both overdependency and self-indulgence must be skilfully handled in work with individual patients. *Prima donna* behavior cannot be overcome by solo featuring but may be tempered, by gradual adjustment, to acceptance of the role of group member. Favoritism of talented patients harms both the performer and other patients. Repetitious playing, with little but steady beat to recommend it, may be hypnotic to an unhealthy degree, or with the addition of sensuous melody encourage sexual drives or narcissism.

Not only the basic characteristics of a music activity but its timing and the way it is conducted have to be considered. If too little time is allowed, an otherwise suitable music assignment may be an annoyance and frustration; if it is too long it may fatigue or bore. If too supportive it may stifle initiative. If too difficult it can end in discouragement and another "closed door" for weaker members. Group work on routine schedule must avoid dullness and stereotype. Large-goal performances must guard against over-pressure and fatigue. In groups of all kinds, where limits as to conduct must be set, it should be stressed that it is not a person but a kind of behavior which must be rejected. If this behavior is destructive either to the activity or to the peace of mind of others in the group, discipline by the group should be favored over authoritative measures by those in charge.

There is a wide gamut of choice in deciding which music activities are therapeutic for different kinds of patients. Music study and practice afford opportunity for helping with personal problems of fear, hostility, and overdependency by encouraging feelings of fitness and well-being. Through participation, increasing frustration tolerance can be built, and acceptance of self and environment encouraged. Self-expression that is appropriate and meaningful to the patient is not only ego-fortifying but also helps him merge his feelings and desires with those of others. He relates. Performance betters his physical tone by improving coordination and by stimulating bodily responses, and helps improve his memory and his powers of concentration. For patients who perform at artist level, it affords the opportunity of keeping up their professional skills and of being heard and appreciated at a time when self-evaluation is low.

Small-ensemble work has its special uses. In playing duets with his therapist at one piano, a patient may learn to overcome the threat of physical closeness. In two-piano, four-hand work, in spite of greater freedom and expansiveness he must cooperate, in sharing responsibility and complementary sensitivity with another person. If he is the accompanist, he must give support to the soloist and play the subordinate role himself. If he is the soloist, then he has to accept this help and support from another, with appreciation of what this entails.

In all *small ensembles,* vocal or instrumental, there are constructive potentials for cutting through isolation by social interaction and adjustments to the group. This may be the first step in "growing outwards" if there is compatibility, fairly equal capacity, and use of material within reasonable limits of achievement. Members share not only in the steady flow of music and in working out special problem-passages but in interpretation of style and meaning. A variety of approaches may influence the choice: study for intellectual and cultural growth; polished performance for emotional satisfaction and achievement; spontaneous playing or singing for socializing, for physiological release through the strong bear and sway, or for nostalgic pleasure from associative content. When special units rehearse and perform for hospital functions, or socially for patient dances, parties, and picnics, each in the group has his place, his responsibility, and his recognition.

Larger groups (bands, orchestras, choruses) demand broader interrelationships, acceptance of leader, subordination to group goal, and conformity to rehearsal routines and composer's intent. Rewards are in feelings of self-worth as a needed member, pride in identification with the group and its performance, and daily growth as each patient works with others toward a mutual accomplishment.

Musicology. From theory and harmony classes come the added security gained in becoming literate in a form of expression which is used by all peoples in our society: the literacy of understanding how to read music; patterns for chords, scales, and keys which clarify what may have been restrictive or tension-creating because unknown or forgotten; the increased enjoyment in listening to music when form, content, and meaning are grasped.

Performance Values. There are special attributes of each of the performance activities: (1) Ward music units can reach all corners of the hospital, bringing variety and "live" entertainment to nonambulatory patients. Planned programs that move smoothly can be informal enough to include request numbers and listener participation, giving patients in the audience recognition. When patients perform in the entertaining unit they share in a feeling of service. (2) More formal auditorium recitals can encourage a maximum achievement potential if greater emphasis is placed on the pleasure of doing than on musical prowess. (3) Music therapy demonstration programs not only give prestige to patients taking part but promote understanding of the field and its goals for in-service training groups and community or professional audiences. (4) Community sings, usually held evenings, to include patients working daytimes, are a great leavener and socializer. Swinging together in a rhythmic experience to a tune that is pleasing and familiar brings people closer in empathy and good will. (5) A big annual show has assets in numbers of patients who can be used in the show itself in some capacity, however small. For these the demands of rehearsing, conforming, meeting the challenge of a major performance, and sharing honors with the total group are dynamic reality experiences. For others who work in peripheral areas on scenery, costumes, posters, programs, there are the stimulus of planning, the excitement of preparation, the final "shared glory" in the performance itself, and a cementing together of feelings of pride and solid satisfaction throughout the institution.

Listening Activities. While taking active part in music making is felt to be the most beneficial way of using music as therapy there is another whole area sometimes called "passive-listening" (if listening can ever correctly be passive.)

For categorizing purposes, listening to recorded music may be divided into three areas. First, patterned after extensive commercial programming elsewhere there is the large use, variously evaluated, of the so-called "to-do-by" recordings: music to wake by, sleep by, eat by. These are broad assignments for whole sections, carefully chosen for mood affect. Short varied music programs broadcast intermittently during the day are also used extensively, often, with patients as "M.C." or performers. Second, there is record listening by a few persons of like tastes who meet together in an intimate setting to play records of their own choosing. Provided this is not wrongly used to fortify exclusiveness and escapism it can be very helpful and relaxing as an assignment for patients who are ready to accept some independence and a simple degree of contact with others. Third, more formally structured programs of recorded music of special kinds can be regularly scheduled for larger groups, for specific purposes. Series of operas, symphonies, musical shows, or study of jazz styles may be planned, or the more general "pops" concert of assorted types of music featured in many communities.

In planning music listening programs — whether records or "live" performance — theme, continuity, and structure should suit the average taste of the group. There is strong, emotional appeal in familiar music although unpleasant associations must be guarded against. Music with steady rhythmic pulse can be used to enhance feelings of comfort and safety; certain styles induce special feelings, as quiet sway for sedation, stirring beat for stimulation, or speed and uneven rhythms for excitement. One well-known theory is the "iso" principle of meeting a group needing mood change with music that matches its own level of emotional and physical activity, and gradually leading it, through changing the character of the music, to one more desirable. Individual taste, temperament, and cultural background will color the degree of enjoyment and response, each person projecting his own private experience into his reactions. It has been said that nonmusical persons can enjoy music only passively, the extremely musical only rarely because they will be too critical, but that the "somewhat musical" enjoy listening most. These make up the vast audience of music lovers — just as they represent the vast number of average individuals.

In "live" performance there are certain additional advantages. Patient-audiences at concerts by other patients share vicariously in the pride of achievement of their peers who are talented, and are warmly responsive. Moreover, while they are enthusiastic about a successful performer, they are invariably generous in applauding patients who do less well. They are also appreciative of guest performers from outside, not only for their volunteer efforts on their behalf, but because they enjoy contact with the community and seeing new faces. Going off the grounds themselves either to give performances or to hear them tends to eliminate the stigma of seclusion and "difference" and builds self-confidence. The anticipation, the dressing up, and the trip itself are all stimulating and patients usually respond with conduct that does the hospital credit, as well as bringing themselves into touch with the public in a way that stresses the "patients-are-people" concept.

Use of Music by Age and Disorders

The Child. In the field of mental illness, there are special approaches for using music for different age groups, and also for large groups of patients with distinctive behavior patterns characteristic of stage of illness and degree of regression. The emotionally disturbed child is an acute problem anytime, anywhere. Whatever the activities used, this type of child, often severely autistic, requires a large amount of individual attention, patience, and "loving care." Here the nonverbal qualities of music for communication and mood influence have significant value. Since he should not be overprotected, or reinforced in his seclusiveness, the socialization values of music-making, either with the therapist or in a small group, can be utilized. The normal instinct of well children to dance and play and to respond to musical sounds and to rhythm can be used to help bring the maladjusted child out of his isolation and to keep doors to reality open for him by using what is normal, though partially dormant, within himself. Dr. Dreikurs[41] urges: children like to make noise, so let these children "bang" away on drums, piano, or on any rhythm instruments, sing lustily, stomp and clap and whirl. Gradually their wildness can be led into quieter, more orderly activity through use of contrasts in volume, speed, and musical style. By using imaginative story suggestions, a music session may become a happy "doing" experience instead of a repetition of resistance.

Music is also recommended as a helpful tool for ventilation and for diagnostic purposes.[42] Improvisations by the music therapist to match a child's mood and his known history, as — "What does this music say?" — "Whom does this sound like?" — "Let's tell a story about it" — will often bring out into the open anxieties, hates, and frustrations, and help the doctor who may use this material to penetrate the child's secret world of fears and fantasies. Later if the child can gradually master sufficient keyboard skill to express his own feelings through music he will have found for himself a safe channel for emotional release.

The Adolescent. The troubled adolescent presents a different kind of problem. If he is very insecure and withdrawn, a non-challenging one-to-one assignment within his capacity, or a group demand at simple level, may gradually lead him back toward accepting people and feeling some sense of personal worth. More often, the adolescent who becomes a problem to himself, his family, or his community is already full of resentments, angers, and frustrations. He may delight in taunting and swagger, or be sullen and negativistic, or even ugly and combative. Above all, he will fight any pressure to conform to the wishes of parents, adults in general, and authority figures in particular. Supervisory personnel and therapist must be permissive of minor infractions, must like and understand these "older children," and yet set limits. They need to be allowed their own choice of music records, be able to play them as loudly, often, and repetitively as they please within the prescribed limits of ward routines. They should be encouraged to dance, the more freely the better for releasing tensions, although again with whatever limits have been set by doctor and psychologist. "Jam" sessions on instruments and song fests should be encouraged, and opportunity for learning to play instruments and sing in solo or group. By accepting their choice of activity and style, respecting their efforts, inviting imaginative planning on their part, and directing their energies unobtrusively most adolescent patients of this type will gradually adjust to the discipline of the activity and required rules of conduct.

The Geriatric. Geriatric patients able to be active can utilize choral singing at various levels. Those with training can and should continue playing and singing. Rhythm-band groups at mature levels, chorus, dancing that is not strenuous, performance programs occasionally and listening opportunities more frequently, records of their own choosing — all these will counteract sedentary tendencies by keeping them alert and interested. It should encourage good grooming, help them substitute satisfaction for resignation, and fortify their feelings of importance and self-confidence. Old-time music and hymns can be used to satisfy nostalgic yearnings. Entertainers with quiet instruments can stroll from bed to bed, play and sing request numbers, and stop for "visiting." Occasionally, an older bed patient can be taught to play a simple instrument like the auto-harp.

The Chronic Regressed. Deteriorated patients can be brought into as many activities as their behavior with other patients allows. They usually enjoy community singing, a variety show, a music circus or a holiday skit. While some may not be able to tolerate a program of more serious music others will enjoy it. It is important that those confined to the wards so much of the time not be forgotten in the overall planning.

The Chronic Ambulatory patient who is well enough to live out a fairly normal life in a large public institution gets and needs maximum benefits of a full activity program. He probably does some ward chores or has part-time work, but his leisure time is usually sufficient to allow him to take advantage of cultural and diversional programs of all kinds. These are made "better patients" not because they obey better, or conform more readily to hospital routines, but because they exist somewhat, at least, in a zone of normality. Instead of constantly feeling that they are rejected by society, they find importance in some group or activity and feed their self-esteem on this small "spot in the sun." These and the challenging group of reception service patients who have passed the initial stage of confinement to the ward make up the bulk of patients on activity referrals.

The Mentally Retarded. In state schools and institutions for the mentally retarded, music is used in regular classroom assignments and widely as diversional activity. Rhythm bands, rote and simple group singing, and music games are suitable. Marked rhythm on percussion instruments can usually furnish an avenue of approach, and a good ear can often be developed. Rote singing with corrective records has been found to relieve stutterers. A kazoo band has proved helpful with other speech defects. Tonettes and harmonicas are assigned to the more adept.[43] The first necessity is to find means of musical expression which can be mastered, even at simple level, in order to allow the success experience which is vital.[44] Seasonal plays and large choral and instrumental groups perform frequently for the school and community as morale builders for the pupils and the institution.

The Alcoholic and Drug Addict. Many music activities are used in rehabilitation programs for alcoholics and drug addicts.

Due to vocational hazards of their professions, successful and talented musicians often become involved in destructive habits and find long hospitalization necessary. When self-esteem is low and feelings of failure and guilt extreme, creative work which brings recognition, but does not expose to temptation in the special weaknesses is invaluable. All kinds of combos, coached or spontaneous, vocal or instrumental, are possible, or writing music, or helping with broadcast programs and planning special entertainment. Personnel must be alert to attempts at manipulation by psychopathic personalities, and to potential professional jealousies. However, on the whole, there is likely to be appreciation of the program and good-natured support of one another.

Music with Medical and Physical Treatment

Adjunct to Shock Treatment. Music as a special adjunct to medical treatment in mental hospitals is used with electro-shock therapy to lessen pre-treatment anxieties and to add sociability to the post-shock period. Where insulin shock is still practiced tempo, volume, and rhythm are manipulated to accelerate withdrawal from insulin coma. Flowing melody with steady underlying pulse may be used with hydro-therapy to fortify relaxation and create a pleasantly restful milieu.

Adjunct to Psychotherapy. Music is sometimes assigned a role in psychotherapy, usually as a preface to group discussion. Since group therapy is not a confessional but a coming together to explore and work out problems, a communal media like music can help promote good social relations and hasten interaction.[45] Patients who have been exposed to soft background music during a session, continuous or intermittent, have said it helped them "stand the silences" and situational developments which became too threatening.[46].

Adjunct to Other Activities. The role of music in support of other activity fields should be touched on. It is inseparable from dramatics in musical shows of any kind, and functions as an additional opening wedge in speech dynamics to free inhibitions and create desired reactions of vocal and emotional control. It can be used with painting to induce relaxation and to influence mood and attitudes for diagnostic purposes. It is an important complement to such physical education activities as baton twirling, flag drills, and precision marching, and is an integral part of all dance forms.

Lessons in social dance can help those who are painfully shy, or low in self-evaluation. It is important that they be pulled in from the role of lonely watchers on the sideline. Folk dancing with its tunefulness and pace can be used to break down barriers and utilize racial associations. It is fine exercise to music as well as being provocative of good will and conversation. There is less threat from hand-touching than in being "held," partners change frequently, and the swing of the music carries the less confident along in a success experience.

Creative dance encourages free uninhibited expression of inner feelings. The choice of music is important in determining responses, from extremes of despair to ecstacy, and from bizarre psychic manifestations to states of relaxation. In addition to the joy of motion, imagination is stimulated by interpreting the music and creating original movements. Under the protective cloak of "art theater," the dancers learn to feel and express beauty without embarrassment.

The use of dance as a therapy agent is being used more and more as an adjunct to other activity treatment programs and as a separate treatment discipline. Therefore, consideration of this specialty will be found on page 100.

With Physical Illness. While music, other than on radio and television, is rarely used in short-term hospitalization, the contrary is true in long-term physical illness. A quietly diversional, morale-fortifying approach is used for patients with functional disorders such as heart disease, tuberculosis, and cancer. Passive-listening activities are recommended: record programs with requests and musical quizzes, or simple nontaxing instruments to play, like tonette, autoharp, and the fretted group — mandolin, guitar, ukelele. In tuberculosis, careful practice on wind instruments under medical guidance is sometimes used to improve respiratory problems. Song-writing, or simple composition, and short periods of small ensemble playing for those with special talents are usually approved by nursing and medical staff. Any pleasant nonfatiguing background music which relaxes and encourages positive thinking is welcomed. Where there is long hospitalization, with stigma of isolation, as in hospitals for leprosy, many music participation activities are in the program to encourage achievement and feelings of self-worth.

With Neurology and Orthopedics. In the fields of neurology and orthopedics, music has broad diversional uses in institutions caring for long-term patients with severely crippling illness and handicap. It supplies hobbies, entertainment, and contacts with other patients and the world of arts "outside." Culturally, it offers opportunity for creative expression and helps meet aesthetic needs. Indirectly, it aids the development of incentive toward health, and perseverence. Singing, playing, acting, games, even wheel-chair dancing have been used successfully. More specifically, it is used on medical prescription in physiological reconstruction problems. This is either as an adjunct to physiotherapy treatments, with music carefully synchronized to exercise, or on direct prescription to a music therapist in treatment centers where qualified musicians have been adequately trained in physiology and anatomy. Compositions are chosen for suitable characteristics to increase co-ordination and mobility, to develop awareness of feelings of tension versus rest, to help relax spasticity and rigidities, and to generally assist in improving tonus, endurance, strength, and control. The enjoyment-of-living aspect of music is emphasized: "Every one can do something with music; find what fits this one"[47] — "The crippled are citizens too, so don't expect trouble; expect cooperation."[48]

A magnificently detailed and comprehensive survey of general and particular techniques in the field of physical disability has been written by a young therapist[49] whose early special training was in music, followed by degree training in occupational therapy and extensive profesisonal experience in use of music on referral in all kinds of physical illness and handicap. She gives many practical suggestions on ways to relate body part, or special problem, to kind of treatment. There are pages of specific joints and muscle groups covering the entire anatomy. Factors of size, shape, heaviness and resistance of materials in the instrument are considered, as well as primary variations in the position of patient in relation to instrument, and to kind of movement medically prescribed.

Various special devices are described which have been developed through imagination and ingenuity to facilitate use of instruments: adjustable tables, chairs, and lapboards; extensions, braces, straps, and special holders to surmount all problems of immobility and weakness. This one article is a textbook of solid resource material for activity therapists working in the field of physical medicine.

With Brain-damaged Patients. There is considerable excellent literature on uses of music as a medium in the treatment of brain-damaged patients. Since such damage is irreversible, development of the patient's maximum remaining capacity for purposeful movement is stressed, and finding ways for him to substitute undamaged faculties for damaged.[50] Carefully planned repetitive movements in music making are used to initiate and reinforce good action habits and management of tension and release, with suitable precautions for guarding against perseveration. Previously acquired inhibitions and emotional defenses can often be ameliorated in music sessions, as ability to concentrate and find interest and enjoyment with others is developed. Music is combined with imaginative, creative approaches of play-acting and story-telling to help eliminate tension and confine excitability to the control-threshold.

With Cerebral Palsy. Music is used extensively in cerebral palsy, the greatest crippler in the brain damage field. Malfunction in blood circulation in the brain does not affect the parts which can receive music, so that through its use improved functioning can be motivated. The basic emphases are on daily success habits, however slow the pace; socio-psychological support from group activity; and use of the instinctive response to music to allay restlessness and break through noncommunicative behavior. The two different types of cerebral palsy behavior require contrasting kinds of music.[51] The tension of spasticity can be shifted or suppressed by stimulating music which gradually increases relaxation and mobility. The disorganization of athetoid motions can be lessened, and the size and indirection of movement brought under control by use of sedative music. A special technique has been developed of beginning the music with the tremor, or immediately preceding the tremor, and guiding it, by the character of the composition through its course. It has been found possible in this way to greatly control the pattern and duration of movement.[52] Calm, flowing music lowers the intensity of the tremor and tends to taper it off; stirring martial music to lengthen it and increase random movement.

Muscular Dystrophy, which strikes early in life and involves the wasting away of muscles with no hope of cure nor halt, causes physical handicap, but not mental, except in the emotional reactions to isolation and helplessness. Here, music activities can only be useful physically, as they counteract effects of disuse, but there is no limit as to how much they can help build morale, and provide stimulation, interest, and enjoyment.[53] Operettas, wheel-chair shows, as well as simple music study and appreciation, can bring to each patient some measure of success. Later, when participation is no longer possible there are memories and residues of the listening tastes cultivated.

With Sensory Handicaps: Blindness and Deafness. Music is used extensively in therapy for the *blind* as compensation for other deprivations and for expanding horizons. It builds self-esteem through achievement, helps to identify in social relationships, and to satisfy emotional and aesthetic needs through self-expression and release of hostilities.[54] It improves bodily co-ordination for the newly blind, by developing sense of balance and rhythm in walking, and counteracts feelings of physical dependency. Music is practiced professionally by many blind people as performers, teachers, and more recently, as therapists. Much music is written and studied in Braille. In the lonely world of blindness, the comforting joys of learning and performing music are emphasized for young and old alike. At the Lighthouse Music School in New York City, over a thousand music lessions are given a month to the blind and partially-sighted by the New York Association for the Blind.

Deafness, like blindness, is a responsibility of special education departments of public schools or separate state and private schools and institutions. Interesting studies have been made of amplifying sounds to penetrate walls of deafness and of learning to "hear" different instruments through their vibrations, either by hand or foot contact. The communication and socialization values of music are particularly stressed for the deaf through singing, music games, and dancing. Instrumental groups feature strong percussion sections. Dancing emphasizes strong beat and sway. The more advanced technical and artistic mastery of performance which the blind can enjoy because of their sensitivity to sound is not usually possible with auditory handicap. Here, a "good ear," so important in music, is lacking.

Adjunct to Speech Therapy. Music is particularly useful in speech therapy since speaking shares with music the physical aspects of rhythm, phrasing, and pitch and volume change. They also equally stress the emotional and phychological factors of self-expression and communication of feelings and ideas.[55] In paralysis, throat thrombosis, and hemipareses, many finely specialized techniques have been worked out for exercises with music for breathing, or for saliva control; lip reading and tone matching to bring back and strengthen voice production, speech, and face and head mobility.[56] Rhythmic speech drills and tape recordings of the patient's efforts are used to develop ear and improve articulation. For cleft palate, playing the flutophone has been utilized to cut off air from the nasal passage and redirect it to mouth breathing for exercise of the soft palate.[57] This is typical of the many imaginative instrumental and vocal devices used as adjuvant therapy in the total field of physical medicine.

With Anesthesia. A final application of music in physical treatment is the use of recorded music in anesthesia. This has been developed in the last dozen years and is now used in several centers. [58] [59] It requires fine mechanical reproduction and careful choice of music for affect. It has been used in childbirth to supplement the natural rhythm of delivery. In the fields of general and dental surgery, usually by earphone, it has been found to quiet apprehension and lessen amounts of anaesthesia needed by utilizing the hypnosis of rhythm. It is used to supplement and potentiate the quieting action of nitrous oxide,[60] and also, in minor operations and dentistry, to provide repetitious rhythmic stimuli for use with ethyl chloride.[61] Doctors who favor its use claim it distracts attention from the unpleasant and painful stimuli of operational procedures, cuts down retching, and increases the pain threshold.[62]

Dance Therapy

Dance therapy embraces all forms, but is much more. The undisputed leader in this field, Marian Chace,[63] who was the first officially appointed dance therapist in the country, in 1942 at St. Elizabeth's (federal mental) Hospital in Washington, D. C., feels "it is inconceivable to separate music and dance." Together they involve the total man: body, emotions, and mind. She holds dance to be the most personal of the arts since it requires no learning of instruments — "just me." It has double-barrelled effects of release, first through instinctive responses to sound, and second through the emotional expression which accompanies them. Free uninhibited body movement satisfies a universal need. Not only does it help the especially gifted but it is for everybody, everyday.[64] Each rhythm can be felt inwardly when awareness and recognition of feelings is developed. Every posture and movement has meaning — the way we walk, for example, whether weary, defeated and slouching, or tall, proud, unafraid.

Our culture stresses intellectual achievement and restraint of emotion with resultant loss in confidence and in easy access to others. The child, wanting and needing unrestricted activity, is taught to control and eliminate it — "Sit still" — "Don't fidget" — yet all life is motion, and inactivity causes physical and psychological withdrawal. If the sick hold on to habits derived from their physiological disabilities and the protective psychological mechanisms which accompany them, then inactivity, unaltered, becomes inertia, and in true inertia lies death.

The aims of dance therapy are to free people through movement so that they can identify with others, communicate feelings, and rid themselves of self-imposed restraints or from those imposed from without. It can be a bridge to reality built on alternating psychomotor tensions and release, making patients more accessible to psychotherapy and awareness of self.[65] The therapist is the catalyst who must accept each patient in the dance group as he is, keeping multiple individual lines of communication open, being aware of individual needs and of responses, however small, and drawing each patient, without forcing, into a relationship of acceptance. Unspoken empathies must be built, and rejections and withdrawals accepted without embarrassment. Attention is paid to relating the whole body to its parts, as well as to relationships in space and time. Meaningful interpretations of individual mood and feelings are invited, and each patient is encouraged to act out any hostility or bizarre autistic behavior he chooses. Discussion is encouraged and effort made to close the session with a general sense of well-being and mutual confidence.

There is growing interest in the use of dance as therapy. One interested psychiatrist,[66] in advocating the use of dance for treatment, urges: "Loosen up — warm up — stride — run! Then fall down relaxed — lie quietly — and listen to the silence." She feels that dance is an expression of human fantasy which involves not only joints and muscles but the whole subjective concept of the body.

Miss Chace summarizes her thinking in the basic concept that the most available, least expensive, and most expressive instruments we have are our own bodies, and that through developing them in free, relaxed movement we can make ourselves feel "live," attractive, and able to respond in warm and natural relationships with others. She refers judgment of the activity to comments by patients: "For a moment we just let go and live!" — "If I could have only kept moving like this, I would never have gotten sick."[67]

PROFESSIONAL STATUS AND QUALIFICATIONS

Since December 31, 1960, a baccalaureate degree in music therapy has been required for professional registration (R.M.T., Registered Music Therapist). The degree may be in music therapy (B.M.T.), or in music or music education (B.M. or B.M.E.) with majors in music therapy. The National Association of Schools of Music (NASM) is designated by the National Commission on Accrediting as the official agency for the approval of degree music therapy courses. The curriculum was developed by NASM with the Education Committee of the National Association for Music Therapy (NAMT).

Of the over 400 Registered Music Therapists in the country, many have music or academic degrees other than in music therapy, or had had sufficient professional training and experience in uses of music in rehabilitation previous to 1961 to qualify for registration by institutional affidavit. While registration is the desirable professional goal, as in all fields, it should be noted that institutions are not limited in their employment of music therapists to the NAMT registration requirements unless so designated by their own or civil service restrictions; also that "equivalency" procedures for making up missing requirements are not yet published. Presently, however, a music therapy degree from an approved school is the only procedure by which the "RMT" coveted by most music therapists can now be gotten.

In the area of hospital music, it is expected that extensive music study will have been a part of precollege-level preparation. The piano is probably the most important single instrument. The ability to teach, perform solos, transpose, improvise, play by ear, and to accompany well are essential even when another instrument or voice is the specialty. The music-therapy course totals 128 semester hours, sixty of these in music. They cover considerable piano and voice, basic training in organ, strings, brass, woodwinds, and percussion instruments, with advanced work in some specialty. Also included are courses in choral and instrumental conducting, theory, and applied harmony, principles of pedagogy (including methods and materials), and music literature and history. The music therapist should be able to arrange music for choral groups and all manner of simple instrumental combinations. Rhythm band, community-sing techniques, and similar types of recreational music activities should be mastered.

The required clinical training consists of a minimum of six months resident internship, in an approved psychiatric hospital with an established music therapy program, and a psychiatric indoctrination course for professional disciplines in which music trainees participate. This is in addition to on-campus hospital-oriented lectures. Thereafter, at least two months training should be taken in specialty hospitals for work in the fields of mental deficiency, physical medicine, or emotionally disturbed children.

RESEARCH

The cry of music therapy for research is the eternal cry of all activity fields: "Which way is better?" — "Exactly what is happening?" Music preference tests tantalize psychologists with potential uses for diagnosis.[68] Seeming relations between kinds of response to kinds of music in specific pathology offer promise for future usefulness. However, how music specifically acts to do any one thing still requires exhaustive investigation. It is difficult to measure a mood, which is transient and personal, by a limit that is intangible; and too easy to let enthusiasm run away with evaluation.[69] Responses are rarely identical or predictable, but rather are altered by individual conditioning and inherent characteristics of all kinds. The present weakness lies in lack of sureness of direction rather than in lack of good intention or of skill in using the specialty. We must rely on more research and many pilot studies with carefully controlled variables for further precision of answer and for time-saving, so that the good that comes out of music therapy assignments will not be by accident but by design.

Actually, there is no dearth of authenticated and validated research in the area of response to music (see extensive research list following reference notes at end of chapter). Moreover, there seems to be strong conviction, rather widespread among doctors, psychologists, and educators, that something unique does happen in the music situation which needs to be further identified. But only through collaboration in further scientific and empirical investigation in which the therapist acts, the doctor helps evaluate, and the scientist analyzes, can specific formulas for treatment be developed with any degree of predictability.

Doctors sometimes say that musicians must learn to function as scientists, and many music therapists make heroic search for criteria to guide them toward effective results. But with the growing demand of expanding hospital populations, and the trend of extending activity treatment to out-patient clinics and rehabilitation centers music therapists can only answer the doctor: "We must do, now, to the best of our abilities, rather than wait until science has confirmed procedures." The latter, however, carefully directed and cautiously evaluated, yet presently remain intuitive and judgemental.

So, in the end, we come back to philosophy. One psychiatrist has said: "Music is a message which everyone understands but nobody can translate — its language an Esperanto of emotions."[70] Another, in discussing music as therapy, comments: "Whether one only touches the fringes of aesthetics as listener or observer, or moves more deeply into a reaction through personal participation great therapeutic potentials are there for the troubled."[71]

Enthusiasts claim it offers a high quality of experience which carries a special quintenssence of enjoyment, either alone or shared, and whether for people in or out of hospital. As we need balanced diet and vitamin sufficiency for physical health, so we need balance in work and play, activity and rest, sports and arts, so that we "wake up and live," availing ourselves of the wealth of our cultural heritage of which music is so integral a part.

The following is a partial list of research bibliography chosen to indicate the variety of aspects of functional music which has been investigated to date.

PARTICULAR ILLNESS

Mays, Thomas: A study of drug addiction: medicine and music. *New York Med. J.*, *105*:832-836, 1917.

Murphy, M.: Rhythmical responses of low-grade and middle-grade mental defectives to music therapy. *J. Clin. Psychol., 13* (4):361-364, 1959.

Shatin, Leo: The application of rhythmic music stimuli to long-term schizophrenic patients. *NAMT Book of Proceedings*, 1957, p. 169-172.

Sherwin, A.: A consideration of the therapeutic use of music in psychiatric illness. *J. Nerv. Ment. Dis., 127* (1):84-89, 1958.

Skelly and Haslerud: Music and the general activity of apathetic schizophrenics. *J. Abnorm. Soc. Psychol., 47:*188, 1952.

Zanker, A., and Glatt, M.: Individual reactions of alcoholic and neurotic patients to music. *J. Nerv. Ment. Dis., 123* (4):395-402, 1956.

PARTICULAR PHYSIOLOGICAL INVOLVEMENT

Crocker, Dorothy Brin: Electroencephalogram response to ultrasonic stimuli. *NAMT Book of Proceedings*, 1954, p. 236-239.

Martin, Edgar J.: Observations on hypnotic effects of rhythmic sounds at Respiratory rates. *NAMT Book of Proceedings*, 1958, p. 177-187.

Misbach, L. E.: The effect of pitch of tone - stimuli upon body resistance and cardiovascular phenomena. *J. Exp. Psychol., 16:*167-183, 1932.

Olichney, Joseph: A Correlation Study of Equilibrium and Kawalwasser-Dykenia Music Test Scores. Unpublished Master's Thesis, Syracuse University, 1942.

Phares, M. I.: Analysis of music appreciation by means of the psycholgalvanic response technique. *J. Exp. Psychol., 17:*119-140, 1934.

Sears, William W.: The effect of music on muscle tonus. *NAMT Book of Proceedings,* 1957, p. 199-206.

Schneider, Carl W.: Effect of Dalcroze eurhythmics upon the motor processes of schizophrenics. *NAMT Book of Proceedings,* 1960, p. 132-140.

Slaughter, Forrest E.: Effect of musical stimuli on normal and abnormal subjects as indicated by pupillary reflexes. *NAMT Book of Proceedings,* 1953, p. 246-249.

Wilson, Virginia Merritt: Variations in gastric motility due to musical stimuli. *NAMT Book of Proceedings,* 1946, p. 243-247.

"STIMULUS-RESPONSE" STUDIES

Alexander, H.: Investigation on the effects of music on personality by way of figure drawings. *Am. J. Psychother., 8:*687-702, 1954.

Arje, F. B.: The fine arts as an adjunct to rehabilitation. *J. Rehabil., 26* (6) , 1960.

Cattell and Saunders: Musical preferences and personality diagnosis. *J. Soc. Psychol., 39:*3-24, 1954.

Diserens, C. M.: Reactions to musical stimuli. *Psychol. Bull.* 20:173-199, 1923.

Fisher, S., and R. S.: Effects of personal security on reactions to unfamiliar music. *J. Soc. Psychol., 34:*265-273, 1951.

Gaston, E. Thayer: *Test of Musicality.* Odell's Instrumental Service, 1958.

Keston and Pinto: Possible factors influencing musical preference. *J. Genet. Psychol., 86:*101-113, 1955.

Lundin, R. W.: The development and validation of a set of musical ability tests. *Psychol. Monog.,63:*305, 1949.

Middleton, Fay, and Kerr: The effect of music on feelings of restfulness-tiredness, and pleasantness - unpleasantness. *J. Psychol., 17:*299-318, 1944.

Morehead, Joan K.: A Study of Sex Difference in Preference for Musical Tone. Unpublished Master's Thesis, Kansas University, 1948.

Riggs, Melvin, G.: The effect of register and tonality upon musical mood. *J. Musicol., 11:*49-61, 1940.

Rubin-Rabson, Grace: Influence of age, intelligence, and training on reactions to classic and modern music. *J. Gen. Psychol., 22:*413-420, 1940.

Scheihing, Geneva R.: A Study of Spontaneous Rhythmical Activities of Pre-school Children. Unpublished Master's Thesis, University of Kansas, 1950.

Shatin, Leo: Influence of music upon verbal participation in group psychotherapy. *Dis. Nerv. Syst., 19* (2) , 1958.

Sopchak, Andrew L.: Individual differences in responses to different types of music in relation to sex, mood, and other variables. *Psychol. Monogr., 69:*397, 1955.

Sunderman, L. F.: Study of some physiological differences between musicians and non-musicians: blood pressure. *J. Soc. Psychol., 23:*205-215, 1946.

GENERAL REFERENCES

1. Gaston, E. Thayer: Factors contributing to responses to music. *National Association for Music Therapy (NAMT) Book of Proceedings,* 1957, p. 23-30.

2. Farnsworth, Paul R.: *The Social Psychology of Music,* Chapter X, New York, Dryden Press, 1946.

3. Dillenger, George E.: Music and music therapy as a patient experiences them, *NAMT Book of Proceedings,* 1958, p. 193-214.

4. Gaston, E. Thayer: Psychological foundations for functional music, *American Journal of Occupational Therapy, XXXVII,* 1948.

5. van deWall, Willem: *Music in Hospitals,* Russell Sage Foundation, New York, 1946.

6. Schoen, Max: Art the healer. In *Music and Medicine,* Chapter XVI, New York, Schuman, 1948.

7. Dreikurs, Rudolph: Dynamics of music therapy, *NAMT Book of Proceedings,* 1953, p. 15-23.

8. Gaston, E. Thayer: Functions of the music therapist, *NAMT Book of Proceedings,* 1953, p. 28-29.

9. Diserens, Charles M.: *Influences of Music on Behavior.* Princeton New Jersey, Princeton University Press, 1926.

10. Diserens, Charles M.: The development of an experimental psychology of music, *Music and Medicine,* Chapter XV, Schulian and Schoen, New York, Schuman, 1948.

11. Mann, James: Dynamics of the music therapy relation, *NAMT Book of Proceedings,* 1954, p. 61-67.

12. Gaston, *op. cit.,* 1.

13. Masserman, Jules: *Principles of Dynamic Psychiatry.* Philadelphia, Saunders, 1946.

14. Kohut, Heinz: Some psychological effects of music and their relation to music therapy, *NAMT Book of Proceedings,* 1955, p. 17-20.

15. Hanson, Howard: The challenge of Music Therapy, *NAMT Book of Proceedings,* 1954, p. 8-14.

16. Meyer, Leonard B.: Learning, belief and music therapy, *NAMT Book of Proceedings,* 1955, p. 27-35.

17. Radin, Paul: Music and medicine among primitive peoples. *Music and Medicine,* Chapter I, New York, Schuman, 1948.

18. Meinecke, Bruno: Music and medicine in classical antiquity. Chapter III, *op. cit.,* 17.

19. Carapetyan, Armen: in preface to *Music and Medicine in the Renaissance,* Chapter V, *op. cit.,* 17.

20. See list of Selective References from 17th to 19th Centuries at end of Chapter V, *op. cit.,* 17.

21. Helmholz, H. E. F.: *Sensations of Tone.* New York, Longmans Green, 1912.

22. Dalcroze, Jacques: *Rhythmic Music and Education.* New York, Putnam, 1921.

23. Vescelius, Eva: *Music and Health.* New York, Goodyear, 1927.

24. See bibliography in Soibelman, Doris: *Therapeutic and Industrial Uses of Music,* New York, Columbia Univ. Press, 1948.

25. Diserens, C. M.: The development of an experimental psychology of music. *Music and Medicine.* Chapter XV, Schulian and Schoen, New York, Schuman, 1948.

26. Diserens and Fine: *A Psychology of Music.* Cincinnati, Ohio, Univ. Press, 1939.

27. Farnsworth, Paul R.: *The Social Psychology of Music.* New York, McGraw-Hill, 1938.

28. Lundin, Robert: *An Objective Psychology of Music.* New York, Norton, 1937.

29. Seashore, Carl E.: *Psychology of Music.* New York, McGraw-Hill, 1938.

30. Mursell, James L.: *Psychology of Music,* New York, Norton, 1937.

31. Schoen, Max: *The Psychology of Music.* New York, Ronald Press, 1940.

32. Gutheil, Emil: *Music and Your Emotions.* New York, Liveright, 1955.

33. Schulian and Schoen: *Music and Medicine.* Chapter IV, *op. cit.*
34. Licht, Sidney: *Music and Medicine.* Boston, Mass., New England Conservatory Press, 1946.
35. van de Wall, William and Liepmann, Clara: *Music in Institutions.* New York, Russel Sage Foundation, 1936.
36. Altschuler, Ira M.: *A psychiatrist's experiences with music as a therapeutic agent. Music and Medicine.* Chapter X, *op. cit.*
37. National Music Council Survey of Music in Hospitals. New York, Russell Sage Foundation, 1945.
38. Annual Books of Proceedings of NAMT 1951-1962, Quarterly "Bulletin" - 1951-1963, followed by Journal of Music Therapy. Beginning March 1954, all published by Allen Press, Lawrence, Kansas.
39. Uses of music in institutions. NAMT Survey, 1954, P.O. Box 610, Lawrence, Kansas.
40. Gaston, E. Thayer: Nature and principles of music therapy. *NAMT Book of Proceedings.* 1954, p. 152-155.
41. Dreikurs, Rudolph: Psychiatric concepts of music therapy for children. *NAMT Book of Proceedings.* 1953, p. 81-84.
42. Crocker, Dorothy Brin: Techniques in the use of music as therapy for the emotionally maladjusted child. *NAMT Book of Proceedings.* 1952, p. 175-180.
43. Smith, Orceneth: Music methods and materials for the mentally retarded. *NAMT Book of Proceedings.* 1952, p. 139-144.
44. Weir, Louise E.: Music therapy at Devereux Ranch School. *NAMT Book of Proceedings.* 1958, p. 22-25.
45. Corsini, Raymond: What is group psychology. *NAMT Book of Proceedings.* 1958, p. 57-64.
46. Sommer, Dorothy Twente: The effect of background music on frequency of interaction in group psychotherapy. *NAMT Book of Proceedings.* 1957, p. 167-168.
47. Breidenthal, Mynatt: Music therapy as special education in the public school. *NAMT Book of Proceedings.* 1958, p. 87-93.
48. Brunner, Olive: Music to aid the handicapped child. *NAMT Book of Proceedings.* 1951, p. 3-6.
49. Denenholz, Barbara: Music as a tool of physical medicine. *NAMT Book of Proceedings.* 1958, p. 67-84.
50. Fields, Beatrice: Music as an adjuvant in the treatment of brain-damaged patients, *Amer. J. Med., 33*:273, 1954.
51. Schneider, Erwin: The use of music with the brain-damaged child. *NAMT Book of Proceedings.* 1953, p. 95-98.
52. Palmer, Martin: Music stimuli in cerebral palsy, aphasia and similar conditions. *NAMT Book of Proceedings.* 1952, p. 162-168.
53. Korson, Frances: Music therapy for children with muscular dystrophy. *NAMT Book of Proceedings.* 1957, p. 192-198.
54. Unkefer, Robert: Progressive report of music therapy study at Kansas Rehabilitation Center for Adult Blind. *NAMT Book of Proceedings.* 1958, p. 185-193.
55. Crocker, Dorothy Brin: Using music in a speech therapy program. *NAMT Book of Proceedings.* 1958, p. 103-108.
56. Harbert, Wilhelmina K.: Music techniques applied in disordered speech. *NAMT Book of Proceedings.* 1953, p. 59-61.

57. Michel, Donald E.: Music therapy in cleft palate disorders. *NAMT Book of Proceedings.* 1960, p. 126-131.
58. Light, Geraldine A., and Willard, Joel: Music for surgery. *NAMT Book of Proceedings.* 1953, p. 171-182.
59. Gatewood, E. L.: The psychology of music in relation to anaesthesia, *Amer. J. Surg.,* April, 1941.
60. Cherry and Balin: *Music as a Supplement in Nitrous Oxide Anaesthesia.* Columbia Univ. Press, 1948, p. 66.
61. Kaplan, B.: Music with nitrous oxide. *Hospital board magazine Anaesthesia.* London, England, April, 1956, p. 160-163.
62. Jacobsen: Effects of sedative music on the tensions, anxieties, and pains experienced during dental procedures. *NAMT Book of Proceedings.* 1956, p. 231-234.
63. Chace, Marian: Physiological aspects of personal gratification. *NAMT Book of Proceedings.* 1952, p. 63-67.
64. Chace, Marian: Dance in growth or treatment settings. *NAMT Book of Proceedings.* p. 119-123, 1958.
65. Chace, Marian: Measurable and intangible aspects of dance therapy sessions. *NAMT Book of Proceedings.* 1957, p. 151-155.
66. Bender, Lauretta: *Child Psychiatric Techniques,* Springfield, Thomas, 1952.
67. Chace, *op. cit.,* #64.
68. Catell and Anderson: Measurement of personality and behavior disorders by the I. P. A. T. Music Preference Test, *J. Applied Psychol., 37* (6) :446-454, 1953.
69. Soibelman, Doris: *Therapeutic and Industrial Uses of Music,* New York, Columbia Univ. Press, 1948.
70. Reik, Theordore: *The Haunting Melody,* New York City, Farrar, Strauss and Young.
71. des Lauriers, Austin: Psychiatric concepts of music therapy. *NAMT Book of Proceedings.* 1952, p. 32-34.

Chapter V

INDUSTRIAL THERAPY

HERBERT GERJUOY, Ph.D., BRUCE FESSENDEN, O.T.R., and
ROBERT GORIL, R.R.T.*

INTRODUCTION

N<small>O SOCIETY CAN CONTINUE</small> effectively unless essential work
tasks are performed. In our society, each person is expected to
fulfill some productive role, but an illness or disability can alter
an individual's capacity to work. The expectation that members
of our society be productive has affected how we treat persons
with physical or psychological disabilities and illnesses: it has led
to the development of a variety of work-oriented therapy programs, all intended to restore pre-illness work capacity. These programs have also had various other objectives, such as provision of
meaningful, ego-supporting daily activities for patients.

Today, work-oriented activity is emerging as a distinct therapeutic entity that deals with the development and provision of
therapeutic work opportunities for patients under medical care,
especially for those under psychiatric care. Generally referred to
as industrial therapy, this activity involves work in both the
hospital and the community and incorporates graded treatment
and rehabilitative experiences designed to meet a variety of patient needs subsumed under the overall therapeutic objective of
normal (or acceptable) social function. Essentially, industrial
therapy is concerned with evaluation, treatment, and restoration
of patients' work capacities.

This chapter first identifies major concerns of industrial
therapy and touches upon its evolution as an activity that is intimately related to, though separate from, the other therapies with
which this book is concerned. Next, this chapter considers the objectives of industrial therapy: evaluation of patients' work capacities and potentials, enlargement of their capacities for normal

*The coauthors wish to thank Sydell T. Carlton, Marilyn C. Durkin, Irma R.
Gerjuoy, Donald F. Mills, and Humphrey Osmond for their editorial advice.

109

interpersonal relationships in the work setting, and gratification of their emotional and social needs by work. These objectives will be dealt with in terms of how industrial therapy helps to attain them.

How an industrial therapy program is developed is next considered. Various medical facilities have established a wide variety of programs; the present chapter deals with their generic characteristics.

The media that are used in industrial therapy are dependent for their implementation upon the therapists who use them. Therefore, some space is devoted to comments on the professional preparation considered essential for the conduct of industrial therapy programs.

Industrial therapy is emerging as a distinct therapeutic specialty at a time when far-reaching changes in medical care are altering basic patterns of treatment and rehabilitation. As a professional entity, industrial therapy has sought a well-defined but flexible identity. Recent trends in psychiatry have emphasized the importance of flexibility in the definition of industrial therapy, since these trends have led to multiple trends in industrial therapy. For example, in psychiatry there has recently been increased emphasis both on the therapeutic hospital community (with patients working within the hospital) and on the integration of all therapeutic services with the general community outside the hospital (with patients working outside the hospital). Thus, it has not seemed suitable to give a highly specific definition of industrial therapy. Instead, this chapter concludes with some comments on current trends in industrial therapy that may suggest the form that such a definition may take in the future.

HISTORICAL DEVELOPMENT, PRESENT DEFINITION, AND LONG-RANGE PROBLEMS

A number of professions are currently involved in efforts to improve the work capacity of ill and disabled persons who are hospitalized. Among these are industrial therapy, psychiatry, social work, vocational counseling, manual arts therapy, occupational therapy, counseling psychology, rehabilitation nursing, educational therapy, and vocational training.

Any definition of industrial therapy should consider its relationship to the various related professional fields but it should also emphasize the core of industrial therapy: provision of work-oriented opportunities for hospitalized patients to experience real situations akin to everyday employment in which they may learn or relearn socially acceptable work patterns. Industrial therapy may, in addition, give patients therapeutic benefits by helping them to meet their emotional needs.

Various mental health professions that are concerned with the work adjustment of patients have come to recognize that if patients are to make long-term adjustments in the community outside the hospital, they need adequate work capacity and ability to appraise this capacity realistically. With the growing awareness of the importance of treating the whole person, work has come to be seen as a vital factor in the life experience of the individual. With the intensified attention to work programming, both in this country and abroad, there have been diverse administrative approaches, great variation in the delegation of responsibility for these programs, and a number of different theoretical bases.

Although the Federal Civil Service Commission has not established a separate classification category for the position of industrial therapist to date, this contrasts with the practices in several state mental hospital systems, and it is in state mental hospitals that most mental patients reside; 839,000 of the 1,240,000 patients on active records in 1957 were in state hospitals.[1] There have been few detailed studies of the use of a separate classification category for industrial therapy; however, a compilation of data on rehabilitation therapy services by Thomas J. Crowe, Chief, Rehabilitation Therapy Services, Anoka (Minn.) State Hospital, indicated that at least 14 states have job classifications whose descriptions of duties and responsibilities suggest a professional position like industrial therapist as the term is used in this chapter. Crowe's survey revealed a variety of job titles under which programs that appeared to be industrial therapy were administered, including, in addition to industrial therapist, occupational therapist, vocational and industrial director, rehabilitation therapist, patient work therapist, and activity program supervisor (industrial) .

Historically, work programs seem to have been part of organized care for the mentally ill since the era of moral treatment in the early nineteenth century.

"In its earlier days, occupational therapy seemed to be synonymous with work therapy and with what was then called 'moral treatment.' It is important to keep in mind the historical relationship between work therapy and moral treatment; for a fundamental premise of the advocates of moral treatment was that work was good for patients, and therefore 'therapeutic,' because work itself was a moral good. Normal people work, therefore sick people, to become well, must work, or at least learn to work again."[2]

The moral therapy basis of work therapy was first expressed by Pinel,[3] writing:

"It is no longer a problem to be solved, but the result of the most constant and unanimous experience, that in all public asylums as well as in prisons and hospitals, the surest, and, perhaps, the only method of securing health, good order, and good manners, is to carry into decided and habitual execution the natural law of bodily labour, so contributive and essential to human happiness. This truth is especially applicable to lunatic asylums: and I am convinced that no useful and durable establishments of that kind can be founded excepting on the basis of interesting and laborious employment. I am very sure that few lunatics, even in their most furious state, ought to be without some active occupation."

Pinel took a progressive position for his time, but the use of work programs with the mentally ill had other roots as well. The emergence in post-medieval society of the total-care institution as a subcommunity into which society relegated its misfits gave rise to powerful economic pressures for intramural work by patients. The new total institutions were given meager support; therefore, in order to maintain minimum custodial services they sought to elicit as many man-hours of labor as possible from their inmates. Thus, work by patients is as old as custodial care and far older than formal rehabilitation programs.

Work programs have also been associated with attitudes even

less reputable than custodialism. Some of these were described by Wittkower and Azima:[4]

"A glance at the history of occupational therapy [sic] shows that its application to the mentally ill long antedated its application to patients suffering from any other disorders and that their employment in the so-called hospital industries preceded any other forms of occupational therapy.

"Impetus to the movement, strange as it may appear, was given by prison reforms early in the nineteenth century. It was indeed a great advance in penology when prisoners were allowed to work. Yet the privilege to work, which may well have boosted the morale of the prisoners, shades so easily into exploitation of cheap labor for the sake of economy and into hard labor imposed as a means of punishment. Attempts followed 'to cheer up the mentally ill and to make them forget their troubles' by keeping them busy and by offering them recreation and amusement."

Another disreputable basis for work therapy was discussed by Kaufmann and Sewall,[5] writing:

"Patient labor is the axis on which many a psychiatric hospital turns. Officials may admit that, were it not for the toils of patients, it would be impossible to operate the laundry or the kitchens, impossible to keep the floors cleaned or the buildings painted. In theory, the goal of such assignments is to help the patient. . . . Yet it is no secret to the sophisticated observer that what determines the assignment, and sometimes the retention of the patients there, is internal hospital efficiency rather than the patient's own needs. Certainly many patients work effectively as gardeners, janitors, kitchen helpers, and in many other capacities for years and even decades without systematic efforts to utilize their well-integrated work behavior for possible advancement into the community. On the contrary, effective performance in the assigned activity may result in such a successful adjustment to hospital living that even, on the part of the patient, there develops a disinclination to leave the hospital and return to the community. Hospitals have not been slow to capitalize on this. As a result, their staffs have been supplemented by a force that comes perilously close to being slave labor."

A decade after Kaufmann and Sewall wrote (a ten-year period that saw major changes in institutional programing and in the attitudes of institutional employees) Bartlett[6] was still able to write:

"The labor needs of the typical state mental hospital are admittedly substantial. Typically, it must exist in isolation from other social institutions, providing as best it can for all the needs of its patient population out of its own internal activities and resources. In the aggregate, the requirements include furnishing and maintaining usual community service needs of town-sized proportions. These can be staggering . . . state hospitals need 'good patients' who are useful, valuable, and expediently indispensable. But these relatively less ill patients, instead of being helped to overcome their illness, as is normally expected on behalf of the patients in any other medical care facility, are doomed by the institutional needs of the state mental hospital to the pathological dependency characteristic of 'good patients'."

With work therapy so prone to serve nontherapeutic ends, it is not surprising that much of the literature consists of reports of attempts to formalize long-standing programs of patient labor and relate them to newer concepts of treatment and rehabilitation. For example, Bryan[7] assumed that some patients would work and urged that assignment of patients to jobs be thought of as similar to the prescription of treatment drugs rather than as akin to placement of workers in industry.

Since, however, work by patients antedates modern rehabilitative programing and was a part of the older and discredited custodial system and of even less respectable systems, there has been a tendency to dismiss the contributions of work programs to rehabilitation because of their guilt by association with nontherapeutic approaches.

Thus, there is, at present, considerable confusion in the United States about the status of work therapy. Olshansky and Unterberger[8] offered a sociocultural and psychological framework that may help clear up this confusion:

". . . in America, where everyone is expected to work, inhospital opportunities for patients to work are not too common or well-planned, in contrast to Europe (Carstairs, Clark, and O'Connor[9]) where even the sickest patient is expected to work, and does work.

"Why this paradox?

"First, it would seem explainable in terms of our great wealth, and acceptance (historically) of unemployment. Even during our recent period of so-called full employment, our country had substantial pockets of unemployment, called distress areas, about which there was much talk but little action.

"Second, since our middle-class professional looks down on menial work, he has little motivation to push patients into activities on which he places a low value.

"Third, being more intrapsychically oriented than their European counterparts, American psychiatrists tend to see recovery in terms of insight following therapy, rather than recovery through the ego-preservative functions of work. Relatedly, psychiatrists—looking at themselves—view work as basically a 'mental activity,' requiring a clear mind.

"Fourth, work is often connected with punishment, required, for example, of prisoners. Kindness requires the indulgence of patients.

"Fifth, implied in the sick role of the mental patient is the image of the physically disabled who, during sickness and hospitalization, is not expected to work.

"Finally, it can be explained in terms of general inertia—the tendency of a system of idleness to perpetuate itself. Moreover, a system of idleness is easier to operate than a system of planned inhospital employment."

Olshansky and Unterberger's[10] discussion of the economic, social, and cultural aspects of work therapy touches upon certain long-range problems: Do patients assigned to work activity believe that work is inherently satisfying? This is a cardinal belief of many managers, professional men, and craftsmen (*e.g.*, Brown;[11] Gurin, Veroff, and Field[12]). If patients do not believe that work is satisfying, does this mean that there is no valid theoretical base for the use of work as a treatment or rehabilitative medium? Increasing mechanization and automation threaten general job security and tend to depersonalize the everyday work situation; how are attitudes toward work affected by these changes? What are the effects of the ongoing transition from a production-oriented to a consumption-oriented society? What are the effects of the increasing importance of leisure time? It is beyond the scope of this chapter to look into these intriguing questions. Rather, we have touched upon them so that the reader may be encouraged to think about them himself.

From the perspective offered by this section, we conclude that industrial therapy has several antecedents and that it is still undergoing development. For the present, it is a diffusely organized rehabilitation movement that is groping with a variety of interpretations of work. Neither theory nor practice is uniform or without contradictions. Consequently, the status of industrial therapy as a legitimate therapy program can best be determined if it is evaluated in terms of the functions it serves and the treatment objectives it helps achieve, rather than in terms of its rationale.

OBJECTIVES AND FUNCTIONS

Medical, psychological, and social evaluations of the patient are well-established procedures which provide data that are used by the therapeutic team as bases for treatment and rehabilitation planning. The activities services, including industrial therapy, are members of the therapeutic team and contribute to the planning process by providing data on the patient's responses to their programs. Thus, *a first objective of industrial therapy is to assess or evaluate the patient's adjustment to work.* Evaluation of the patient's work performance in industrial therapy provides data that may be particularly useful for prediction of his long-term adjustment after the current illness has subsided. For example, industrial therapy may expose educational deficiencies that interfere with social and vocational adequacy.

Evaluation is not, moreover, a time-limited function confined to the first phase of treatment. For many patients, long-term adjustment outside the hospital will depend largely on their success in finding and holding jobs. Since there is no generally accepted indirect measure of a patient's potential for work adjustment, the best solution to the problem of measuring work-adjustment potential is to place the patient in a typical work situation and observe how he performs. Consequently, work-adjustment evaluation continues to be appropriate through all phases of treatment and is particularly important just prior to discharge.

When they leave the hospital, hopefully most patients will have to deal with situations like the industrial therapy situation. In the hospital work setting, then, the patient may practice adaptive social behaviors he will need outside the hospital. *A second objective of industrial therapy is to help the patient develop acceptable interpersonal relations in the work situation* with other workers, with the work group as a unit, and with other persons who are outside but related to the work group, such as customers, administrators, and clients. This objective will be best achieved when the hospital work setting most closely resembles work settings encountered outside, since the patient's work experiences and habits at the hospital will then generalize or transfer to work outside.

A third objective of industrial therapy is to satisfy ancillary needs such as development of self-reliance, development of social responsibility, enhancement of self-esteem, training of basic work habits, training of specific vocational skills, and exploration of alternative vocations or work settings.

Finally, it is a moot question whether *satisfaction of institutional needs* should be included among the objectives of industrial therapy. There is ample evidence that whether or not this *should* be an objective, it *is* an objective, and that it is dictated by the practical realities of the economic situation of most government-operated institutions (Bartlett;[13] Kaufmann and Sewall[14]). Furthermore, activities that actually have this last objective are often easy to rationalize as having therapeutic purposes.

Satisfaction of institutional needs is not necessarily incompatible with achievement of therapeutic goals. For example, for work to be therapeutic, it should appear meaningful to the patient, and that his work contributes to the economic or social well-being of the hospital community may provide the necessary meaning.

An industrial therapy program needs built-in checks and balances, however, to ensure that the institution's needs do not outweigh the patients' needs. For example, there should be a reversal of the typical hospital's dependency on patient labor for economic survival. Such a reversal would make the industrial therapy program dependent on the production and service departments of the hospital (instead of vice-versa) ; these departments would provide work opportunities for the program. There should be a backlog of patients ready for placement as soon as vacancies occur in the hospital job roster. If the industrial therapy program is under pressure to find jobs for patients, then it will be less difficult to move a patient out of the hospital even though some hospital department or employee has become dependent on his services.

There should be a detailed and continuously updated review of the hospital jobs available for patients and of the job requirements with respect to skills, capacity for assuming responsibility, and ability to act effectively interpersonally. With such information, each patient may be placed so as to fit his needs and capacities to job demands. Furthermore, the program must stress movement of patients through successive levels of job assignment. Any hospital has many levels of available work assignments that have distinct degrees of responsibility and interpersonal commitment. Although many patients who work never leave the hospital, hope should not be abandoned for any given patient. Instead, his contribution to the hospital community should be conceived of as a temporary one, as one step on the graded series that will move him into transitional institutional structures away from the hospital. Thus, the series of levels of job assignment in the hospital should be thought of as continuous with and part of the succession of levels of autonomy that the patient moves through on his way toward discharge.

PROGRAM DEVELOPMENT

A hospitalized psychotic is, *ipso facto,* an individual who has failed to meet society's demands for conformity to social norms. Therefore, if his appraisal of himself is at all realistic, it is reasonable that he be concerned about his social adequacy. In order to encourage and maintain acceptable social behavior in such an individual, without excessively arousing his natural anxiety about his capacity for normal interpersonal behavior, it is usually necessary to use an adroit schedule of reinforcements to shape his social behavior through a series of successive approximations to acceptable behavior.

Since past interpersonal failures are likely to have a patient unusually ready to perceive himself as rejected and to have made him unusually sensitive to rejection, a single untoward incident may have considerable unfavorable influence on the course of his recovery; it may undo the therapeutic influence of many favorable experiences. Consequently, if a single individual or a single situation in a patient's social environment persistently arouses feelings of social inadequacy, this may block progress toward recovery despite an otherwise ideal treatment program. Because a patient's treatment program is likely to be no more effective than it is in the least favorable social situation to which he is exposed, it is difficult to appraise the contribution that any treatment or rehabilitative program makes to the hospital's overall program, since an anti-therapeutic component in the program may mask potential positive contributions by all the other components.

A corollary of the foregoing is that the best possible industrial therapy program will accomplish little unless it is part of a well-administered overall treatment program that deals with all facets of patient life. Unfortunately, because of economic considerations, expansion of one phase of a hospital's treatment program has at times been at the expense of other phases. When the industrial therapy program has been enlarged at the expense of other programs, this has rarely led to noteworthy improvement among the patients. Evaluation of work programing under such circumstances can hardly be fair.

Because a patient in industrial therapy is commonly shifted from job to job and is therefore exposed to many different staff members, industrial therapy is unusually dependent on favorable attitudes throughout the hospital staff. If work by patients is regarded by the hospital personnel as part of the patients' treatment or rehabilitation programs, the personnel may be expected to act more therapeutically toward the patients than if patient work assignment is seen as punishment or as a device to cut labor costs. What attitudes the personnel have, however, depend largely on what they see the industrial therapy program accomplish day by day.

Those responsible for treatment and care in a particular hospital should see that each patient's industrial therapy program is planned in the context of his overall individual treatment requirements. Decisions about how the work or vocational aspects of treatment should be integrated with the rest of the treatment program should be decided by the full hospital treatment-planning staff, although the industrial therapy staff should take particular responsibility. Prior to planning the industrial therapy program for a specific patient, the industrial therapy staff should assess his vocational problems and potential. It may be useful to assign him to one of a set of categories of patient types. Baur[15] presented a list of the most common categories; it is given below with some modification:

1. Patients who were successful on the job before their illness but who need help to retain skills or to brush up.
2. Patients (most often adolescents or young adults) who have had no work experience but who are able to learn. Many of these patients have no skills and have had no job training or job-selection guidance.
3. Patients who were not suited to their former vocations or who are in need of training or adjustment to other work because residuals of their mental disorders make return to their previous work inadvisable.
4. Patients with a poor prognosis for discharge who may, nevertheless, benefit from vocational activity.

To deal with the various types of patients, an industrial therapy program should have four components, each of which should be involved in the treatment of each type of patient:

1. Ongoing Job Survey. As Baganz, Namen, Hall, and Swickle[16] pointed out, a survey of the jobs available in the hospital should provide information on the positions open to patients and on the attitudes of relevant hospital personnel about working with patients. Ivany and Rothschild[17] and Willard and Spackman[18] have described methods of conducting such a survey. It is also desirable that the work activities be graded with respect to the physical exertion they involve: *e.g.,* (a) strenuous; (b) heavy; (c) moderate, and (d) minimal. It may be useful to group the jobs in the hospital in the same way they are grouped in the *Dictionary of Occupational Titles.*[19] Such a grouping facilitates comparison between positions in the hospital and ones in the outside community. It is important that psychological factors be taken into account in the job survey; for example, the industrial therapist should be sensitive to the status connotations that different jobs have for both employees and patients.

Since the attitudes of hospital personnel and the work needs of various hospital departments change from time to time, the job survey should be a continuing task for the industrial therapy staff. The survey should be conducted with the current needs of the patient population of the particular hospital in mind.

It is not always practicable or even possible to use existing hospital positions to provide jobs that meet the needs of every patient. This is especially true for chronic patients, for whom the purpose of industrial therapy is primarily to improve morale (the third objective of industrial therapy, discussed earlier). For such patients, the job survey should be extended to include investigation of the feasibility of creating new hospital jobs—not occupational therapy—that are under industrial therapy staff supervision. For example, patients may be assigned to key-punch jobs in which they prepare cards for data processing; several patients may be given the same key-punch assignment, so that errors may be eliminated by collation. Such jobs differ from jobs in departments such as the kitchen, farm, or laundry that are subject to relatively inflexible service demands and cannot easily be manipulated to meet individual or group work needs of patients; such jobs also differ from those typically given to recently admitted patients in active psychotherapy, whose work assignments may be direct adjuncts of their psychotherapeutic programs.

At the opposite end of the rehabilitation continuum from chronic patients are those who are nearing discharge and need work experiences that are even more realistic than those typically provided by the hospital industry situation. The job survey should seek to identify those job situations in the hospital that are particularly suitable as transitional or pre-discharge work experiences.

The remaining three components of the industrial therapy program all pertain directly to the treatment and rehabilitation of patients.

2. Evaluation and Basic Training. Through specialized tests, interviews, and on-the-job observations, the patient's emotional and vocational capacities for work adjustment are evaluated. The results of this evaluation contribute to decisions concerning industrial or work assignments. They may suggest that such an assignment is contraindicated.

Basic training is part of this component because an important factor in the evaluation of a patient is his response to basic training in work habits, general work skills, and attitudes toward work.

For on-the-job observations by members of the industrial therapy staff, a "trial" work task may be set up. The trial task is usually a group work activity, but an individual (*i.e.*, solitary) work assignment may also be used. Any work assignment can ordinarily serve both evaluation and treatment objectives.

Aspects of patient behavior to consider in evaluation include: (a) responsiveness to direction; (b) effectiveness in relations with fellow workers; (c) responsibility for materials and tools; (d) punctuality, and (e) thoroughness of general work habits. These are social-conformity aspects of job adjustment. Martinson[20] has discussed them and has also dealt with patient awareness and acceptance of general social imperatives such as taxes, unions, social security, savings funds, checking accounts, insurance, income budgeting, job application procedure, and interview behavior.

Merker, Vehlow, and Nelson[21] discussed patient reaction to the initial work assignment:

> "The initial attempt to place the patient in the industrial therapy program produces a variety of reactions. He may deny his ability physically to do work with outbursts such as 'I am in a hospital. I am sick. I am unable to work or I wouldn't be here.' This denial may also take the form of physical illness

which requires careful checking by his physician to determine its etiology. Other patients become aggressive towards the person in charge, usually expressing verbal hostility 'Do your work yourself if you want it done. Don't take out your feelings on the patients,' etc. Passive aggressiveness is often seen, with the patient saying nothing, doing nothing, and giving no indication of his feeling. Some aggressive patients will take the role of seeming to shield a more passive patient, and thus keep themselves and their more passive partner from becoming involved. For these reasons, kindly and persistent insistence on patient participation is often needed to establish for the patient a newly prescribed daily activity program which involves the industrial therapy projects.

"For the schizophrenic patient assigned to industrial therapy, an attitude involving a minimal amount of demand is essential with reward and praise, meaningful to the patient, forthcoming the instant any initiative or interest on the part of the patient is observed by the therapist. Otherwise, if the patient is pushed at a speed not established by himself, he seems to retreat beyond recall."

Since interviews conducted for other purposes may also provide data pertinent to work program planning, records of interviews conducted by the medical, psychological, and social service departments, for example, should be readily available to the professional industrial therapy staff, provided there is no violation of the confidentiality of a psychotherapeutic relationship. Specific aptitude and achievement tests pertinent to work assignment may be administered by the psychology staff. Such tests need not be administered or scored by industrial therapy personnel; the industrial therapy department, however, should be permitted to conduct its own interviews or tests if the staff members are competent to do so. This may be particularly convenient when the interview or test procedures have been developed by the industrial therapy staff for industrial therapy purposes.

Some basic work-adjustment training should be part of the earliest preliminary-evaluation phase of treatment. This training should seek to give the patient a healthy orientation to the industrial therapy program. For this purpose, group activities seem most suitable. Such activities may be used to help heighten motivation to contribute to production or service; subsequently, such motivation may be used to encourage social conformity with respect to responsiveness to direction, punctuality, and so on. It is important that such industrial-therapy-orientation groups be supervised by industrial therapy staff members trained for this function. The group activities should be realistic and meaningful, but they should not necessarily be essential to the hospital economy. Pressures for production should be under the control of the industrial therapy department and should be adjusted to the patients' capacities to respond to them. Housekeeping, furniture repair, and grounds maintenance are examples of suitable activities, since in each of these there is an obvious effect that patients can see when they finish a job and since it is relatively easy to have other personnel finish the job if the patients are not able to do so.

3. Work Conditioning. In this program component, the patient is given diverse work assignments that provide a series of graded social-vocational situations designed to help move him toward his overall treatment goals.

Patients may be given group or individual assignments. Group assignments may be similar to those used for basic training or they may include more complex or important tasks, such as typing, mimeographing, producing the hospital newspaper, or operating a "washmobile" for washing and polishing autos and other vehicles. Refurbishing furniture and operating a personal laundry service are further possibilities.

Such programs should be the responsibility of the industrial therapy department and should be supervised by industrial therapy personnel. This administrative arrangement is recommended for two reasons: first, because it is desirable that patient work be supervised by persons whose primary concern is not production itself but rather the growth and development of patients' productive capacities; second, because it is desirable that patient work be supervised by persons who are best qualified to compare the work behavior of patients with the standards expected outside the hospital.

Pay-for-work projects are included in this program component as well as in the next and last component. Denber and Rajotte[22] have considered the responses of various types of patients to a work conditioning program involving paid labor in an intrahospital workshop similar to a factory:

"The prospect of a daily occupation appeals to those patients who are either relatively symptom-free and soon to leave or to the chronic patients, and least of all to the sickest and the psychopaths. In the latter groups, the negative feelings reflect directly the underlying psychopathology.

"Work has meaning mostly to those who have done factory labour before and to housewives, and least to those with secretarial background or one of higher education. For those patients, we try and find work elsewhere in the hospital or assign them to help with the secretarial work in the ward.

". . . It has been found that acutely ill patients who begin to hallucinate in the shop (particularly with ideas of destruction of self or of others) usually spontaneously ask to be returned to the ward.

"On the other hand, depressed patients can be integrated into the shop setting. At times, this required urging on the part of the staff, and more often than not was successful. While the output was low, at least the social set, the work, and group support were of value to the patients. From an administrative standpoint, it was easier to keep these patients under observation in the group than on the ward.

"It has been surprising to find how easily the long hospitalized patients adapted. They were among the most eager workers at the outset, still are, and sometimes in spite of incapacitating psychopathological symptoms perform well and earn a reasonably good salary.

"The major difficulty was with the younger patients (sixteen to twenty-three years) who either never had worked before, or had been intermittently hospitalized and knew only the custodial institution where patients 'sat all day' or when given honour cards 'walked on the grounds.' To them, the hospital was a place 'to rest'."

Assignment to an intrahospital factory job is made on an individual basis, and patients residing in the same ward may be sent to a variety of different projects; unlike work assignment in earlier phases of the industrial therapy program, a patient's work group and his ward group may overlap only slightly. Nevertheless, in the hospital factory the work itself is often organized as a group project. Patients are individually assigned to intrahospital factory jobs so that their ability to meet production standards may be taken into account and so that consideration may be given to the personalities of prospective fellow workers and work supervisors.

The industrial therapist does not have as much control of the intrahospital factory work situation as he has of work settings directly supervised by the industrial therapy department (as discussed above). He may, however, have a variety of intrahospital factory jobs to choose among, any one of which may be more akin to jobs in the outside community than are jobs directly supervised by the industrial therapy department. This is because production demands are pivotal in the outside community, and only under exceptional circumstances are concessions made to emotional disturbance.

4. Work-readiness Preparation (Transition). Finally, the patient is placed in a work setting that is as realistic as possible. This situation provides the final dress rehearsal before the patient leaves the hospital and starts (or starts again) to work on his own in the outside community. The transitional work experience may be in a special transitional workshop in the hospital or it may be outside the hospital; the patient may continue to reside in the hospital or he may reside in a halfway house or in some other transitional agency. An example of a transitional work program is the community employment plan discussed by Stem,[23] in which the patient works in a community job while maintaining his hospital residence; this is a day-work, night-hospital plan.

In this final phase of the industrial therapy program, responsibility for the patient's work activity starts to shift away from the hospital industrial therapy staff. It is particularly important, therefore, that there be a close liaison with the physician, social service worker, psychologist, vocational counselor, and (when there is one) community employer.

This completes the description of the components of an industrial therapy program. The description implies, correctly, that such a program should have a beginning, a middle, and an end, and that the end may be ill-defined since it is commonly part of a transition that points toward the successful reintegration of the individual in a productive role in the community. However, a given patient may not need the entire program sequence. An appropriate individualized work plan can best be developed if the patient is given an early vocational assessment and if there is continuous reappraisal of his vocational potential.

There are four classes of professional techniques that are used in conjunction with the implementation of an industrial therapy program. These are referral, selection, placement, and follow-up.

1. *Referral* is the means whereby the patient secures a work assignment. The initiative may come from various sources, including the patient. However, final responsibility for review of a proposed assignment must rest with the professional person or group (usually a psychotherapist or physician) in overall charge of the treatment program for the given patient. Recently, this has become most commonly a treatment team responsibility.

2. *Selection* involves the traditional methods of personnel psychology, including interviewing and testing. There should be special consideration given to the social and emotional significance to the patient of a contemplated work assignment.

3. *Placement,* too, is a procedure that superimposes on traditional industrial methods an overlay of psychotherapeutic considerations. Placement requires familiarity with the various available jobs. The industrial therapist should know the skill requirements, psychological and social aspects, difficulty and strenuousness, and physical work conditions of each job; he should also know the labor needs of various potential placement settings, the patient's current clinical status, prognosis, treatment plan, and treatment objectives.

4. Finally, in *follow-up* the patient is observed in the work situation in which he is currently placed. His response is evaluated in terms of his treatment or rehabilitation goals, and the therapy plan may be adjusted in the light of this response. The patient's

response may also be used to help guide successive steps in an on-going work-adjustment training program that may involve either counseling and guidance or manipulation of his work environment, such as placing him in contact with work supervisors who have particular personalities.

PROFESSIONAL PREPARATION

Administrators of superior work therapy programs have generally not been successful in ensuring the continuity of their programs across generations of personnel change. With the death or retirement of the first generation of individuals who have set up a therapeutically effective industrial therapy service, such a program has often lost its effectiveness.

One important cause of the difficulty in perpetuating successful industrial therapy programs has been the rarity of persons qualified to cope with the extraordinarily broad range of problems with which an industrial therapy supervisor is concerned. The service obligations of an industrial therapy program make it necessary for its director to be qualified to assign patients to work in many different divisions of the hospital. Not only must he be skilled in personnel placement if he is to make these assignments properly, but he must also be well informed about clinical diagnosis, the theory of personality disorder, and the relationships between personality disorder and work environment.

No one curriculum provides training in all the various skills and knowledges needed by industrial therapists, and in no curriculum is there a course on the influence of work environment on behavior pathology. Therefore, it is difficult to find or to identify persons with the appropriate educational background for work as industrial therapists. Moreover, individuals who do possess the necessary broad qualifications are usually qualified for much better-paying positions outside the hospital.

Gerjuoy[24] has discussed the professional preparation and standards for industrial therapists. For the proper direction of an industrial therapy program, there are special technical skills and knowledges that must be acquired. No other professional group is presently trained to have these necessary specialized skills and knowledges. Therefore, the future industrial therapist should be given specialized technical training in an industrial therapist training curriculum distinct from other curricula; industrial therapy should be recognized as a distinct profession that requires its own unique program of academic professional preparation.

Academic training of industrial therapists should include a course in clinical job analysis and worker placement. In this course the industrial therapist should learn how to analyze a job systematically in order to establish personnel specifications for it with respect to the industrial therapy program. He should learn how to recognize the therapeutic possibilities and training potentials of a vocational context. The emphasis in such a course should be on job analysis procedures and on the preparation of job descriptions for use in industrial therapy program planning. Unlike the job analyses and job descriptions that are the concerns of personnel and industrial psychologists who work in the outside community, industrial therapy job analyses and job descriptions should emphasize the emotional-clinical aspects of work environments and their influences on individuals with various behavior pathologies.

It is evident by now that industrial therapists are coming to be regarded as co-professionals with workers in other, better established, activity therapies. There is a kind of Gresham's law in the training and selection of therapists: Graduates of bad training programs tend to drive out graduates of good ones. Moreover, students tend to gravitate toward programs that make minimum demands on them. Administrators, too often handicapped by financial limitations and a general shortage of trained professionals, tend to hire those who will accept the lowest salaries and the poorest working conditions. Such persons are usually graduates of programs that accept the least qualified persons for training and that teach their students the least. Therefore, in the interest of the professional integrity of all the professions that border upon industrial therapy, we must make certain that industrial therapy training does not become a haven for individuals who are not up to the rigorous training given to those who prepare for careers in better established rehabilitation fields, in which standards of education are already well defined and well maintained.

We ought not to expect another specialist (*e.g.,* a physician) who has not had the necessary specialized training to be able to make the same informed decisions that would be made by a trained industrial therapist. This is precisely the line of reasoning that has led to the recognition of every one of the other specialties now established in mental hospitals as distinct professions. For example, the medical profession has come to recognize that social work requires special training. Therefore, a physician carefully and respectfully considers recommendations made by the hospital social service department when matters arise that pertain to that department's special competence. Of course, the physician, in his role as executive coordinator of the various services that are brought to bear on an individual case, may overrule a recommendation from one department in the light of information provided by other departments or in the light of knowledge that comes from his own specialty, medicine.

Unless the industrial therapist is regarded in the hospital as a professional specialist on a par with other hospital specialists such as psychologists, social workers, or occupational therapists, his usefulness to the hospital may be nearly negligible. It may be too much to ask of the social flexibility of that status-conscious institution, the hospital, if we ask that a person who is regarded as a subprofessional technician be taken seriously when his views oppose those of professionals from other departments. Therefore, if we wish the industrial therapist to contribute an independent point of view to the staff decisions regarding patient care, we must train the industrial therapist so that he is recognizably a professional person with status comparable to that of other hospital specialists.

Discussed earlier was the danger that an industrial therapy program may be used merely to provide hospitals with a class of cheap (or wageless) laborers. It may be doubted whether elaboration of protective regulations will have much practical value in safeguarding patients from abuses, since patients are hardly in a position to protest effectively against violation of a labor code. Their protests are likely to be like the gesture of a patient in one large state hospital, who painted the words "Garbage Therapy" on the cans that he was required to empty.

If, however, we can help create conditions in which industrial therapists, the persons who are in charge of and actually administer work programs, are intelligent and enlightened persons who have been trained to be tolerant and to respect human dignity and have been given a broadening and liberalizing education, and if we select persons for this profession whose personalities make such enlightened attitudes and behavior ego-syntonic, then we can look to the nascent professional ethics of industrial therapy to provide its own bulwark against abuse of industrial therapy programs. This is exactly the sort of protection from abuse relied upon in other medical and paramedical specialties. For example, the real protection that the average citizen has from being unjustifiably incarcerated in a mental hospital is not the ponderous legal machinery whereby he may seek release if so held; rather, it is the high morale and the high morals of mental hospital physicians that protect him, since these physicians would not think of unethical abuse of their legal authority to hold persons in the hospital by force if neecssary.

Consequently, the need for broad liberal training of industrial therapists as a professional group rather than merely as a technician class need not be justified solely on the narrow basis that an industrial therapist with professional status will be in a better position with respect to the intramural professional rivalries in his hospital. We must train the industrial therapist to be an educated and responsible professional person because his work involves important ethical considerations and requires nice judgments concerning the relative weights of institutional and individual needs. We want the industrial therapist, therefore, to be educated to a maturity of ethical commitment that will make him oppose any tendency for his program to be corrupted to a cost-cutting dodge that may do therapeutic harm. We also want him to be educated to the personal and social sophistication that will help him find his way through the years of compromise that will be necessary before the obligations of industrial therapy to patients and to the institution itself are fully defined.

CURRENT TRENDS

Since the publication of the report of the Joint Commission on Mental Illness and Health in 1961, there has been a considerable increase in efforts to involve the community in responsibility for treatment and rehabilitation of the mentally ill. Major long-range planning now envisages comprehensive community responsibility for comprehensive community services. The increased concern with early detection and early treatment of mental illness has fostered planning of community-based programs that may be more readily available to patients in the early stages of mental illness than are outpatient services at mental hospitals. There has also been increased interest in preventive measures and in after-care and follow-up services in the community. These trends have jointly encouraged more interest in and experimentation with a variety of interrelated community mental health services that have tended to blur some of the previously sharp boundaries—or actual gaps—that have existed between formalized institutional settings and the mainstream of community activity.

This chapter has been mainly concerned with industrial therapy as administered in a hospital setting; the point of view of this chapter, however, is compatible with a comprehensive community-based program. Such programs are now evolving: Day-hospitals that provide vocational programs already exist; some long-established institutions now take day patients into their activity programs; and a number of community-supported work-adjustment centers that accept after-care referrals or provide pre-admission services have recently been established.

The burgeoning popularity of one particular type of industrial therapy program is perhaps the most significant recent trend. This program involves giving patients monetary rewards for their labors. Programs of this type have had various names, such as pay-for-work program, compensated work therapy, and subcontract project. Impetus for pay-for-work programing has come in part from successful European experiences. In this country such programing has been encouraged by the development in many hospitals of a system of subcontracts for the intrahospital factories with local industries; such subcontracts have provided the hospital workshops with sources of steady income. Thirty-two of 114 hospitals that responded to a questionnaire on vocational rehabilitation in 1960 indicated that some patients were compensated in one way or another for their services.[25] In some institutions monetary compensation has been an established practice for many years; it has, however, generally been little more than token payment. More often, some other reward has been substituted for actual cash or credit: common substitutes have been tobacco or cigarette rations, canteen chits, and ground privileges.

Nagler and Kirkland[26] speculated that "a survey of institutions across the country would disclose a variety of practices in regard to payment for work done in the institution. There are various combinations of the basic methods, and some are used exclusively by some institutions. There are four basic methods: equal pay regardless of the amount and kind of work; a differential pay scale, with some jobs earning higher wages than others; a universal allowance, equal for all patients and provided without regard to work contributions; and no pay at all." Barton[27] has presented an interesting account of the economic and therapeutic arguments for and against paying patients for work they do; he endorses neither approach but recognizes many values in monetary reward as a strong incentive and as a reality factor.

McGrath and Burke[28] contended:

"Within an institution, compensated work therapy must have as its primary purpose the rehabilitation and training of a patient to return to the community as a contributing member of society at his highest capacity. The aims and objectives of this program include the opportunity to learn new skills or to relearn factory-type piecework and the opportunity for practice in adjusting to realistic job situations prior to returning to the community. The money earned, in addition to providing a motivating factor, also affords the individual initial security upon his release from the hospital.

"Evaluation of the patient in this realistic work setting can be made as to his use of money, his productive ability and his relationships with others in the shop. This evaluation provides valuable information for the medical staff and social service."

Since compensated work therapy appears to have so many advantages, if paying a particular patient is inadvisable at a particular time, it may be best to place his compensation in a special reserve account. He need not even be informed of this payment until he can benefit from the knowledge.

Compensated work therapy may give rise to pressures on other parts of an industrial therapy program. For example, patients who are not paid may complain, or hospital personnel may resent allotment of part of the hospital budget to paying patients. The positive contributions of compensated work therapy to the overall treatment goals of the institution should be weighed against any unfavorable impact it may have. Moreover, if compensated work therapy is viewed as a means to the end of patient recovery rather than as an end in itself, it will be easier to justify *not* compensating a particular patient when this is best for him.

There is, finally, yet another trend. This chapter has not stressed industrial therapy programs for nonpsychiatric chronic diseases, for emotionally disturbed adolescents, for geriatric patients, or for physical disability. A specialty parallel to industrial therapy has developed in these areas, primarily under the aegis of occupational therapy. See, for example, Jones and Kandel.[29] Workers in these areas have evolved traditions relatively independently of those that have evolved in the psychiatric area, despite the fact that the profession of occupational therapy has members in both areas. Recently, however, occupational therapy has been restructuring its internal professional organization so as to bring these parallel endeavors together.

It is not clear, however, that psychiatric industrial therapy should be administered by occupational therapists; this is presently a moot point. The administrative format of industrial therapy should depend on the availability of professional personnel qualified for this important task. Few workers in related professions such as occupational therapy, manual arts therapy, or educational therapy presently have the specialized training or experience in clinical vocational assignment that seems requisite for administering an industrial therapy program at a professional level. It does not seem likely that the education of individuals for specialties that border on industrial therapy will be modified to provide the necessary specialized training. Therefore, it seems best that industrial therapy programs be administered by industrial therapists. *i.e.*, by professional specialists trained for this kind of work. It is abundantly clear that this is professional level work and that training to perform it adequately is a sufficiently complex educational task that it ought not be superimposed on other professional training programs. On the other hand, the experience that many occupational therapists have had with work programing for nonpsychiatric patients suggests that the formal title of occupational therapist may be the most suitable one for industrial therapists and that industrial therapy may best be regarded as an unusually specialized specialty within occupational therapy. Regardless of the administrative format of industrial therapy, however, it can and does provide its own unique program element in the activity-therapy spectrum.

An excellent bibliography appears in Appendix E on Industrial Therapy.

REFERENCES

1. Joint Commission on Mental Illness and Health: *Action For Mental Health.* New York, Basic Books, 1961.
2. Landy, D., and Raulet, H.: The hospital work program. In *Rehabilitation of the Mentally Ill.* Greenblatt, M. and Simon, B. (eds.) Washington, AAAS, 1959, p. 71-87.
3. Pinel, P.: *A Treatise on Insanity.* London, Cadell and Davis, 1806. (Facsimile ed: New York, Hafner, 1962.)
4. Wittkower, Ed., and Azima, H.: Dynamic aspects and occupational therapy. In *Rehabilitation of the Mentally Ill.* Greenblatt, M., and Simon, B. (eds.) Washington, AAAS, 1959, p. 103-111.
5. Kaufmann, P., and Sewall, L. G.: Hospital industrics: Honest therapy or slave labor? In program guide; Physical Medicine and Rehabilitation; G-2; M-2, Part VIII. Washington, Department Medicine and Surgery; Office of the Chief Medical Director, VA, 1955, p. 21-23.
6. Bartlett, F. L.: Institutional peonage: our exploitation of mental patients. *Atlantic Monthly, 214* (1) :116-119, 1964.
7. Bryan, W. A.: *Administrative Psychiatry.* New York, Pageant Book Company, 1936.
8. Olshansky, S., and Unterberger, H.: The meaning of work and its implications for the ex-mental hospital patient. *Ment. Hyg., 47:*139-149, 1963.
9. Carstairs, G. M., Clark, D. H., and O'Connor, N.: Occupational treatment of chronic psychotics. *Lancet, 269:*1025-1030, 1955.
10. Olshansky, S., and Unterberger, H., *op cit.*
11. Brown, J. A. C.: *The Social Psychology Of Industry.* Baltimore, Penguin Books, 1958.
12. Gurin, G., Veroff, J., and Field, S.: *Americans View Their Mental Health.* New York, Basic Books, 1960.
13. Bartlett, F. L., *op. cit.*
14. Kaufmann, P. and Sewall, L. G., *op cit.*
15. Baur, A. K.: Hospital vocational rehabilitation. *Ment. Hosp., 12* (8) :9-10, 1961.

16. Baganz, C. N., Namen, J. M., Hall, R, and Swickle, J A.: The industrial therapy program at Lyons. In *Program guide; Physical Medicine and Rehabilitation; G-2; M-2, Part VIII*, Washington, Department Medicine and Surgery; Office of the Chief Medical Director, VA, 1955, p. 3-8.

17. Ivany, E., and Rothschild, D.: Relationship of the occupational therapy department to hospital industries. *Amer. J. Occupational Ther.*, 5:16, 1961.

18. Willard, H. S., and Spackman, C. S.: *Occupational Therapy*. Philadelphia, Lippincott, 1947.

19. *Dictionary of Occupational Titles*. Part IV. Entry Occupational Classification. (Rev. Ed.) Washington, U. S. Government Printing Office, 1944.

20. Martinson, M. C.: General considerations basic to a work experience program. Educational Rep., 1961, p. 2.

21. Merker, F. F., Vehlow, E. L., and Nelson, A. V.: Patient treatment possibilities of industrial therapy at Winter VA Hospital. In *Program guide; Physical Medicine and Rehabilitation; G-2, Part VIII*. Washington, Department Medicine and Surgery; Office of the Chief Medical Director, VA, 1955, p. 12-15.

22. Denber, H. C. B., and Rajotte, P.: Problems and theoretical considerations of work therapy for psychiatric patients. *Canad. Psychiat. A. J.*, 7:25-33, 1962.

23. Stem, M. A.: Springfield State Hospital's Program for Community Employment. *Psychiatry Study and Project*. Mental Hospital Service, American Psychiatric Association, 1963, 1 (1). Washington, APA, 1953.

24. Gerjuoy, H.: The industrial therapy curriculum. *American Arch. Rehab. Ther.*, 10:25-33, 1962.

25. Durling, D.: State hospitals make a new start in vocational rehabilitation. *Ment. Hyg.*, 44:105-110, 1960.

26. Nagler, B., and Kirkland, M. H.: Institutional work programs-boon or bane? *Amer. J. Ment. Def.*, 66:375-380, 1961.

27. Barton, W. E.: *Administration in Psychiatry*. Springfield, Thomas, 1962, p. 53.

28. McGrath, V., and Burke, B. B.: Compensated work therapy programs in the New York State Department of Mental Hygiene. *Amer. Arch. Rehab. Ther.*, 11: 48-50, 1963.

29. Jones, M., and Kandel, D. Eds.: *Work Adjustment As a Function of Occupational Therapy*. Study Course V. Third Internat. Cong. World Fed. Occup. Therapists. Dubuque, Ia., Brown, 1962.

Chapter VI

BIBLIOTHERAPY AND PATIENT LIBRARIES

LUCILLE K. LEUSCHNER*

THE GROWTH OF HOSPITAL LIBRARY SERVICES

A LIBRARY IS ONE OF THE SERVICES in a hospital which, in addition to medicine and other treatment, aids in the recovery of patients. In the modern concept of medicine, the patient is treated as a whole personality and with that concept in mind, the library as an aid in the rehabilitation of the ill cannot be overemphasized.

The subtle powers inherent in the written and spoken word have been obvious since ancient times. The inscription on the front of the ancient library at Thebes read "Medicine for the Soul." Our next introduction to the use of books in hospitals was in the great hospital at Cairo, built by Calif Al Mansur in 1200, where priests were provided to read the Koran night and day in addition to performing medical and surgical care.

The first knowledge of libraries for the sick in the United States dates back to 1811. At the first meeting of the Corporation of the Massachusetts General Hospital in that year "it was decided that the visiting committee take care that the patients in each ward be supplied with a Bible and other religious books as they deem suitable."[1] In 1823, a gift of $50.00 was donated and books of a religious nature were purchased. A few titles which were judged to be most suitable were: *Afflicted Man's Companion, Art of Contentment, Blair's Sermons, Brown's Remains, Balm of Gilead,* and *Christian Philosophy.* Years later, one of the hospital's physicians, Dr. John C. Warren, established a fund of $1,000 for the "purchase of publications, religious and moral description, to

*The author wishes to acknowledge the secretarial help of Mrs. Rose Davies, Agnews State Hospital, the editorial assistance of Virginia Kline, San Francisco; Ruth Tews, Hospital Librarian, Mayo Clinic, Rochester, Minnesota; and Mildred Moody, Librarian of Glenn Lake State Sanatorium, Minnetonka, Minnesota.

be given to the patients while in the hospital and upon leaving." When the committee submitted a report describing the manner in which books had been circulated, it "emphasized the advantage the institution might receive from a well sustained library" and suggested that the reading not be restricted to books on moral and religious themes and "would recommend an annual appropriation of $50.00 for the purchase of amusing and interesting books."[2]

During the same period, hospital libraries had their start in England. The Chaplain suggested a library in the Worchester Royal Infirmary. The committee contended that the circulation of Bibles among the patients was sufficient. The Bishop was in accord with the Chaplain's recommendation, so the library was started.[2] However, it is to religious endeavor that we owe the first institution of patient's libraries all over the world, which Walton McDaniel[2] states "is founded on the principle that reading can make us better men." By 1904, Massachusetts General Hospital was providing regular book service to bed patients. By 1910, a cart for carrying large numbers of books was in use. It was the forerunner of hospital carts used today, small enough to pass between cots and low enough for patients to see the books. Also in 1904, McLean Hospital, a private hospital for mental patients in Waverly, Massachusetts, came under the administration of the Massachusetts General Hospital and was first to insist on the value of a carefully selected library with a trained librarian for its patients. Dr. McDaniel[2] states that psychiatry may have recognized the natural affinity existing between bibliotherapy and psychiatry. The principles formulated by the first library for the mentally ill are the principles which are in effect today. "First, an organized central library, as charming and homelike as it can be made; second, a librarian with personality, knowledge of books and library technique; third, an annual appropriation sufficient for the purchase of new books as they are published; fourth, the exclusion of morbid, gruesome and unwholesome literature."[3]

At about the same time, Miss Alice Tyler of the Iowa Library Commission visited one of the state hospitals for the insane in that state and was appalled by the hopeless, aimless way in which the patients just "sat around" with nothing to occupy their minds. She was responsible for having books issued by the state library to institutions, but discovered that books alone are useless unless there is an intelligent and experienced person to guide the collection so she interested the legislature to authorize appointment of an institution library supervisor. Vermont, Minnesota, Nebraska, Indiana, and one or two other states quickly followed Iowa's lead, some of them operating through the state board of control and some through the library commission.[3]

During World War I, libraries were established in large Army and Navy Hospitals by the American Library Association. Hospital libraries as we know them today had their beginnings in World War I. The librarians report that "Zane Grey and Harold Bell Wright were the favorite authors."

"When men became convalescent they became interested in navigation, machine guns, aviation engines, and automobile trucks, but were interested in nothing between the two extremes."[3] It is interesting to note one difference in reading tastes of those wounded in battle, brought home to convalesce. "The merry, light-hearted boys who were sent overseas returned men."[3] More than ever they called for books. Adventure and romance were chosen to erase the memory of battle and pain, then books on every trade and profession so as to prepare them to make a living in a changed world. They also wanted inspirational and educational books.

In November, 1919, the American Library Association gave up its work with the Army and the Navy, turning over to them all libraries, books and personnel in those departments. It continued its service in the U. S. Public Health Service hospitals for disabled soldiers. In the spring of 1921, Congress appropriated $100,000 for the purchase of books and magazines. When the U. S. Veterans assumed the care of the disabled soldiers, the libraries were taken over by that organization. To the present day, the Veterans Hospitals provide excellent libraries for the sick and disabled veterans of foreign wars.

Remembering what organized libraries, selected books, and bedside service meant to wounded and ill service men, the librarian in Sioux City, Iowa, started the first library service in civilian hospitals. This is known as the "group" plan whereby the hospital and public library combine and furnish books to patients as opposed to the "unit" plan, the term applied to libraries in hospitals where the librarian is attached to the staff and both general and medical libraries are maintained and supported from hospital funds.

During the Twenties and the Thirties, the hospital library movement gained momentum. World War II saw the rapid mobilization of library facilities and libraries. Librarians from all over the United States were called to serve in libraries, including hospital libraries, for all branches of military service. In order to give the quickest and best service to the wounded service men, technical processing was simplified and streamlined.

Organization of hospital libraries within the American Library Association occurred in 1944. A study on goals and the means of achieving good service in hospital libraries was a joint project of the American Library Association, the Medical Library Association and the Special Libraries Association. This resulted, in 1952, in the definition of objectives and standards of hospital libraries "which was approved by the library, medical and hospital association."[4] These standards present a working basis for, and the minimal requirements of, good library service in medical, nursing school and patient's libraries."[5] Since the adoption of the standards, "the status of the hospital librarian is equivalent of heads of other departments and the value of libraries is more firmly established."[5]

Many institutional libraries have a long road to travel to reach these standards, both in holdings and in the number of personnel employed.

The objective of the patients' library, as stated in Objectives and Standards of Hospital Libraries is to furnish reading material for all patients, for the purpose of contributing to their recovery and welfare.* This would necessitate an adequate budget to furnish books of all types with good print to all patients, and adequate personnel to administer library services. According to studies of the joint committee of standards, one professional librarian and one clerical assistant are needed for a 300 bed hospital, a

---

*The Objectives and Standards of Hospital Libraries are currently being revised by a joint committee of the ALA, MLA, and SLA with the addition of the Catholic Library Association.

minimum of two to five professional librarians is required in hospitals where more than 500 beds are serviced.[4]

At the 1958 workshop for institutional librarians, conducted by the Library Extension Division of the New York State Library, University of the State of New York, it was concluded that the minimum number of people needed to staff Institution Hospital Libraries of 2,500 is as follows:[6]

> If patient, medical and nursing schools are integrated:
>> 1 librarian (trained and experienced).
>> 1 full-time assistant librarian.
>> 1 clerk-typist.
>> 1 technical aide (to oversee book collections deposited in various parts of the hospital; to help with book cart, etc. [a college graduate is desirable]).
>
> If medical, nursing school and patients' libraries are separated and in various parts of the institution:
>> 1 librarian (trained).
>> 1 full-time assistant librarian.
>> 2 full time clerks (at least one clerk-typist).
>> 2 technical aides (college graduates).
>
> For the 5,000 patient population hospital (integrated):
>> 1 head librarian.
>> 1 assistant.
>> 3 clerks.
>> 2 library aides with a college degree.
>
> The patients' library staff at the Mayo clinic consists of:
>> 1 head librarian (trained and experienced).
>> 1 assistant librarian.
>> 2 library assistants.
>>> Clerical and page help.

In many hospitals having several thousand patients, only one librarian is provided to administer the medical library as well as the patient's library. Only inadequate service can result from this. Even if good library programs are inaugurated, only a small percentage of patients needing this type of library program can be accommodated.

Bibliotherapy

It is acknowledged that the sick man's mind is affected during illness and that reading alleviates anxiety and worry. That the value of bibliotherapy in the treatment of the ill, the neurotic, and the psychotic has impressed many non-medical authors is evidenced by the fact that 84 per cent of the literature on bibliotherapy has been written by non-medical people and 62 per cent of the items published has appeared in non-library journals. Bibliotherapy has also been used in the treatment of emotionally disturbed children. T. V. Moore,[7] of the Catholic University, Washington, D. C., has used books to help children reconstruct their thinking, books which touched upon the children's specific problems and illustrated conduct that they might absorb or be guided by in their own behavior. Moore's use of bibliotherapy is based on the fact that the mind stores ideals and principles which may be a force in influencing conduct.

Constructive reading programs are conducted with successful results for delinquent children and for children needing guidance.[8] That books console the bereaved and impart strength to face reality is indicated in a thesis, *Bibliotherapy for Orthonasia: Books for the Bereaved*, by Florence Grannis.[9]

The term "bibliotherapy," which is used to describe hospital library service, was coined in 1919. Reverend Samuel McChord Crothers[10] is credited with the first use of the term in an article describing the "Bibliopathic Institute" of his friend Bagster.[10] In case histories, Bagster stated that he prescribed reading of the Congressional Record. Bagster stated,[10] "Bibliotherapy is such a new science that it is no wonder that there are so many erroneous opinions as to the actual effect which any particular book may have." The word appeared in print again in an article by G. O. Ireland in the periodical, *Modern Hospital*.

Drs. Will and Karl Menninger began using what was called "bibliotherapy" with their patients many years ago. Dr. Will presented a paper on the subject before the American Psychiatric Association in 1937.

Bibliotherapy has as many variations of meaning as there are people who use the term. Even librarians disagree in the concepts. Dr. Jerome Schneck,[11] formerly with the Menninger Clinic, says it "may be defined as the use of books, and other reading material, in the treatment of patients." Kenneth Appel[12] defines bibliotherapy as the "use of books, articles, pamphlets, as adjuvants in psychiatric treatment." Alice I Bryan,[13] of the Columbia University School of Library Science, a pioneer in the study of bibliotherapy, states "the field of bibliotherapy might — be defined as the prescription of reading materials which will help to develop emotional maturity and nourish and sustain mental health."

Dr. Bryan[14] states in her article on the psychology of the reader "I see no reason why bibliotherapy, as a technique of guidance, should not be extended scientifically to include types of literature other than that specifically related to mental hygiene. Why should not novels, poetry, plays, works on philosophy and ethics, religion, art history, and science be placed in readers' hands for the specific purpose of helping them to face their life problems more effectively and to gain greater freedom and happiness in their personal adjustments?"

Dr. Lewis Wolberg,[15] Director, Postgraduate Center for Psychotherapy, Associate Clinical Professor of Psychiatry, New York Medical College, firmly believes that assigned reading by certain patients may help change faulty attitudes and influence poor motivation. They may be helped to understand how personality evolves, why and how adaptation breaks down, and how psychotherapy may help. Advice on handling specific problems may also be obtained from reading. The doctor contends that bibliotherapy is valuable primarily for individuals who are not yet motivated for psychotherapy and need more information about emotional illness before they can recognize its presence in themselves and their need for treatment.

To arrive at a definition understood by all, one of the projects assigned to the Bibliotherapy Committee of the Association of Hospital and Institution Libraries was to "formulate a definition which would be acceptable, valid, and workable."[16]

To accomplish this, questionnaires were distributed to sixty people chosen from hospital librarians, psychiatrists and members of the disciplines active in the field: (1) to determine current thinking of a selected group of individuals who were actively engaged and interested in bibliotherapy and who possessed knowledge of the potential for the use of reading in a therapeutic way; (2) to obtain a consensus of what bibliotherapy is and what it can do, and (3) provide a basis for the formulation of a definition.[16]

A month after the first questionnaire was mailed, the questionnaire was sent to an additional sixty individuals who served as a control group. These names were selected at random from the membership list of the Association of Hospital and Institution Libraries. When the survey was closed some eight months later, in February, 1962, replies had been received from everyone in Group 1 to whom the questionnaire had been mailed, and from 93.3 per cent, from Group 2. Miss Ruth Tews, Chairman of the Committee on Bibliotherapy, prepared the following tables to show results of the survey:

TABLE III

Question 1. Bibliotherapy is any form of library service offered by a librarian to patients.

Answer	Group 1* with comment			Group 2* with comment			Total with comment		
	Total	No.	Per Cent	Total	No.	Per Cent	Total	No.	Per Cent
Yes	14	7	50	20	14	70	34	21	62
No	38	27	71	30	27	90	68	54	79
Total	52	34	65	40	41	82	102*	75	73

*In Group 1, eight, and in Group 2, six did not answer this question.

TABLE IV

Quesion 2. Bibliotherapy is any form of reading for character formation (in hospitals, schools, etc.) .

Answer	Group 1* with comment			Group 2* with comment			Total with comment		
	Total	No.	Per Cent	Total	No.	Per Cent	Total	No.	Per Cent
Yes	17	11	65	19	10	53	36	21	58
No	35	20	57	31	18	58	66	28	58
Total	52	31	60	50	28	56	102*	59	58

*In Group 1, eight and in Group 2, six did not answer.

TABLE V

Question 3. Bibliotherapy is a group reading activity with patients, initiated and conducted by a librarian (or other) not in association with a member of the medical staff.

Answer	Group 1* with comment			Group 2* with comment			Total with comment		
	Total	No.	Per Cent	Total	No.	Per Cent	Total	No.	Per Cent
Yes	22	15	68	21	12	57	43	27	63
No	29	17	59	28	16	57	57	33	58
Total	51	32	63	49	28	57	100*	60	60

*In Group 1, nine, and in Group 2, seven did not answer.

TABLE VI

Question 4. Bibliotherapy is group reading activity with patients, conducted by a librarian in association with a member of the medical staff.

Answer	Group 1* with comment			Group 2* with comment			Total with comment		
	Total	No.	Per Cent	Total	No.	Per Cent	Total	No.	Per Cent
Yes	45	30	67	44	23	52	89	53	60
No	5	3	60	5	3	60	10	6	60
Total	50	33	66	49	26	53	99	59	60

*In Group 1, ten, and in Group 2, seven did not answer.

TABLE VII

Question 5. Bibliotherapy is a request for a specific title or type of reading for a patient by a medical staff member to the librarian, who fills the request and reports back to the physician.

Answer	Group 1* with comment			Group 2* with comment			Total with comment		
	Total	No.	Per Cent	Total	No.	Per Cent	Total	No.	Per Cent
Yes	40	25	63	45	27	60	85	52	61
No	11	10	91	6	4	67	17	14	82
Total	51	35	69	51	31	61	102	66	65

*In Group 1, nine, and in Group 2, five did not answer.

Not all answered all of the questions. Almost all added qualifying comments. To many there was no clean cut "yes" and "no" answer. Miss Tews[16] summarized the survey:

The complexity, intangibility and elusiveness of the subject were mentioned as reasons for the difficulty in answering the questions. The questionnaire was not intended to present an exact definition; the purpose was to elicit responses which might be indicative of the trend in thinking from which a definition could be framed. The committee's conclusion was:

Analysis of the responses was that good library service is beneficial, effective, and valuable in the overall treatment and rehabilitation program of the patient. It cannot be considered bibliotherapy, however, unless it is an adjunctive activity which is planned, guided, and controlled by skilled, trained librarians working in close cooperation and consultation with the medical team which usually included the physician, social worker, occupational therapists, nurse and others. To be considered bibliotherapy, library service must have the specific purpose of furthering or supporting the therapeutic program as it related to the needs and problems of the particular patient.

"Bibliotherapy," explains Miss Tews—if one uses the analysis of the comments and definitions of the questionnaires as a basis, a composite statement can be attempted—is a program of selected activity involving reading materials, planned, conducted and controlled as treatment under the guidance of the physicians for emotional and other problems. It must be administered by a skilled, professionally trained librarian the prescribed purpose and goals. The important and dynamic factors are the relationships which are established, the patient's reactions and responses, and the reporting back to the physicians for interpretation, evaluation and directions in follow-up.

In 1945, Jerome Schneck, M. D.,[17] formerly with the Menninger Clinic, pointed out that "rarely is one person sufficiently well-versed in general literature and experienced in psychiatric work to permit him to bear full responsibility in a program of bibliotherapy. A team of workers is more effective, with a psychiatrist as captain of the team."

The busy librarian, responsible for extending library service to all patients in the hospital, the selection of books, then classifying and cataloging, processing, organizing and conducting discussion groups, training and directing patient assistants and volunteers, and in some instances also processing medical works and supervising personnel in the medical library, would have little opportunity to be a true bibliotherapist. Margaret Hannigan[18] suggests that eventually we may have specialists to practice bibliotherapy with no responsibility for administration of the library.

Training and Qualifications of Bibliotherapist and Hospital Librarians

Preparation for hospital librarianship should include a basic broad academic background with emphasis on the natural sciences, the humanities and social sciences (especially psychology) which will contribute to the breadth of knowledge and understanding which is needed to fulfill his charge as a librarian. Possession of the widest possible acquaintance with all types and kinds of literature suited to all reading levels and as deep a reading knowledge as possible is essential. A reading knowledge of at least one foreign language is required for admission to most library schools.

The first library school was opened at Columbia University in 1887. At the present time, there are thirty-two accredited library schools offering courses in librarianship on the graduate level leading to a master's degree and, in a few cases, to a Ph. D.

Until the 1930's, admission to the school of librarianship was granted in the senior year of college and the library science and B.A. degrees were combined, if the applicant had a scholastic average of B— or better. Only three years of an academic background were required, with one year of specialization. However, educators and librarians themselves became cognizant of the fact that a broader liberal arts education is essential in the broad field of librarianship so graduation from an accredited college or university became the minimum requirement for admission to an accredited library school. Prior to 1948, the library student who was a college graduate received an additional bachelor's degree for a fifth year in the professional school. Beginning in 1948, several library schools modified programs to provide for a master's degree after the fifth year of college work with the last year being at the graduate level.

Courses in library science are offered in almost 600 colleges and universities primarily in training for school librarianship, but these courses are considered as inadequate preparation for employment in any other type of library.

Basic courses offered in accredited library schools present a knowledge and methods common to libraries of all types. Between thirty and thirty-six semester hours of approved courses are required for graduation with an MLS degree.

The required basic courses are: Administration of Libraries; History of Books and Libraries; Reference; Books and Materials Selection; Classification and Cataloging. Elective courses which would be beneficial for the hospital librarian are: Audio-visual Materials in Libraries; Children's Literature; Story-telling; Selection of Books for Young Adults; Library Methods with Young Adults (methods of guiding and stimulating the reading of young adults would be most important to help guide the youth in their reading habits); Literature of the Humanities; Literature of the Social Sciences; Library in the Community. The latter course, which is offered by some library schools, emphasizes the public library as a basic adult education institution and offers methods of working with individuals and groups. This course would prepare the new librarian for working with groups of people in a setting which is just as appropriate in a hospital library as in any other as it helps pave the way for patients to participate in adult education classes in the community.

At the present time, specialized training in hospital library work, especially with patients, is offered at Western Reserve, in Cleveland, Ohio. The course in hospital library work which includes organizations and techniques which apply to different types of hospitals, institutions and public library extension services, stressing bibliotherapy and the library's contribution to rehabilitation is offered here.

With the exceptions cited above, there is no specific training for bibliotherapy in the professional library school. In the reading courses in graduate, undergraduate, or library school, there is little emphasis on the effect of reading on the individual.

Miss Margaret Kinney,[19] Chief Librarian, Veterans Administration Hospital, Bronx, New York, States:

> The bibliotherapist is, primarily, a librarian who goes further in the field of reader guidance and becomes a professional specialist.
> "It is necessary that the bibliotherapist have an understanding of the principles of clinical psychology and learn some of

the basic skills of the psychologist, for the bibliotherapist must know both the reader's clinical status and his abilities and interests. It is imperative that the bibliotherapist be able to evaluate the emotional significance of the patient's responses, to relate the reading assignments to the patient's mental and emotional needs and to make valid interpretations of his reactions to reading. Other training should include elementary psychiatry, psychology of the physically handicapped, psychology of reading, techniques of rehabilitation, techniques of diagnosis and counseling, medical and social problems of illness, basic anatomy and physiology, rehabilitation of the aging, principles of motivation and remotivation and the rehabilitation of different kinds of patients as well as the psychology of different kinds of ethnic groups. Courses in the techniques of clinical psychological testing should be included for background knowledge of this field, along with training in the interpretation of test results. Training is needed in report writing and group dynamics."

The librarian must, in addition to training, possess understanding and a genuine interest in people, tact and sympathy for others. She must know the psychology of the sick. Good grooming is an asset. The hospital librarian must "shift gears" quickly to meet the varied demands made of her, so a certain flexibility in her nature is a desirable trait.

Duties and Functions of a Librarian in the Hospital Setting

The librarian is responsible for the administration of the library, the proper selection of books, the cataloging and classification and circulation of books to patients in the library, to bed patients, and to those confined to wards; she must be proficient in reader's guidance and reference, and must subtly and gently stimulate interest in the ill person to read. She must have a broad knowledge of books and people and know instinctively what books will appeal to certain classes or types of patients. A librarian works with books and people and must know how to bring the two together. She should try to suit books to the mental and emotional needs of the patients.

If the librarian works with patients who are hospitalized for long periods of time, she should watch for every opportunity to introduce books to people who have not had the opportunity before; to further stimulate and direct reading interests to divert mind and thoughts from themselves to events, people and places outside of themselves with the hope and goal that this new discovery will continue as a lasting source of enjoyment and knowledge to effect a healthy and wholesome attitude toward themselves, relationship with others and life in general.

Bibliotherapy may well be a science of the future which cannot be practical in many libraries because of limitations of staff and training, but the library as an activity is therapy and can be a dynamic factor in the rehabilitation of the physically and mentally ill. One of the major duties would be to be alert to any and all effective means and uses of books in the rehabilitation of patients.

A librarian must conform with rules, regulations, and routines of the hospital and correlate library programs and services with nursing service to enlist interest and assistance of the department.

The librarian must publicize the library to stimulate interest in it by use of bulletin boards, talks, reading lists, book reviews, news items and reviews of new books in the hospital paper, reading and hobby groups; and also conduct story hours where there are pediatric wards, train and supervise patient employees in clerical work and the many housekeeping duties in the library, supervise volunteer workers who may distribute magazines to patients, conduct group discussions, book reviews, or assist in story telling, read to the bed-ridden or geriatric patients or to groups of patients, and operate the record machine on which talking books are played. When possible, the librarian should meet with members of the treatment team to discuss and provide the best therapy for the patient. Attendance at professional library meetings to represent the hospital or institution and to share ideas with others in the field is a stimulus to the librarian to strive to better the situation of the hospital library and librarian and to provide better library service to a greater number of patients.

Administration and Organization

The basic knowledge and techniques required in a public and hospital library are similar, but the division of labor inevitable in a modern public library is a complicating factor which may rob the individual of a chance to survey the whole and to understand his particular duty in relation to the entire operation. Very few comprehend the scope of a special or hospital library. Any small library is a general library extending over a smaller area. It has the same multiplicity of tasks, often requiring one person to cover several specialized areas. The book selection, ordering, cataloging and classification, reference, supervision of employees or patient assistants, supervision of library discussion groups, ward programs, book-cart service to wards, is done by one person.

If the hospital has a medical and nurses' library or both, all the library service should be combined under one supervisor. A trained librarian can handle the work of the three divisions. As the library grows, more assistants are needed.

In some instances, a library committee is appointed to meet occasionally with the librarian to discuss problems and ideas, and to help correlate the work of the library with the activities of the hospital. The members should be the hospital administrator or his representative, a physician, a nurse, and a member of the activity therapy. The librarian should set up policies.

Collection. The number of volumes in a general hospital library is in relation to the size and type of hospital. A minimum of eight books per patient should be purchased, if a hospital contains 500 beds or less. If a hospital is larger, fewer books per patient are necessary. In a 1,500 bed hospital, or over, the minimum of books should be four books per patient. In special hospitals, such as orthopedic, children's and 200-400 bed mental, at least 25 per cent more would be needed, and a larger mental hospital would need fewer.

Budget. An annual budget should be allocated for books, salaries of library staff, library materials, supplies and equipment. Funds should be provided for a turn-over of one fifth of the book collection annually. The budget should be flexible for future expansion. It may be supplemented by various means; volunteer groups may donate funds or books; special funds and proceeds from canteens might be available.

If the hospital operates under the group system, where the public library provides library services to the hospital, the public library may pay the salary and furnish the book collection; the hospital provides a room for books and one book cart. In some instances, the hospital contributes to the book budget.

The Library Room. The library should be housed in a pleasant room which is conducive to reading and browsing. It should be cheerful, attractively furnished and conveniently located for patients so it will be easily accessible to them. There should be ramps for wheel chair patients.

Colorful draperies and plants make it cheerful. Pictures, ceramic articles and other forms of art work, products of the patients in the occupational therapy clinic, add interest. The furnishings should be planned for comfort and relaxation, with arm chairs, reading tables and lamps. Good lighting is a necessity. The book cases should be preferably, four to five feet tall, with open, adjustable shelves. Here is one place in the hospital where a patient can find a retreat from his ward, recapture moments of pleasant reading of his daily newspaper or favorite magazine, as at home, without the distraction of television or the chatter of his ward mates.

The library should be equipped with a charging desk and chair, card catalogue, typewriter, bulletin board, magazine racks, newspaper racks, book trucks and library carts, and tables where books can be sorted and prepared for delivery to the wards. A workroom for the librarian's use in processing books and a space for book repairing should be separate from the library, if possible.

Selection of Books. One of the most important duties of the librarian is the selection of books. Since the people in the hospital represent a cross section of a community, books appealing to various social, educational and religious backgrounds should have a place in the hospital library. Discrimination, not censorship, should prevail. Some authorities are of the opinion that depressing books, those containing suicides, or those derogatory to the nursing and medical profession should be eliminated from the collection of any hospital. Others contend that books for mental patients should not be restricted.

The librarian, by careful selection of books, can correct and eliminate dangerous mental attitudes and create good ones by a judicious prescription of books. The right book at the right time can help a patient regain confidence and self-reliance.

That the printed word has great impact on the well mind, as well as on the sick mind, was evidenced by the fear which Rachel Carson's book, *Silent Spring,* instilled. Further evidence is presented in Robert Down's book, *Books Which Changed The World.* How many teen-agers, a generation or two ago, inspired by Gene Stratton-Porter's books became interested in moths and butterflies? A great naturalist and authority on moths and butterflies says that he first became interested in them after reading *Freckles* and *Girl of the Limberlost.*

It should be the goal of hospital librarians to purchase the best books on any given subject. Several excellent aids are available which are invaluable in helping determine library acquisitions. One such aid is the *Booklist,* published by the American Library Association. The books are reviewed and selected by librarians. A number of titles are suggested, especially for the small public library. *The Library Journal,* published by R. R. Bowker, is also a bi-monthly publication which estimates books, and is invaluable for its comments. General book review journals are the *New York Times, New York Herald Tribune Book Review Sections,* and *Saturday Review.* The bibliography, *One Thousand Books for Hospital Libraries,*[20] by Perrie Jones is very helpful. The *Fiction Catalog* and the *Standard Catalog of Books for the Public Library,* published by H. W. Wilson Co., are also useful for the selection of adult books. *ALA Booklist, Horn Book,* and Fenner's *Proof of the Pudding,* and the *Children's Catalog,* are useful aids in the selection of books for children. Factors to be considered also are the size and weight of book, the print and illustrations, especially in regard to children's books and the post-operative and geriatric patient.

The *AHIL Quarterly,* published by the Association of Hospital and Institution Libraries, frequently includes bibliographies.

Patients sometimes have an additional problem with which to cope such as blindness, deafness, or a language barrier. In some states, there are teachers for the blind, employed by the state to teach braille to the blind throughout a given county, with whom arrangements might be made to teach braille to the patients. You may write to Library of Congress, Division for the Blind, Washington, D. C. 20540, for information about service to the blind and for the address of one of the thirty-one regional libraries which will supply your hospital with materials for the blind. The regional libraries will provide you, upon request, with catalogs of braille titles and a mimeographed list of talking books available. Selections may be made from this list. Books in braille and on records are also available for children from the age of five up and consist of old favorites as well as new titles.

Deafmutes and those patients unable to speak English are doubly handicapped by not being able to communicate with patients or staff. A book on sign language is helpful to the patients and to friends who have the desire to learn the language in order to converse with the deaf patient. Collections of foreign books are usually obtainable from state libraries to supplement those in the hospital library to furnish reading for those patients with a language barrier.[22] Inability to communicate sometimes aggravates the mental condition of patients and books may be their only solace. If the patient has not had the opportunity to learn the English language, the librarian may be able to furnish him with an English book for the foreign born or a picture book so that he may learn enough English to enable him to communicate.

Reserve Books and Inter-library Loans. In the library possesses a book which is in circulation at the time a patient requests it, it may be reserved for the patron and he is then notified when the book is returned to the library. When a patient or staff member requests a book which the library does not possess, the librarian usually makes an effort to borrow it from a local or state library. The only exception to this would be in the event the patient is too ill to accept the responsibility of a book which belongs to another library. The librarian would then suggest a substitute for the one originally requested. If possible, the librarian would attempt to procure what the patient wants so his feeling of isolation which he may have while in the hospital is not intensified, and to convey the idea to him that his library is statewide.

Book Orders. Orders for books may be placed with a local vendor. Placing your order with the same dealer will result in a larger discount. To extend the budget, good used books may be purchased at a sizable discount from lending library companies. All types of books are offered, but careful perusal of your tools for book selection will aid you in selecting the best of the titles offered. Paperback books are useful for additional copies of a recommended title. They can be made more durable by using the plastic covers made especially for paperback books.

Procedure. All routine duties should be simplified. A simple system of cataloging and classification is recommended. Assistance in assigning Dewey decimal class numbers may be found in the aids to book selection, which classify every recommended title. An author, subject, and title card, and a shelf list card should be sufficient. The catalogue must be uniform, consistent and accurate.

Catalogue cards may be purchased from the H. W. Wilson Co., or from the Library of Congress.* If the budget will permit, a cataloging service[+] would be recommended.

Plastic covers on the books are recommended. The collection should look new and clean to appeal to readers.

Gift books are usually accepted on condition that they may be disposed of if they do not meet standards or if they are not in good condition. Arrangements might be made with a used book dealer to exchange such gift books for good used editions of recommended titles. Weeding the collection should be done regularly. Old, worn books should be removed from the shelves.

Current periodicals are greatly in demand. About 10 per cent of the budget may be used for magazine subscriptions. The local post office may donate undelivered magazines which may be distributed to the wards.

---

*Catalogue cards may be purchased from: (1) H. W. Wilson Co., 950 University Avenue, New York 52, New York, or (2) Library of Congress cards to be ordered from Card Division, Library of Congress, Building 159, Navy Yard Annex, Washington, D. C. 20541.

[+]At additional cost, these companies will provide processing and cataloging service for books purchased from them. (1) Alanar Book Processing Center (a subsidiary of Bro-Dart industries), Box 921, Williamsport, Pennsylvania, and (2) Alesco, Harristown Road, Glen Rock, New Jersey.

The Library as Industrial Therapy. Patients may be assigned to assist in the library. It may help them to renew their skills, relearn responsibility, redevelop self reliance, build self confidence and ready them for the routine in work outside the hospital. In hospitals where there are industrial therapists, a patient is assigned to work by the therapist for the mutual benefit of the patient and the job to which he is assigned. In other hospitals, the doctor or ward personnel can assist in selecting the right person. Filing, dusting, shelving, reading shelves, sorting magazines, mending, charging and discharging books, arranging displays, typing catalog cards, doing secretarial work, and writing overdue notices may be very therapeutic. Some may become adept at reader's advisory service in helping other hospitalized patrons in the selection of books. The *Fiction Catalog* (Published by H. W. Wilson Co.) as well as the card catalog may be helpful as a guide in finding stories written in a certain period of history or on a certain subject. Such an assignment would instill in a patient the confidence to communicate with other individuals.

Schedules. It is desirable to keep the library open during the day when the patients are free to use it. Regular hours should be established. Where there is sufficient staff, ward visits are recommended at least once a week. Arrangements should be made with ward personnel to establish a convenient time for cart service to a particular ward. Ward meetings and other ward activities must be considered in making schedules.

Patients are encouraged to attend library group activities if permission is granted by the doctor and if the patient's schedule is correlated with his other therapy assignments. If a choice must be made, the doctor's decision is based on which activity is most therapeutic for the patient involved.

Books are charged out for the specificd loan period and may be renewed. There is no charge for overdue books.

Records. Daily circulation records are kept as well as record of attendance in the library. Records of reference questions are helpful. A simple charging system is most feasible. The patient's name and ward number are written on the book card. Records of a patient's reading and his participation in library programs should be kept whenever possible.

The Patient and His Reading. Miss Tews[5] points out:

A library program for the patients, has a threefold purpose: (1) recreational—to provide a pastime and relaxation, a change of activity, and a source of gratification for the patient; (2) educational—as a means of acquiring new interests and information of the world about him, so furthering and maintaining his contact with reality, and (3) inspirational and therapeutic—to contribute to the well-being of the patient, through the elevation of his morale and assistance in identifying himself with the social group, to instill confidence in himself and to encourage him once more to concentrate.

The librarian should be perceptive in recommending books which will meet the patient's mental and emotional needs. A depressed person may need a book which will serve as a tonic, whereas an anxious or overactive person may need one to sedate him.

The right book for the hospitalized person would depend on the type of hospital, the kind of patient and the difficulties involved. Whether the hospital cares for the acutely or chronically ill, young patients with long term illnesses, or geriatric patients, medical or surgical cases, would be a factor in determining the kind of bibliotherapy to be offered. The physician and nursing staff tend to the physical needs of the patient, but his psychological needs must be considered also. Books for the hospitalized person should be informative, inspirational, comforting or amusing to alleviate anxiety as to the effect of his illness or to allay apprehension caused by impending surgery. Even the well person fraught by the pressures of his work, or with anger, may forget his feelings in the reading of a mystery story. In identifying with the characters, he sublimates his feelings and his emotions are released. In so doing, he derives enjoyment and satisfaction. Reading is therapy when it provides emotional balance.

Every hospital patient afflicted with a physical ailment is beset with some anxiety. His emotional state can aggravate the physical disorder. Bibliotherapy can make it easier to endure his sojourn in the hospital.

Each person reacts differently to illness and hospitalization. One patient may dread the separation from his family and be anxious about children or other members of the family at home who are normally dependent on the hospitalized patient. Anxiety for another may be based on fear of death or a lingering convalescence. Other patients may worry needlessly over a trivial illness and so magnify his symptoms to the extent that his emotional state could complicate his illness. On the other hand, some patients may regard their hospitalization as a rest or a welcome change from the daily routine and enjoy the attention received.

For books to be therapeutic, every patient must be treated as an individual patient, as each patient's needs are different from any other patient. In the selection of books for the individual patient, the education, age, sex, social, ethnic and religious background, the seriousness of the illness, intelligence and personality, must be considered. An illness often changes personality functioning. The librarian may need the help of the medical staff in providing this information to guide her in the recommendation of appropriate books. The patient should be provided with the books he wishes to read, from within the collection.

Light reading appeals to most patients, even those who, in good health, may read books with more depth. Those hospitalized with an acute illness, whose recuperation is short may be content with reading the newspapers or current magazines. Romantic novels, westerns, mysteries, adventure, travel, or biographies may bring contentment and distraction from his current setting and to help relieve the boredom. A person soon to undergo surgery may be distracted by a mystery, a humorous book or even a book of cartoons. One of the many pictorial books would be an excellent choice.

Hospitalization may mean a different way of life for many patients. The heart patient, previously active, must now curtail his activities; a paraplegic, as a result of an accident, may have to make radical adjustments. Illness may mean a change of career for some. A child injured in an accident or operated on for heart surgery may not be able to romp and play as he formerly did; an older person may realize that he cannot return to normal living; a neuro-psychiatric patient may be so confused that he cannot approach life realistically. Bibliotherapy for those people may help them in adjusting to their new way of life. Books about people who have overcome handicaps can be a source of inspiration to others so afflicted. Many patients ask for books about their specific illness to understand their illness and how to learn to live with it. These books are not carried on the book cart, but may be available in the library. They are loaned to patients upon consent of the doctor.

Mental patients, obtaining ground privileges for the first time, head for the bibliotherapy or "self-help shelf" which includes books on general psychology, mental hygiene, personality problems, marriage, sex, care of children; problems of teen-agers; problems of the senior citizen; and the problems confronting the one-parent family. These books, written for the lay person, help one to gain insight into his illness.

Care should be taken in the recommendation of certain types of literature to certain types of patients. It would be imprudent to suggest a highly exciting book for a heart patient or one with a history of high blood pressure. Morbid books or those containing suicide, or those critical of the medical profession should be eliminated. A busy housewife may look forward to hospitalization as an opportunity to catch up on reading. She may select Michener's *Hawaii;* perhaps a classic or a current best-seller. However, the sensational best-sellers would not be prescribed.

In the case of mental patients, paranoids tend to read themselves into literature, so a work of an impersonal nature, or one concerning obstacles that have been overcome, would be suggested. A schizophrenic patient living in a world of fantasy should be offered a book of non-fiction to help him face reality.

Religious or inspirational reading may be of solace to some. Man is affected by physical, spiritual, mental and social factors and in illness the whole man must be treated. Books of a spiritual nature within the realm of the patient's belief, by recognized authors, would be a definite contribution to his well being. In recognition of the fact that the religious belief of a patient affects his treatment and cure, the American Medical Association has established a new committee on medicine and religion to bring about the closer relationship between the physician and clergy for the benefit of the patient. From this, it would naturally follow that books of a spiritual nature would be recognized as therapeutic. However, reading of the Bible and other religious material would not be recommended for the psychotic patient. Bible reading often is a symptom of a patient's mental state. The patient's doctor should be consulted before a religious work would be given to a mental patient.

A person with a long convalescence often prefers more serious reading. In many instances, a patient confined to a hospital for a long period of time, will pursue one subject until he has satisfied his need to learn all he can of the subject. A long-range reading program can be guided by the librarian. Books to aid in rehabilitation, and vocational books are in demand and the library should be prepared to meet the demands of people who may be exploring the possibility of changing vocations or need to renew skills lost through illness. Hobby books would encourage a new interest for the adult or child who may be confined to a hospital for a long time. The subject matter may be of interest, but the books on the cart must be attractive and colorful to appeal to the patient.

Illness may interfere with concentration. For those people and particularly mental patients who find difficulty in reading or whose interest span is short, the excellent books now written for young adults, including the Newberry Award books, well written and with a high interest level, have proven to be a fine introduction of books to the adult non-reader, as well as to the young adult.

The library should be prepared to serve people from all walks of life. Patients, as any other library patrons, have diversified interests and books in the library should encompass all subjects. As you recall, the wounded men returning from World War I read books with more depth than those who had not been overseas, and those librarians who had the privilege of working with returned Army and Navy men in World War II also found this to be true. The same is true of a patient with a long convalescence as a result of an injury or physical illness or of a long term neuropsychiatric patient. Books may also open up new horizons for the patient, or he may wish to pursue an interest opened up to him prior to his hospitalization.

Miss Helen Haines[23] in her *Living with Books* states:

"Librarianship is the only calling that devotes itself to bringing books into the common life of the world. The materials librarians work with are materials which furnish the understanding, knowledge and reason that can inform the mind and direct the will to meet the challenge of time."

The resources of a hospital library may aid in the direction of a patient's perspective and interest outside of himself. The purpose of the hospital librarian is to divert the attention from the patient to the world outside.

Patients are hospitalized for much shorter periods of time than previously, but even for a short period, in which time stands still for the hospitalized patients, many changes are taking place outside the hospital. Consider the fact that new knowledge is discovered daily, and that it becomes obsolescent just as quickly.

In these days of continuing education, where the trained person is continually being reeducated to further his development, it is necessary that the librarian make available materials to the patient so he does not return to his community feeling like Rip Van Winkle, which could be detrimental to his feeling of security, and add to his fear and anxiety. The librarian should exert an effort to expose patients to resources of the library especially those who may not have had the opportunity heretofore.

The life of the patient should be enriched by books available in the library. The librarian may be intuitive in combining her knowledge of books and people in recommending the proper book to fit the mood and need of the patient. The books may divert him momentarily; it may awaken a new interest or revive a former interest. If the book disgusts him or upsets him, it should be reported to his psychiatrist if he is a neuro-psychiatric patient, or to his physician if he is a medical or surgical patient. It will enable the doctor to understand the patient's conflicts.

Dr. Allen[24] states "the patient may also gain insight into the vulnerable spots in his personality structure. The background, however, should be considered, as a more sophisticated book can be recommended to those with a broader or more cultural and tolerant background." Principles of reader's advisory service in a public library may well be applied, to a certain extent, in a library for hospitalized people.

Dr. Gerald Lawlor,* psychologist at Agnews State Hospital uses books successfully in therapy with neuro-psychiatric patients. He considers reading a good adjunct to any therapy and one which can be therapeutic in itself. Dr. Lawlor states in a paper he is writing:

> The reading serves to keep alive the urge to change, and stimulates patients with a continuing flow of ideas concerning new ways of looking at themselves and their world and feeds them suggestions about new attitudes and ways of behaving.
>
> A survey of the aims of psychotherapists today indicates that whereas all are interested in producing CHANGES in patients, the type of change stressed varies. Some emphasize producing in the patient a change in his relationship to the world wherein the patient is encouraged to see his world differently and make more adequate adjustive responses toward it. Others put more stress on changing the person's relationship to himself wherein the patient is encouraged to get a different picture of himself and to develop himself to the point where he feels more adequate and more comfortable in living with himself. The distinction here seems to be in terms of an outward versus inward orientation. A third emphasis is now appearing in which the patient is encouraged to break through the outer-inner dichotomy and to experience himself as part of the world as it is at the moment with all its fluidity and changingness.
>
> Reading can serve all of these aims if only the material is sufficiently descriptive and contains enough bridges into varied experential areas to reach not only different types of readers but many experience regions within a single reader. It appears now that means will have to be devised to prepare the reader before he can benefit from the printed word.
>
> Specifically the question is, how can the patient be intellec-

---

*Lawlor, Gerald, Ph.D. Paper in two parts: Part 1, WHAT IS THERAPY: Part 2, HOW READING HELPS. (unpublished paper).

tually and emotionally sensitized so that he can *co-experience with* the fictional or biographic character. To produce contact with the life space of another there must be something within the reader that matches the experiencing in the other. If, at first glance, there appears to be no common elements, bridges may be offered by the author and used by the reader. The bridges are areas of experiencing which have footings in both the experience of the reader an the experiencing of the fictional character. For example, if the author is writing about the love of a girl for her dog, the reader, particularly if he is a city-bred male, may have considerable difficulty reproducing within himself the feelings of the girl as she interacts with her dog. If, however, the author describes the girl's loneliness, . . . (he, too, has felt lonely) , the girl's desire for touching something warm and alive (this he has a longing for), the girl's hunger for affectionate responses (this is part of his yearning) , and the girl's need for assurance that the object of her affection will not reject her (this has been his concern) , our city-bred male reader may find himself entering the world of the girl and her dog and be able to release and partially gratify some of his own uncoordinated and perhaps unacknowledged feelings.

Recently, the prescribed reading for Dr. Lawlor's groups have been Eric Berne's books. *Transactional Analysis in Group Psychotherapy* (Grove, 1961) alerts the patient to watch and get control of himself. This helps in training him to observe his relationship with others. *Games People Play, The Psychology of Human Relationships* (Grove, 1964) help him to identify the "games people play," which Berne states people tend to do either consciously or unconsciously.

Dr. Lore Hirsch[25] also uses books as clues to a patient's problems and considers them important. She writes, "I can almost diagnose the patients from the choice of books which they have at their bedside. The more intellectual neurotics frequently read about personality, inner conflicts, and problems of living, while the more antisocial psychopath are likely to choose books whose gruesome titles appeal to them, such as *The Corpse Comes Home* or *Blood on the Hatchet.*" Dr. Hirsch further states that people need to identify or to find themselves or part of themselves in every piece of art or literature, in order to be able to enjoy and appreciate it—that the individual preference and reaction can be meaningful. Many novels that are discussed and enjoyed by patients, such as *Wasteland* by Joe Sinclair, or *Mine Own Executioner,* by Balchin, are psychiatric case histories in novel form; others are novels with psychiatric implications such as Somerset Maugham's *Of Human Bondage* or *Razor's Edge* or Marquand's *Point of No Return.* Dr. Hirsch believes, like many others, that "one can read a novel and live through the same experience." This, she feels, is therapeutic. However, she feels almost any book, even a book on budgeting, can be therapeutic if read at the right psychological moment and can start an individual on a new road toward a new goal. Dr. Hirsch states that "the therapeutic value of a novel or biography is greater than that of any purposeful educational book."

Patients may want to read books on the "best-sellers" lists and in a review of the book *I Love You Honey, but the Season's Over,* by Clausen, a book about the circus, the reviewer quoted a circus performer who stated that he never indulged in liquor, as performers wish to attain a perfection in their performance which could not be achieved under the influence of liquor. A patient remarked afterward that this had impressed him and had a great effect on his determination to overcome this habit.

Patients may want to read books on the "best-sellers" lists and some of them may be in the patient's library. The selection would be left to the discrimination of the librarian.

It has been observed that a depressed patient does not always want to be "cheered up." He may select a sad book or a rather depressing book so he can identify with the characters. This may bring him out of a depressed mood more quickly than a cheery book. Sometimes, if a book with happier overtones is recommended, the comment will be "but life isn't like that" and the patient will look for one that is more realistic.

The book, *The Lonely Passion of Judith Hearne,* by Brian Moore, was recommended by her psychologist to a patient who had an alcoholic problem. It may not have been therapeutic for every patient, as there was no solution to Judith Hearne's case given in the book, but this particular patient could see a solution and she ceased to feel as sorry for herself after reading the book, because the main character seemed to be much worse off than she was.

Non-fiction as well as fiction should be included for the ward bookshelf in a hospital. Travel and biography are always enjoyable reading. Sometimes a neuropsychiatric patient who is sufficiently ill to need shock treatment may be able to comprehend a book of profound nature. One young woman was delighted with the book *Atlas of World Affairs* by Boyd. After she read it, world news and politics had more meaning to her. To another person, to whom this would have been dull, perhaps only a light novel would appeal. So the collection on the ward should be diversified.

LIBRARY SERVICES

Ward Service

The goal of the hospital library is to provide library service to all patients. Book cart service is available in hospitals where there are ramps and elevators. Open and closed wards should be serviced at least once a week. Where book-cart service is not feasible, rotating collections of books should be placed on the wards and changed regularly by the librarian or by volunteer workers. Even if there is book-cart service, it has been found beneficial to leave a collection of books in the day room so patients who cannot get to the library will have something to read when the mood strikes them. There should always be current magazines available. If the library is too far from hospital proper, small libraries could be set up in small rooms, wherever possible, to offer a large selection of books.

If escort service can be arranged, it is more satisfactory to have the non-ground privileged patients escorted to the library, where they can choose books from the larger collections. It is more to the patients' benefit and a welcome change of environment.

Library Programs

In addition to a library of well-selected books for patients, a dynamic library program to motivate and stimulate interest in the contents of the books is recommended. If a program is to be conducted on a ward, the climate of the ward would determine the type of program which would be most feasible. Even the most regressed patient will respond to a simple program. It is the librarian's duty to prevent "mental starvation" during a patient's enforced residence in a hospital. "Mental starvation" could very well perpetuate mental illness, in permitting the patient to dwell unduly on his problems.

The program is best conducted by a librarian. However, a dedicated volunteer well-versed in books, who would not merely "accept" the patient, but treat him as a person, may do a fine job. The relationship established is important. After arranging the hour and the day with the ward doctor and nursing personnel, the meeting must be held at the regular time each week. The patients will be anticipating the librarian's visit on the day designated.

Anyone conducting a group discussion should greet each patient warmly to create a comfortable atmosphere. A few introductory remarks will prepare the group for what is to follow. Poetry, short stories, and plays may be read, with patients reading the part; or a talking book may be played. A poem may stir the memory of a patient who might chime in with the reader and then recite the poem to the finish. Short stories are excellent to read to those with a short interest span; also selections from the *Readers Digest* or chapters from books in which the characters are the same throughout the book, and there is no continuity of plot—but in which the chapters are episodic.

Talking books may vary the program. The professional voice of the reader commands attention, perhaps, more than an untrained voice. One installment of "talking books" may be played at a meeting and the story may continue for several weeks. Whether the programs consist of reading poetry or prose, or listening to someone else read, it is well to choose material which will evoke discussion. Play reading can furnish fun and stimulation. Role playing has been found to be beneficial. There are many excellent plays from which to choose. To those who read before they were ill, this program would be enjoyable because they are getting a small dosage of what they like and it is a continuation of something they would like to do, but their illness does not permit. To others, it is an introduction to the pleasures of reading. When these people gain ground privileges, they find their way to the library immediately because of their introduction to it by means of the library program. Such a program could pave the way for bibliotherapy. Since many are not readers, they must be motivated to read, and the joys of reading introduced to them before they would read a book prescribed to them.

To send "just anyone" to read to a group on a ward would be helpful to patients by helping them to pass the time, but hardly any benefit would be derived from spasmodic and desultory programs. The person who has the inclination to conduct a program should know by training and experience how to approach the patients and should have an understanding of their needs—just as competent people trained in methods of teaching are employed to teach our children although most adults have mastered grammar school subjects.

In reviewing the "remotivation technique," which was introduced in Philadelphia State Hospital by Dorothy Hoskins Smith, we find the approach very similar to that which librarians would use and have used in ward programs. Mrs. Smith's[23] program is a "technique of simple group-interaction to enable the psychiatric technician to reach his patients in a meaningful and constructive way." To achieve this, Mrs. Smith uses five steps: The first one is "Climate of Acceptance" in which each patient is greeted warmly to create a comfortable atmosphere; the second is "A Bridge to Reality," in which objective poetry is read and the same kind of reaction is evoked as in the library program; the third is "Sharing the World We Live In," in which pictures, plants, magazines or other props are passed around; the fourth is "An Appreciation of the Work of the World," in which the skilled leader guides the discussion into the value of work; and the fifth step is "Climate of Appreciation," at which time the leader expresses his enjoyment of the group and his pleasure that the patients attended the session. Steps three and four would be omitted in the library program but this could be a pattern easily followed by a beginner in reading group programs.

Discussion Groups. Discussion programs scheduled may be on Great Books, an American Library Association sponsored American heritage program, or one of the packaged programs (although the librarian should be alert to ideas for discussions). These may be held in the wards or in the library. They may be moderated by a patient, which is excellent experience and instills confidence. In some instances, a volunteer experienced in the field of adult education or in a specific field of endeavor may act as a moderator or may be a resource person. The participants may attend voluntarily or by referral of the ward doctor. Patients may often express their desire to study or explore specific subjects. During an election year, for example, they may express their need to know about the organization of the party conventions; how the candidates are chosen; how delegates are selected; the workings of the electoral college; or the qualifications of the prospective candidates. After the candidates are chosen, the party platforms may be explored. A moderator may be chosen among members of the group, but no one is an authority. The librarian gathers book and pamphlet material. She may need to supplement material by inter-library loans from the local or state libraries.

Discussion groups are excellent means to stimulate interest in the world outside and to return the patient to reality. The mentally ill tend to magnify the ills of the world and confuse the facts. To discuss the facts as they are substantiated by reliable source material sometimes stills their fears. To be a member of a group instills a feeling of "belonging" and helps to restore their dignity. They also meet people with interests in common. Here again, books have been a means of relating to people.

Adult education is important. "The scope of bibliotherapy includes the aims of the field of adult education and also the skills, knowledge, understanding, appreciation and insight which affect the reader culturally, vocationally, intellectually, and spiritually."[19] The library is the ideal place in which to hold discussion. Source material is readily available when needed.

Book Reviews. The library patron sometimes responds eagerly to suggestions that they share their favorite book or books with others. Others may volunteer to review books. In this way, the library may serve as a proving ground for people who wish experience in expressing themselves.

The audience is introduced to new authors and books. Many senior citizens attend reviews. It is like bringing in a little of the "outside" world into the hospital. It may simulate a weekly afternoon activity they might have attended if they were at home. This mental stimulation could also be a means of preventing or delaying senility. Book reviews and group discussions sometimes have a "carry over" on to the ward where the patients continue to discuss the book reviewed or the topic discussed in the afternoon. An outgrowth of the library programs has been organization of small groups on the wards. This is encouraged for resocialization and to make constructive use of leisure time.

Neuropsychiatric patients usually have a problem of relating to others and participating with others in activities. Book reviews, and discussion groups are a very effective way of getting the patient to "relate to" something and to aid in communication with others.

Audio Visual Aids

Films. Educational and documentary films are a source of enjoyment and education. These films, which embrace every subject, expose the culturally deprived patient to ideas, places and people unknown to him. For the more alert, interested patient, it offers an opportunity to continue to reach out to new horizons. These are used in the library and on the wards not only for pleasure and information in themselves, but as an opening wedge to introduce further reading on certain subjects. The films do inspire some of the viewers sufficiently to incite in them a desire to explore the subject further, which leads to requests for books of that nature. The hospital librarian should make an effort to have books available on subjects introduced by film. Not only travel, history, biography, etc., are popular, but also the "how to" films, such as *Flower Arrangement, How to Set a Table,* and *How to be a Better Hostess,* are met with delight by women patients.

Additional Audio Visual Aids. View masters are inexpensive and enjoyable to look at as well as easy to handle. Children and adults would welcome these to help pass the time. Talking books have been mentioned for the blind, but these have been used successfully also with regressed mental patients, those too physically or mentally ill to want to make the effort to concentrate on reading.

Bulletin boards, posters, and pictures do much to arouse interest in books and reading. One need not spend a great deal of time in making posters, as colorful pictures or book jackets in conspicuous places, used with mittens or plastic letters, are most effective in advertising books. In each issue of the *Wilson Library Bulletin*, are pictures of effective poster displays which can be adapted to any library.

Mechanical aids for those who can read but need help are: automatic page turners, reading tables, prisma glasses, mechanical readers and reading projectors. There are two types of page turners, a small, light one useful for bed patients unable to turn pages which can be adapted to magazines and books of varying size, and another, which is known as the turna-page, is designed principally for respirator use.

Prisma glasses are a boon to the paralyzed and to those with casts. The reading projectors are books on microfilm that can be projected on the ceiling where they can be easily read by bedridden or by a post-operative patient. They can be operated by a push button.

The book stand is available in both a stand model and a clamp model. The stand can be used from either side of a couch, bed or chair and the book holder adjusts to any desired reading angle. It can be used by a patient who must remain flat on his back, by one reading in a reading chair, as a conventional book rest, reader's use with mouth-stick, as an easel, music stand, or podium.

Other Library Activities

Quiz games are fun and stimulating for both children and adult groups. Story hours for the children's wards and reading programs in geriatric patients help while away the hours and give the patients something to which to look forward.

Essay contests have proven to be a stimulus for the longer term patient. National Library Week is generally considered an appropriate time for such a contest. For several months, patients may think about and search for ideas. The Library Week slogans have been thought provoking and can be used as titles. Some may choose to write about a favorite book, character or author, or on what reading has meant to them.

If there are any authors in your community, invite them to a hospital program. For the past several years, Agnews has invited authors from the Bay Area to a "Meet the Authors" program during Library Week. Patients, staff, and authors mingle and chat with each other. Some patients do not have an opportunity to participate in community functions so this part of the community is brought into the hospital. This is a rewarding experience for all concerned. Prizes for essays are awarded to winners at this program.

Conclusion

Librarians have demonstrated that they are applying their knowledge, training, and skills in the use of reading material to divert the mind of the patient from himself and thus speed the healing process; to instill in him the desire to get well, to stay well, and to maintain his health once he bridges the span from the hospital back into the community.

REFERENCES

1. Washburn, F. A.: *The Massachusetts General Hospital: Its Development, 1900-1935*. Boston, Houghton, 1939.
2. McDaniel, W. D.: Bibliotherapy - Some historical and contemporary aspects. *A. L. A. Bulletin, 50:*584-589.
3. Jones, Edith Kathleen. *The Hospital Library*. A. L. A., 1923.
4. Joint Committee on Standards for Hospital Libraries: *Hospital Libraries: Objectives and Standards*. Chicago, American Library Association, 1953.
5. Tews, Ruth: The patients' library. In *Applied Medical Library Practice*, Keys, T. E., Springfield, Thomas, 1958, pp. 97-134.
6. New York State Library - Library Extension Division: *Proceedings of Workshops for Institution Librarians*. St. Laurence University, Canton, New York, 1957 and 1958. The Division, 1958, p. 48.
7. Moore, T. V.: *The Nature and Treatment of Mental Disorders*. Bibliotherapy, 2nd Ed., New York, Greene, 1951, p. 217-232.
8. Sharp, E. Preston: Philadelphia - team - free library and youth center. *A. L. A. Bulletin, 55:*10-14, 1961.

9. Grannis, Florence Sprague: *Bibliotherapy for Orthonasia: Books for the Bereaved.* University of Southern California, School of Library Science, 1960.
10. Crothers, S. McChord: A literary clinic. *Atlantic Monthly 118:*291-301, 1916.
11. Schneck, Jerome: Bibliotherapy in neuropsychiatry. In *Occupational Therapy: Principles and Practice,* Dunton and Licht: Springfield, Thomas, pp. 197-233.
12. Grannis, Florence: *Bibliotherapy for Orthonasia: Books for the Bereaved.* University of Southern California, School of Library Science, 1960.
13. Bryan, Alice I.: Can there be a science of bibliotherapy? *Library Journal 64:* 773-776, 1939.
14. Bryan, Alice I.: The psychology of the reader. *Library Journal 64:*11, 1939.
15. Wolberg, Lewis: *Techniques of Psychotherapy.* Grune and Stratton, 1954, pp. 578-579.
16. Tews, Ruth M.: The questionnaire on bibliotherapy. *Library Trends, 11:*217-228, 1962.
17. Schneck, Jerome M.: Studies in bibliotherapy in a neuropsychiatric hospital. *Occupational Therapy and Rehabilitation 23:*316-232, 1944.
18. Hannigan, Margaret C.: The librarian in bibliotherapy: pharmacist or bibliotherapist? *Library Trends 11:*184-198, 1962.
19. Kinney, Margaret M.: The bibliotherapy program requirements for training. *Library Trends 11:*127-135, 1962.
20. Jones, Perrie: *One Thousand Books For Hospital Libraries.* Minneapolis, University of Minnesota Press, 1944.
21. Fenner, Phyllis R.: *The Proof of the Pudding: What Children Read.* New York, John Day Company, 1957.
22. Dooley, Kathleen: Library service international style. *Hosp. Prog.,* December, 1958, p. 69-102.
23. Haines, Helen E.: *Living With Books: The Art of Book Selection.* Columbia University Studies in Library Service, No. 2, 2nd ed., New York, Columbia University Press, 1950, p. 10.
24. Allen, E.: Books help neuropsychiatric patients. *Library Journal, 71:*1671-1675, 1946.
25. Hirsh, Lore: How a doctor uses books. *Library Journal, 75:*2046-2049, 1950.
26. Robinson, Alice M.: *Remotivation Technique.* A. P. A. Mental Hospital Service, Smith, Kline and French Foundation, Remotivation Project.

Chapter VII

EDUCATIONAL THERAPY

DARYL B. ADRIAN, M.A.

INTRODUCTION

Educational therapy is only one of the therapeutic disciplines which the physician may prescribe to help treat and rehabilitate the ill or incapacitated person. Not too many years ago, physicians and the various activity therapists seemed to feel that patients could benefit most from such therapeutic activities as arts and crafts, manual arts, recreation, gardening, or special work assignments. It was felt that the patient needed to have something to do with his hands during the time that he was not on the hospital ward or in the physician's office. In some cases, the patient presented unique information about himself and his illness by the manner in which he performed his assigned task with his hands. In other cases, the patient was able to express his delusional feelings of grandeur or extreme emotion, find external release for his pent-up feelings of anger at someone, or keep himself so busy that he at least would not become more involved in his inner world of depression or fantasy.

During the past decade, however, physicians have become aware of the fact that the hospitalized person needs more than treatment or psychotherapy sessions with a physician and work with his hands. The hospitalized patient is not necessarily incapacitated in a way which precludes that no intellectual activity can or should be attempted. Perhaps the fact that outpatients usually were able to carry on their businesses or academic programs at school has contributed to helping the hospital physicians realize that the hospitalized patient need not necessarily refrain from intellectual activity. In fact, some inpatients seemed to become stagnant intellectually if they were not engaged in activities which exercised these faculties. Thus, gradually more hospitals, especially Veterans Administration hospitals and some state hospitals, began to develop educational therapy departments which planned discussion group meetings, special concerts, etc., to engage the intellects of those patients whose earlier lives had required an active intellect in their regular life situations.

Also, during the last ten years, more and more elementary and secondary-age children have needed to be hospitalized. If the hospitalization was not too long, the child lost only a semester or a year in his school program. However, child psychiatrists, physicians, and teachers who were called on to tutor a child who had been hospitalized before the end of the semester, became aware of the acute need for a realistic, accredited school program for these hospitalized elementary and secondary children. Thus many psychiatric children's hospitals have added educational therapy to their activity programs. The addition of educational therapy has been slower, however, in hospitals where patients of all ages are admitted.

DEFINITION OF EDUCATIONAL THERAPY

Educational therapy may be defined as a form of milieu therapy which uses educational materials, methods, and procedures in the medical treatment and rehabilitation of a person. It is a particularly useful form of milieu therapy in the treatment of persons who are confined to a hospital setting as either inpatients or day patients. This is true for both those patients who are college-age or younger and those adult patients who are not interested in any formal, academic courses. If carefully prescribed by the patient's physician and properly carried out by the educational therapy staff, educational therapy may be one of the therapeutic activities which will contribute significantly to the recovery of the patient.

Educational therapy is more than teaching formal classes in a hospital setting, similar to those which the patient may have been attending prior to his hospitalization. On the other hand, whereever possible, the educational therapists should be qualified, certified teachers in the educational fields in which they are "teaching" at the hospital. This is particularly true if an educational therapist is teaching a course for which the patients-students are to receive academic credit. Unfortunately, however, this is not always possible in many hospitals. There simply are not enough certified teachers who are interested and motivated to teach students who are patients in hospitals. Thus certification of the entire educational therapy staff may need to be a goal and not a reality for some time in some hospitals. Nevertheless, a goal toward which to strive it ought to be. As Robert Browning, a 19th-century poet, once wrote: "A man's reach should exceed his grasp." This reach, however, does not become a reality by merely waiting, but by rigorous working to achieve it.

Educational therapy, like the other activity therapies, has as its primary *goal* the treatment and rehabilitation of patients. It naturally differs from the other activity therapies in its content, structure, and inherent purpose. The inherent purpose of every educational therapy activity must be to engage the patient's intellect in a learning process within a structured program. While it is true that a discussion group (which generally is considered an educational activity) will be more informal than a class in algebra or English composition, both types of activities must follow a definite format, progress toward a definite goal, and adhere to definite classroom decorum—if the activity is to be considered to be both therapeutic and educational. A discussion group meeting (whether on current affairs or some general-interest topic) in which one member or several members are permitted to monopolize the discussion probably has gone beyond the point of a learning activity and has become instead a personal exhibition of argumentation for argumentation sake. Hence the discussion group probably has lost much of its therapeutic benefit as an educational activity. One would not say that a basketball game in which one player is permitted to run, charge, and shoot without any regard for the rules or the other players would still be considered a basketball game. A basketball game must be controlled and played according to pre-determined rules. The same is true of a class in algebra or English composition, or a special concert by a visiting orchestra. Even the more loosely-structured discussion groups and reading and writing clubs must insist on decorum and orderliness if the participants are to benefit most from the activity.

If intellectual activity is necessary for an educational activity to serve a therapeutic purpose, then perhaps educational therapy ought not be considered as simply one of the activities to which every patient is assigned to have a well-rounded program of activities that will keep him busy all day. A withdrawn, unmotivated person who is assigned to an algebra class probably will not benefit either intellectually or therapeutically from this activity. Later maybe, but not at this time. His sitting at his desk while not participating would only afford additional opportunity for him to escape into a world of fantasy. And to send him to the blackboard to attempt to work some problems would only humiliate him before his peers and thus tend to increase his withdrawal. School would become a part of his already unrealistic world, just the opposite of what should happen in the healthy, therapeutic environment of the hospitan's milieu program. As Dr. Gunter Ammon states in *Theoretical Aspects of Milieu Therapy:* "The healthy response of the milieu program toward the individual patient does *not* [must not] fulfill his predetermined sick expectations."[1]

Finally, the overall structure of the educational therapy program in most hospitals probably could be divided into three different types: (1) formal academic classes on the elementary, secondary and college level; (2) adult education classes, and (3) extra-curricular or cultural activities. These types obviously will overlap in some cases, but a division of this kind or a similar one probably would be helpful to both the staff and the patients in helping them decide the exact purpose, structure, and content of these activities in educational therapy. For example, a forty-five-year-old man wants to learn to type so that he can type his own letters whenever his office secretary is not available. He needs to follow the same basic instructions in learning to type as the sixteen-year-old boy who wants to study typing for high school credit. The manner of learning to type will be essentially the same and the textbooks probably will be the same for both persons, but the emphasis obviously will be different for each. For this reason, they should attend the course at different hours, together with others who are interested in the course for the same reasons as they. Also, the sixteen-year-old boy will need to be graded for his performance, but the forty-five-year-old man has no need at all for grades.

The same point can be exemplified by the patient who writes an article for the patient newspaper about the concert by a visiting orchestra. If the patient is writing the article as a reporter for the newspaper (extra-curricular activity), the educational therapist probably will thank the patient for faithfully completing the assignment but himself will make all the needed corrections on the article before it is published. However, if the patient is receiving academic credit for this article, the educational therapist probably will discuss the faults and weaknesses of the article in more detail with the patient. The therapist might even require the patient to rewrite the article. Finally, the therapist will need to record a grade for the quality of the patient's work on this assignment.

Thus it is evident that educational therapy, as a form of milieu therapy which is prescribed by the patient's physician, uses educational materials, methods, and procedures in such ways that the patient will experience not only learning but also treatment and rehabilitation. Various realistic requirements and demands are made of the patient "enrolled" in this structured program. These are in accordance with the particular type of educational activity and the exact prescription of the patient's physician.

BRIEF HISTORY OF EDUCATIONAL THERAPY

A complete, accurate history of the field of educational therapy is difficult to find. This is particularly true of educational therapy as it is utilized in psychiatric hospitals. Numerous Veteran Administration, state, and private psychiatric hospitals are known to have educational therapy departments as a part of their milieu activity programs, but seemingly few of their educational therapists or supervisors have published histories of the development of this treatment milieu.

Mr. Edward R. Belknap has made one of the most complete historical studies of the profession that is in print. His findings, however, are based primarily on the following sources: Dr. Sidney

Licht's two books, *Occupational Therapy Sourcebook* and *Occupational Therapy, Purpose and Practice*,[2] and Dr. Christina Zubaithis's unpublished doctoral dissertaion, *Educational Services in Rehabilitation*.[3] Most of the information concerning the history of the profession of educational therapy which is presented below is based on these sources for Belknap as well as on Belknap's lecture which he presented at the Tri-Scientific and Clinical Annual Conference in July, 1957, as it was printed in *American Archives of Rehabilitation Therapy*.[4]

Dr. Caelius Aurelianus, a 5th-century physician of North Africa, seems to have been the first physician to have prescribed educational therapy for patients. His prescription differed from the modern physician's in that he specifically recommended reading "books with incorrect passages." The purpose of the incorrect passages was to stimulate the patient's intellect, ". . . to arouse interest in finding errors . . ." but that, on the other hand, ". . . neither conversation nor reading should be sufficiently exciting to cause mental strain." His prescriptions for educational therapy activities also included such activities as theatrical performances based upon the particular humour dominant in the patient and special lectures illustrating adherence to the best rules of rhetoric.[5]

Although mental hospitals became established in the 16th century and were rather popular by the end of the 18th century, it was not until the middle of the 19th century that educational therapy became an integral part of their treatment programs. In 1843, hospital schools were established at Hanwell near London and at Utica, New York, so the patients could attend regular classes while hospitalized, usually in small groups no larger than fifteen. Classes in reading were most popular and successful: "Among the readers may be seen some who were formerly looked upon as among the most troublesome patients in the asylum, and several who are liable to occasional attacks or maniacal excitement; but they attend the classes with gratification, and observe a remarkable order and decorum. . . ."[6] It is interesting to note that the instruction was "designed to excite, relieve, and recreate as well as inform their minds." Instructors were hired full time to instruct these patients, without any extra charge to the patients

—at a time when free public education was not widely accepted. Many of the adult patients learned to read and write for the first time during their hospitalization. At Utica some of the patients were given the responsibility to teach some of the classes.[7]

In 1858, Ireland added an educational program to the Richmond District Asylum at Dublin. It offered "a curriculum similar to that of the best schools in the kingdom." The patients were grouped in classes on the basis of their capabilities and proficiencies. Rewards and disciplines were used to motivate the patients.[8]

With the gradual development of the various occupational therapies (which often included the manual arts, recreational, work, and music therapies in their early stages of development), educational therapy seemed to drop out of the limelight. It obviously continued to be used to some extent in most hospitals, however, published findings about the details of these educational therapy programs are most difficult to locate.

The first hospitals in the United States to realize the need for educational therapy along with the other activity therapies were the federal hospitals established immediately after World War I. In fact, educational therapy (although not called by that name at that time) played a large role in the activity programs at these hospitals. Academic subjects, commercial subjects, and drawing and painting were the three major categories of activities. The academic subjects included English, spelling, arithmetic, mathematics, penmanship, foreign languages, and Civil Service. The commercial subjects ranged from typing and shorthand to business letter writing, commercial law, and bookkeeping. The same type of activities program for veterans was continued and expanded greatly in the Veterans Administration hospitals during World War II and later, even to this day.[9]

Various studies of limited scale and scope have been made in the last two decades or so of the use being made of educational therapy as a part of the treatment programs in Veterans Administration, state, and private hospitals. Most of these studies, however, include not only psychiatric hospitals but also mentally retarded, tuberculosis, general medical and surgical, etc. Mr. Belknap, in his lecture at the Tri-Scientific and Clinical Annual

Conference in 1957, referred to two of these studies.[10] Miss Patience Sanderson, in a study of 317 psychiatric, tuberculosis, and children's hospitals, ascertained that 54 per cent of these hospitals had some type of educational therapy program for their patients. Dr. Christina M. Zubaitis, in research for her doctoral dissertation based on a sampling study of certain selected private, city, and state hospitals, noted that a large percentage of these hospitals included educational therapy programs as a part of the medical rehabilitation of their patients.[11]

Educational therapy has made its greatest gains in growth and importance during the last decade. More and more hospitals have added educational therapy activities to their activity therapies department. In some cases, these educational activities have been of the general type which have been classified above as adult education and extra-curricular activities, hence they have not always been identified with educational therapy activities. In some cases, a separate department for educational therapy has not been added until such time as an aggressive academic program for elementary- or secondary-age patients was initiated. In some of these cases (e.g., The Menninger Clinic, Topeka, Kansas), even this formal organization of this new milieu therapy was preceded by a year or more of individual and small-group tutoring by local teachers who were hired by the hour, and thus not considered as official members of the activity therapies department.

The field of educational therapy definitely is experiencing a new Renaissance. More psychiatric hospitals are adding it to their milieu treatment programs. General medical and surgical hospitals as well as hospitals for the mentally retarded also are utilizing educational therapy as part of their total treatment programs. In some general medical and surgical hospitals, this includes informal reading and writing groups, music listening, discussion groups, special lecturers, etc. If the patient is too ill to read, the staff still can use educational therapy by reading to the patient or playing musical or literary records for him.

In the hospital for the mentally retarded, the possible use of educational therapy is not only limitless but also an inherent necessity for treatment of these persons. Educational therapy in conjunction with the other activity therapies can be one of the unique tools to help rehabilitate the mentally retarded person as much as possible. Understanding, patience, and acceptance coupled with creativity and challenge on the part of the therapist can motivate and rehabilitate the mentally-retarded person to an extent that pity and sympathy never can. This fact some hospitals and community groups have begun to realize in the last few years. One recent example of this new interest is the Workshop on the Mentally Retarded which was conducted by the Mennonite Mental Health Services, at Newton, Kansas. This church-sponsored organization, which operates psychiatric hospitals in California, Kansas, Indiana, and Maryland, conducted this workshop for Mennonite leaders in church, school, and community activities to examine the possible role (s) that the church and its members should play in the field of mental retardation. The conclusion of those attending was that the church and its members definitely should become involved both by supporting existing local programs and by assisting in research on retardation.[12]

Thus, a new interest definitely is developing in the field of mental retardation on all levels and in all hospitals and communities that should revolutionize the trends in this field during the next decade. Educational therapy, to be sure, will play an important role in this revolution.

EDUCATIONAL THERAPY AND THE TOTAL TREATMENT PROCESS

Educational therapy, as one of the activity therapies of the broader field of milieu therapy, plays an important role in the total treatment process of a patient. While the general structure and content of the academic classes, adult education courses, and the extra-curricular or cultural activities seems to be designed for groups of patients whenever possible, the carrying out of the activity is still based upon an individual therapeutic process. This is one of the factors which makes the activity therapies' role in the milieu therapy process so unique. As has been stated earlier in this chapter, the patient's physician is the chief leader and controller of a team of trained staff whose chief concern is the treatment and rehabilitation of each individual patient. The activity therapist—just as the nurse, social worker, or psychotherapist—very possibly may need to approach and respond to each of the patients in his group in a slightly different manner. The secret to this concentrated, consistent approach by the team lies in a feeling of rapport and team-work between all members of the team. These members, in turn, must communicate the thinking, observations, and recommendations to their colleagues in each of their respective areas of interest. Thus, through such carefully planned sharing of observations, findings, and suggestions, the patient will be treated in the exact same manner (ideally) in the educational therapy department as in the manual arts department or the nursing department. The only differences will lie in the tools which the various milieu therapists will employ in this treatment process. One department may use physical activities; educational therapy uses intellectual activities.

The tools of the educational therapist, however, are not restricted to the various educational materials, methods and procedures. With public schools and state universities becoming more and more crowded during a period in history when education seems to become a "union card" to a job, it is possible for a high school or university instructor to present information in the form of a boring lecture without any concern for the students who are sitting before him and taking copious notes. The instructor can easily rationalize and say that the motivated students will study and learn, and the others will flunk out. For the instructor who is also an educational therapist, this approach is not proper. The chief reason for this is that the educational therapist is not concerned primarily with presenting a rhetorical lecture which will display his profound knowledge on the subject. The educational therapist is first and foremost a member of various therapeutic teams which are working together to attempt to treat and rehabilitate people. Just as the physician must do more than prescribe medications or some type of activity to keep the patient busy the entire day, so the educational therapist must do more than lecture and give homework assignments. Educational materials and methods are tools which the educational therapist uses and the quality of performance is the realistic measure to indicate the progress of the patient, but the performance or the grade is not the chief concern or goal. If knowledge and absorption of facts becomes the prime concern, then perhaps the patient should not be assigned to the particular educational activity.

Thus, it is evident that the role of educational therapy in the total treatment process is no greater than that of any of the other activity therapies. Educational therapy is just an adjunct to the other activities which aim specifically in treating and rehabilitating patients. While the educational therapist ought to be most aggressive in the use of the latest methods and materials in the field of education on all levels, he must remember that his primary attitude and concern must remain more focused on therapeutic benefit than on academic achievement by the patient.

STRUCTURE AND CONTENT OF EDUCATIONAL THERAPY

Formal Academic Classes

The structure and content of any educational therapy program will depend upon both the ages of the patients and their primary interests. Educational therapy with children is in the unique position of being able to restrict its program to academic classes and extra-curricular activities similar to those in the public schools. The reason for this is that school seems so natural for a child. It is what all children do; it is the exception for a child not to attend formal classes. Hence, it seems that educational therapy automatically should be an essential part of the activity program for children who must be hospitalized. In some hospitals, it is the main activity program with the other activity therapies as adjuncts. Again, as in life outside the hospital, it is the exception for a hospitalized child not to be attending classes for academic credit. Even art and manual arts usually are considered more as classes than activities.

This tendency to speak in terms of classes instead of activities in the educational therapy program for the children's section of the hospital, however, does not mean that education is primary and therapeutic benefit is secondary. Not at all. Rather, it simply points out the fact that it seems more natural to refer to the activities as classes and the entire educational program as a school program. This borrowing of terminology from the public school system seems justifiable when one considers for a moment the ages of these patients and what their primary, natural interests in life are at that age.

If the above logic is valid, it is natural that the structure of these classes should be rather similar to that of their public school counterpart. Subject matter, grading forms and standards also should be similar to those in the local public schools. In this way, the hospitalized child will not feel his classes in the hospital school program teach him less or demand less than he would experience if he were not hospitalized. In fact, this realistic experiencing of life in the hospital school program, as it is manipulated and controlled by the educational therapists to meet its primary goal of treatment and rehabilitation, is part of the secret which makes this program therapeutic for the child.

For the secondary-age patients who are admitted to the same wards and the same activity therapies as other adult patients, the educational therapy program must receive a different emphasis than on the elementary level. On this level, the program of activities must carefully be integrated with the entire activity therapies program. Formal classes might seem more important to the adolescent in the hospital than to the adult, but formal classes cannot become so important that academic knowledge pre-empts therapeutic benefits. A secondary-or college-age patient can avoid facing his emotional problems rather successfully by losing himself in his school work. This fact is a potential danger also when the patient begins attending the local schools again. If this occurs, education has become a symptom of the disease instead of a tool to treat the disease.

Assuming the proper emphasis is placed on educational activities for the secondary-age patient, one is ready to examine the structure and content of such activities on this level. As is the case on the elementary level, the materials, methods, and procedures in conducting formal, academic classes should be basically the same as those in the local schools. This would include the textbooks, length of class periods and semesters, regular attendance, punctuality in assignments, etc., which are part of the routine of the public schools. Only if the standards in the hospital school program are realistic and the same as those in the local schools will the patients feel that they are, in reality, attending school. (Beginning and ending the semesters of the hospital school program the same time as the local school also facilitates a patient's transfer to these schools for some or all of his future courses.) Patients who play basketball must abide by the rules, whether it be a physical educational class for credit or a recreational therapy activity or a social game just for fun. Without the rules of the game, the activity would be a farce; it would lose its meaning. The same is true in a so-called academic course if those enrolled only play school. Being ill may affect one's performance but it does not make a poor performance good. If a patient is to recover and again live in the outside world in a realistic manner, he must experience realistic activities while in the hospital. Busy work is not therapeutic; it is not work; it is merely wasting time. For the school-age patient, formal classes are the most realistic activities which could be prescribed for him. To this age patient, school is life in the most realistic sense.

The courses to be offered to these patients will depend primarily upon two factors: (1) the academic needs of the patients, and (2) the staff and time available to fulfill these needs. In addition, some patients cannot function properly in a group, especially if Miss X also is in the class. Group classes obviously are more economical, but the educational therapy staff must carefully consider all the factors before it decides which classes can be offered. The physician may write the prescription of a class in nuclear physics for Joe B., but this does not mean that the class can be offered this semester, or ever, in the hospital's educational therapy program. The patient may need to delay studying a certain subject until he is well enough to attend classes at the local schools.

Another factor to keep in mind, in planning the academic program in the hospital school, is each patient's physical, emotional and intellectual capabilities at that time. If a patient, for example, is severely disturbed to the extent that he is unable to follow regular assignments in one class, perhaps he should not be scheduled for formal educational classes until the next semester. While some hospitals automatically schedule formal classes for all patients of elementary or secondary age, one might question such routine procedure. One might wonder whether this is properly using educational courses for either academic or therapeutic purposes, or if it is rather a distortion of reality. If a child has a broken leg, he is not expected to attend football practice and attempt to learn the game of football as best he can under the circumstances. This is particularly true if the child needs to take medication for the pain, which would, in turn, affect both his physical equilibrium and his mental alertness to understand the game. Then, why should a similar struggling performance be expected from a patient who is severely ill emotionally? Would it not be much more realistic and therapeutic either to delay the patient's attending a formal class or to enroll him in a correspondence course in which he can work as he is able?

For the patient who is severely disturbed but still desires to study, a correspondence course often may serve as an interim link between him and the formal classes offered by the educational therapy department. The nature of the correspondence courses implicitly suggests that the enrollee need not feel under pressure to complete the course within one semester. He can work as he has time, interest, and motivation. Most schools allow a person two years to complete the course, often with a possibility of a year's extension for a small additional fee.

Having removed the pressure of time for the severely ill patient, the educational therapist can use the correspondence course as a treatment tool. Whether or not the patient accomplishes much, or anything, on the course is of little importance. Therapeutic benefit remains primary, and this cannot be ascertained by pages completed or grades received.

Several possibilities exist to make the correspondence course a genuinely therapeutic tool for the withdrawn or severely ill patient. One of the initial concerns of the educational therapist probably should be the establishment of an external structure for the course by scheduling a regular time to work on the course. At such scheduled times, the patient's favorite aide or nurse on the ward could help the patient work on the correspondence course as best as he can on that particular day. The educational therapist should stop by regularly (preferably daily or on alternate days) to check with the patient to see if he has any questions concerning the course. The patient could also be encouraged to feel free to request a special visit by the therapist if some problem or question about the course should arise between visits. This interest and willingness to help the patient would be more therapeutic for the patient than attempting to force him to attend a formal class in the same course with other students. In some cases, a private, tutored class with the educational therapist might be preferable to the above arrangement, if adequate staff time is available.

Another point to keep in mind in planning the academic schedule of these ill patients is that the patients should not be overloaded, especially during the first semester in attendance at the hospital school. The same thing should be noted when the patient returns to the local high school. The patient probably has already experienced enough failures in school without compounding them in his present circumstances. The patient also may have built up a resentment toward school and all teachers. Thus, the first return to school and teachers should be as favorable and successful as possible. The success undoubtedly will not damage his academic record, and it probably will be therapeutic in his treatment program. Of course, it is assumed that the educational therapist will not alter or lower the academic standards for any of the patients, regardless of their illnesses. To be understanding and to give the patient a little more time to complete a course is perfectly correct, but to award a grade of *A* or *B* for academic performance which is inferior and poor is unrealistic and unjustified. The patient is at the hospital to recover his health, not to be given a diploma because the therapist feels sorry for him. Furthermore, the patient would some day probably suffer from his lack of knowledge in an area or subject in which he had been "given" a grade. Attendance and effort are not enough to receive credit for a course, even if the grade would be a *C* or lower.

On the other extreme, neither should an exceptionally intelligent student be given various achievement examinations and then given course credit for the areas in which he scored exceptionally high. If he failed to receive credit earlier in these courses, either because he had not attended these courses or because he had failed to meet the requirements set up by the teachers, giving him credit on the basis of an examination would be ethically wrong. If his intelligence is adequate so that he could be admitted to college on the basis of some type of state equivolency certificate, then perhaps he should be assisted in applying for such examinations and in enrolling in the local university. This type of exemption for a student is completely different, because the state department of education in some states has established such provisions for those persons above age twenty who are capable of college work but are not qualified with adequate credits. The former procedure is cheating; the latter is therapeutic assistance with a person's academic program.

One final point concerning the structure of the formal classes for secondary-age patients needs to be stated. The patient who is able to attend a full academic program in the hospital setting should be governed by academic load limitations similar to those at the local schools. For example, some secondary schools require one scheduled study hall for every two courses that the student is attending. Thus the average student is permitted to enroll in only four courses plus two study halls; he may enroll in five courses if not more than three are considered "solids" and he has made several *B's* during the past semester. Only the exceptional, straight-*A* student is permitted to enroll in six courses without any formal study halls. The requirements will vary with the school located near a particular hospital, but the requirements and standards of the local school definitely should be followed by the hospital's educational program for these patients.

Perhaps it should be clarified at this point that the above emphasis on formal classes does not mean to imply that the educational therapy staff are the only ones involved in educational activities offered to patients in a hospital. The educational therapy staff does tend to have a monopoly on the patient's time each day, but this monopoly gradually declines from the elementary level to the secondary level to the college level to the adult education level. The older and more academically advanced the patient, the more need he has for the other activity therapies. Even on the elementary and secondary levels, however, the other activity therapists play important roles in the hospital life of these younger patients. In some of the activities, the patients may be receiving regular academic credit; in others, they may not. The structure, content and demands might be varied somewhat for the patient receiving academic credit for his performance in manual arts, arts and crafts, or softball, but the overall, primary objective of the therapist in charge of the particular activity is to use that activity as a therapeutic tool to treat and rehabilitate the patient. It is to guide the patient, to teach him "ways of living, better ways of living . . . of expressing instinctual urges," as Drs. Karl Menninger, Paul Pruyser, Martin Mayman, and Marietta Houston state in "The Prescription of Treatment."[13] In this sense, then, all activity therapists are "teachers" and all activity therapies are "modalities of living, structured in a didactic program . . . as an *educational* program, a school in 'practical living'."[14]

For the college-age patients who are hospitalized, the need for formalized classes on the hospital campus also exists, but several factors make this an impossibility for most hospitals, whether general or psychiatric. First, the interests and academic status of the patients tend to vary so much that it is difficult to find a course in which at least ten patients would be interested and qualified to study, much less several courses. Secondly, unless the hospital population is large, the demand for the same course (s) probably would not be repeated for a semester or so. Thus, it would become rather inefficient and too expensive to hire a therapist to teach college courses, unless he could be used to teach secondary classes also. This last possibility, of course, is one practical way of solving the problem; but because of its dual nature, it probably tends to be overlooked in some hospitals where such a need exists. One practical example of such an arrangement would be for the secondary English and history instructor-therapist to offer freshman or sophomore college courses in these areas whenever adequate interest for such courses exist.

Another possible way of using education as a therapeutic tool for treating and rehabilitating the college-age patients who are not too ill is to enroll them in correspondence courses from one of the state universities. This avoids the problem of needing a certain number of patients interested in a course before it is economically feasible to offer such a course. Each student may be enrolled in a different correspondence, if necessary. If several patients do enroll in the same course (e.g., Introduction to Sociology, History of Civilization, Survey of English Literature), then arrangements can be made so these patients will study on the same course, at the same hour and place each day. This would tend to add a little classroom atmosphere to the course.

For the correspondence course program to be a success on either the college or secondary level, proper structure is a most important necessity. A suggested procedure would be to schedule each patient for one hour per day per correspondence course, in a supervised study hall in the educational therapy department. This would give a positive emphasis to the course as a regular, therapeutic activity for the patients. The results should be more completed assignments and better grades on these assignments than if the patient were left to his own whims and mood to govern his productivity. At least such were the results of the two-years' experiment with college correspondence courses at The Menninger Clinic, Topeka, Kansas.[15]

Adult Education Courses

A second type of educational activity which needs to be developed in more hospitals might be labelled adult education courses. On the surface, it might appear that no great need exists in this area, but the opposite probably is true. Intellectual stimulation should not be ignored for the patient who either has graduated from college or is not interested in college. The ever-increasing enrollments in the non-credit evening college courses is evidence to the contrary. Even the person of retirement age probably could benefit from this type of activity during his hospitalization.

The obvious latitude of such courses should make this type of activity one of the most popular and most therapeutic educational activity on the hospital campus. Furthermore, this should be one educational area in which staff from all services of the hospital as well as patients could work together in a unique way in suggesting, developing, and conducting courses. If enough patients would show interest or practical need for a certain course, the best-qualified staff member could be relieved from other duties for the necessary hours to "teach" this course. Or, a patient might be asked to accept this responsibility, or, a volunteer from the community might be called on to assist in the treatment program in this way. The latter arrangement would also help establish a better rapport with the community as a whole.

A place to begin in planning adult education courses on the hospital campus might be to consult some of the nearby universities which are offering adult education courses in their evening college programs. In order to make the first such course in the hospital setting as successful as possible, one might arrange for an experienced adult education instructor to teach a course on the hospital campus. This would give the new program a fair chance as well as encourage the patients to take advantage of this special course.

Most Veterans Administration hospitals and some state hospitals already have educational therapy programs which include adult education courses. These include classes in typing, business English, political science, business finance, discussion group meetings with guest lecturers, and various vocational training classes. These hospitals and therapists deserve much praise for their efforts to make these courses therapeutic and beneficial to the patients.

It seems appropriate here to add one word of caution to all activity therapies departments considering adding adult education courses to their activity program. It would be advisable not to begin too many courses without careful forethought and preparation by qualified or experienced staff. Also, the central control of these courses probably should not be distributed to numerous supervisors. Having too many people involved will not permit even a carefully planned program in adult education to develop as it might. Many staff and patients have good ideas for such new courses, but not everyone is qualified to teach or supervise them. Ambition is not enough. Besides the probability that the courses will not be strong in content, the patients attending such classes soon discover the fact that the teachers really do not know very much about these courses. This, in turn, may cause these patients and others in the hospital to begin to question the entire educational therapy program.

The area of adult education courses on the hospital campus presents a unique opportunity and challenge to not only the educational therapy department but also all the departments and services in the hospital. This is one area in which the creativity and resources of persons from all areas of the hospital can contribute to the treatment of patients through intellectual stimulation. The educational therapist possibly may be the least qualified to teach some of these courses. He can, however, play a tremendous role in developing this aspect of the treatment program if he is able to elicit and coordinate the ideas and energies of other interested staff and patients.

Extra-curricular Activities

Some activities are educational in general scope and nature but usually cannot be included in either formal academic courses or adult education courses. These activities, for lack of a better label, might be referred to as extra-curricular, or cultural, activities. They are similar in numerous ways to regular courses but generally tend to be more unlimited in scope and purpose. Often, they are more cultural or entertaining in immediate purpose than strictly learning. For this reason, it is most difficult to define and discuss these activities in detail in terms of content, structure, and educational goal. Educational activities which belong in this category include the publication of the patient newspaper and patient literary magazine, discussion group meetings (if not already included in the adult education category), educational tours, special cultural programs and concerts on and off the hospital grounds, and guest lecturers. Some of these activities naturally would be under the direction of staff in other areas of the activity therapies department, social work department, nursing department, or even the patient body itself. Here, as in the case of the adult education courses discussed earlier, proper cooperation and coordination between various staff and patients can result in therapeutic benefits not otherwise realized.

One final word needs to be mentioned about the key to the success of an educational therapy program on any level. That key is *motivation.* In educational therapy, probably more than in any of the other activity therapies, motivation is tremendously important. The patient may still benefit from pounding out an ash tray even if he hates every moment of it, but the same patient probably would not receive much therapeutic benefit from a course in algebra if he were not motivated to learn algebra. He may be forced to attend the course for six months and still not know much more algebra than when he enrolled. Furthermore, when his emotional health improves, he will probably have some misgivings about the validity of educational therapy as a therapeutic activity. He can understand how working on an ash tray when he was severely depressed was a help, but how was his sitting and fantasizing when a teacher was explaining algebraic formulas?

This motivation to a large extent must come from within the patient. It must be there before he can benefit very much from the educational activity. On the other hand, the educational therapist in his attitude toward both the patient and the subject matter can do much to stimulate and develop this motivation in the patient.

ADMINISTRATION OF EDUCATIONAL THERAPY

The initial responsibility of the administration of the educational therapy program naturally rests on the supervisor or director of the educational therapy department. Besides scheduling and coordinating the activities under the direction of his own staff, he often is responsible for assisting in coordinating all the various educational activities which are offered by the various activity therapy departments. Thus, he usually will be concerned directly with the planning and functioning of all these activities, even though many of them will be directed or taught by other activity therapists, other hospital staff, or volunteers from the community.

The educational director will not be the originator or supervisor of all these activities, but he usually will be directly involved because of the nature of his position.

This coordinating of the educational activities with each other and with the other activities in the hospital's activity therapies program requires the coordinator to be an administrator with responsibilities and problems very similar to those of a high school principal. Besides being able to administrate properly and efficiently, he will also need to be well informed on academic standards, requirements, etc. For this reason, it seems most important that this person should be an experienced teacher who currently is certified by the state board of education. Active participation in local, state, and national educational and activity therapy associations probably should be considered next in importance. Finally, if he at present does not have a Master's degree, he might be encouraged to work toward such a degree, preferably in education and a basic teaching field. This would both add prestige to his office and better qualify him as teacher and administrator.

Some of the functions of the administrator of the hospital's educational program for patients have been discussed in the section concerned with the structure and content of educational therapy. Thus this section will be concerned primarily with the administrator's role in such matters as arranging official accreditation of the courses taught in the hospital school program, obtaining transcripts of patients' former academic performances, deciding which classes to schedule for each semester, and determining the teachers' work load.

If the educational activity is one in which official, academic credit is to be given, the supervisor of the educational therapy department has the responsibility to make the necessary arrangements so that the patients actually will receive credit for the course (s) when completed. This would include, first of all, making certain that as many as possible of the therapists or volunteers teaching these courses have valid teaching certificates to teach these courses, or are working toward such a goal. As was stated earlier in the chapter, a fully-certified staff usually is not possible, but it still should be a goal toward which to strive. Secondly, the supervisor's task would include making certain that the standards, requirements, textbooks, etc., are the same as those of the local schools. Finally, most importantly, the supervisor should make appropriate arrangements with either the state department of education or the administrative staff of the local schools so that the patients would have legitimate, transferable credits in these courses when completed.

Several possibilities exist which would facilitate the transfer of credits earned by the patient-student. These possibilities range from institutionalizing the hospital school program so that the patient would receive an official transcript indicating that he has completed the courses with the designated grades at this particular hospital. Usually, however, this is not desirable because of the social stigma which still exists concerning certain illnesses. A more preferable possibility is to make arrangements with the administrative staff of the local schools for the transfer of credits from the hospital school to the local schools at the end of each semester. This arrangement would, in effect, mean that the hospital school would operate as a type of annex to the local schools. This procedure has been followed very successfully by the hospital school program at The Menninger Clinic, Topeka, Kansas. In fact, this arrangement was initiated at the suggestion of the officials of the local high school. They not only were willing but also eager to help in this way in the rehabilitation of these young people who were hospitalized.[16] Similar arrangements could also be made with the Extension Department of the nearest college or university for the courses to be taught on that level.

Obtaining proper transcripts of the patients' earlier performances is another administrative procedure which might become the responsibility of the supervisor of the educational therapy department. In some hospitals, the case social workers request official transcripts for all patients of college age or younger. Sometimes the patient himself is asked to write for his transcript. It is not at all important who writes for it (from the administrative point of view), as long as it is done. The supervisor of the educational therapy department might desire to request that this be made a part of the routine data which is collected on patients upon admission to the hospital, and that a copy of the transcript be on file not only in the patient's medical file but also in the educational file in the educational therapy department for convenient reference.

The practical need for having an official transcript on file in both the medical records and educational records cannot be stressed too heavily. The following case illustrates what can happen if the need for an official transcript is temporarily ignored: The patient had stated in a sincere manner that he was enrolled in several courses at an out-of-state university, but that he had made arrangements with the professor to receive a delayed grade until such time when the work could be completed. This reasoning appeared logical to both the physician and the educational supervisor, so no transcript was requested. Instead, the patient was encouraged to write for his books and assignments so that he could complete them during study hall hours in the hospital school. To save time and confusion, the patient was assigned immediately to the study hall, assuming that he could read a few books for leisure while he was waiting for his books and assignments from his home university. To be brief, the books and assignments never arrived—he was not, in reality, enrolled in either the course or the university as he had told the physician and educational supervisor. They had accepted his story as fact, and the results were both embarrassing and antitherapeutic. This example should not be interpreted as suggesting that a patient should not be trusted; it rather makes the point that official transcripts should be just as routine case information for most school-age hospitalized patients as it is for the student who plans to attend a university. Official records avoid errors, embarrassment, and keep the focus on the realistic aspects of the situation.

Besides requiring transcripts, some educational supervisors prefer to have the prospective patient-student take a brief series of achievement tests. This gives the educational staff an opportunity to meet the patient in a more academically neutral situation, while at the same time collecting data which may say more than grades on a transcript can. These findings often can be helpful to the hospital team as they discuss and plan the treatment program for a patient.

The matter of deciding which classes to schedule for each semester is another administrative procedure which must ultimately be resolved by the educational supervisor. In this case, he probably would do well to inquire what the interests and desires of his staff are in this regard before he attempts to elicit the same information from the patients' own comments and official transcripts. Obviously, not all the desired courses can be taught each semester. At times, the patients will have to attend courses other than their favorites, just as the educational therapists will need to teach some courses which they are not very fond of. However, if the educational therapists are directly involved in this scheduling and if their desires and suggestions are carefully considered, it will be surprising how many courses a small staff can offer. Furthermore, the enthusiasm and creativity of the staff will become contagious to both patients and other staff.

Obviously the educational therapists will need to examine the patients' transcripts and attempt to arrange a class schedule which will include not only courses which the patients consider as their preferences but also courses which the students have failed or have not completed. Furthermore, this planning should attempt to predict which courses the patients might attend the next semester or two either at the hospital school or the local schools. For example, if Algebra II is offered only the second semester at the local high school and if any possibility exists that a certain patient might be able to attend the local high school during the second semester, this student should be enrolled in Algebra I during the first semester, either in residence at the hospital school or by correspondence. If by correspondence, a schedule should be made out so that the student will be able to complete the first semester course by the time the second semester course begins at the local high school. If he is unable to progress that rapidly, however, the prospects of the entire schedule for this patient will, of course, be changed completely.

A final consideration concerning the administration of the educational program of any hospital school concerns the educational therapists' teaching load. If quality teaching is to be practiced by the educational therapists, they cannot be expected to have a total work load that is heavier than that of their colleagues in the local schools. In most cases, the educational therapists have fewer patients per class, but this does not excuse assigning an educational therapist to six different preparations per day, as sometimes happens. The supervisor of the hospital school, in cooperation with the other activity therapy supervisors and the coordinator of the activity therapies, has the responsibility of planning a schedule that will involve as many patients as possible (for economy reasons). He also must plan a schedule which will permit him to expect quality performance from his staff. In addition to their teaching load, the supervisor must allow time for such vital matters as (1) writing reports on the patients in one's milieu area; (2) giving achievement tests to new patients and writing reports on them; (3) attending staff conferences on patients involved in one's area; (4) attending special meetings with staff of the other activity therapies, and (5) arranging to meet a patient's physician to discuss a particular problem which has arisen with the patient that day.

The general type of curriculum which seems the most adaptable to the type of academic program just described depends upon the academic level of education concerned. On the elementary level, obviously, the educational therapy department will have to have adequate staff to handle all levels and areas of courses with a sense of adequacy. On the college level, staff qualified to teach in the fields of English, history, and social sciences probably would be adequate for the average-sized psychiatric hospital. On the secondary level, two teachers can offer a fair-sized curriculum to approximately thirty patients, if one teacher has a major in English and the other in social science. The third teacher probably should have a major in mathematics, with a minor in recreation, spending half his time in the recreational therapy department. With careful planning and the aid of correspondence courses, these two or three teachers could offer enough courses to suffice until the patient is able to attend the local high school for the sciences, languages, etc. Of course, without a qualified, enthusiastic, pleasant supervisor for this department, even a large number of educational therapists would not be able to meet the most needs of these patients in the best way possible.

It is not always easy for the educational supervisor to keep all of these needs and factors in perfect balance. He can only strive to do his best, learn from the errors, and ambitiously push forward to face the next challenge of the day. With adequate ambition and courage, he probably will be able to perform his task adequately. Strange as it may seem, a man's ambition generally seems to parallel his capacities. Or as Dr. Samuel Johnson has said: "Providence seldom sends any into the world with an inclination to attempt great things, who have not abilities likewise to perform them."[17]

EDUCATIONAL THERAPY AS A CAREER

The professional preparation required to become an educational therapist cannot be stated so explicitly as it might be for an occupational or recreational or music therapist. The main reason for this is the fact that educational therapy is relatively new as a recognized profession. While it is true that educational therapy has been practiced for many years (as discussed earlier in this chapter), it did not become professionalized until the last decade or so. As a result, two conditions currently exist: (1) a shortage of persons working as educational therapists, and (2) a large percentage of educational therapists not meeting the academic background suggested by such organizations as the American Association for Rehabilitation Therapy (A.A.R.T.). Consequently, it would be rather impractical to insist suddenly on certain academic preparations and clinical training as prerequisites to becoming an educational therapist. On the other hand, if educational therapy is to grow professionally, it will need to set definite requirements and standards as the goal for every educational therapist to attain within a certain, reasonable period of time.

The American Association for Rehabilitation Therapy suggests in one of its recent brochures that the would-be educational therapist should prepare for a career in educational therapy by either (1) earning a Bachelor's degree in educational therapy from an accredited college or university, or (2) earning a Bachelor's degree in education from an accredited teachers college or university and then getting the clinical training at the hospital where the person will begin his employment. Several colleges and universities have established affiliations with Veteran Administration and state hospitals for such training in clinical practice for the therapist trainee. Details concerning a career as an educational therapist and registration are stated in Appendix A.

Teaching experience in the public schools, prior to working in the hospital as an educational therapist, also might be considered a preferable way of preparing oneself for this career. Such experience, to be sure, would be a valuable asset, but it should not be considered a prerequisite. Similar experience should be encouraged, but it can be obtained later by teaching an evening class or summer school class in the local schools. This continued contact with the local schools can help the therapist keep informed about the latest educational materials and methods and maintain requirements and standards in the hospital educational activities which will be compatible with similar ones in the local schools. Also, in a more general way, this "outside" contact can give the therapist new ideas of how to use certain educational activities more effectively, both academically and therapeutically.

Creativity, ambition, and enthusiasm are essential qualities which an educational therapist needs to possess and to practice in his career. Primarily, these qualities will be reflected in his daily performance as therapist-teacher. Secondarily, and of great importance, these qualities should "overflow" and result in active research by the therapist in the field of educational therapy. This is necessary if educational therapy is to advance as a therapeutic modality. As Mr. Arthur A. Sorenson so succinctly states in his article, "Research in Educational Therapy": "Research means growth; growth implies wider horizons, acquiring new facts. . . . It helps to develop newer and better therapeutic procedures."[18]

Unfortunately, according to several surveys in recent years, there seems to be a present lack of interest and activity in research among educational therapists. Mr. Arthur A. Sorenson, for example, sent out questionnaires to 210 educational therapists, but only seventy-four questionnaires (or 33 per cent) were filled out and returned. This meager return of seventy-four questionnaires seems to suggest either apathy among these educational therapists or embarrassment about their inactivity in this area. Furthermore, the findings in the returned questionnaires point out the apparent lack of active research even more clearly. Only six hospitals responding had completed or were working on research projects in educational therapy; twenty-five hospitals had no research in process and none was planned.[19]

The above findings should not frighten or discourage the educational therapist. Rather, they should challenge him to become a crusader in this area. His efforts and actions could reform and revitalize the educational activities in his hospital and also serve as an encouragement for educational therapists at other hospitals. The motivated and enthusiastic educational therapist will not wait for his supervisor or hospital administrator to suggest research. The urgency for constant research, evaluation, and reevaluation of the educational therapy program will be felt so strongly by the educational therapist himself that he will not be content unless he is planning or engaged in some professional study and research. As a result, he will become a leader-teacher not only of the patients in his activity area but also of his colleagues in all the activity therapies. Finally, he himself "can be assured of growing professionally, of being a better therapist each time he works with a patient."[20]

REFERENCES

1. Ammon, Gunter: Theoretical Aspects of Milieu Therapy. Unpublished manuscript written while a resident physician in psychiatry in The Menninger School of Psychiatry, Topeka, Kansas, June, 1959, p. 6.
2. Licht, Sidney, (Ed.) : *Occupational Therapy Source Book*. Baltimore, 1948, and *Occupational Therapy, Purpose and Practice*, Springfield, Illinois, 1950.
3. Zubaitis, Christina M.: Educational Services in Rehabilitation. Unpublished doctoral dissertation, Teachers College, Columbia University, New York City. (The exact date of this dissertation is not cited by Mr. Belknap. He only states it was written in the decade prior to his lecture in July, 1957. See next reference.)
4. Belknap, Edward R.: Retrospect and prospect in educational therapy. *Amer. Arch. Rehabil. Ther.*, *V*:101-109, 1957.

5. *Ibid,* p. 102.
6. *Ibid.*
7. *Ibid.* This practice was not again commonly practiced until recently when physicians began to realize that the teaching experience itself could be therapeutic for the patient. The experiences of this type of educational therapy at The Menninger Clinic, Topeka, Kansas, during the past several years has been most successful.
8. *Ibid,* p. 103.
9. *Ibid,* p. 103-104.
10. *Ibid.*
11. Unfortunately, I was unable to obtain a copy of either Miss Sanderson's report or Dr. Zubaitis's dissertation.
12. The findings of the workshop are summarized in the following article: Maynard Shelly: Study Committee Says: Church Should Develop a Conscience on Needs of the Mentally Retarded. *Mennonite Weekly Review,* XLII, December 3, 1964, p. 5.
13. Menninger, Karl, Paul Pruyser, Martin Mayman, and Marietta Houston: The Prescription of Treatment. *Bull. Menninger Clinic, XXIV:*233, 1960.
14. *Ibid.*
15. Adrian, Daryl B.: Correspondence study proves effective adjunct. *The Alumni News,* a publication of the Kansas State Teacher's College, Emporia, *XLI:* 5, 1961. See also: Correspondence study is useful tool to help re-orient mental patients. *The Alumni News, XXXIX:*6, 1960.
16. Adrian, Daryl B.: Patients go to school. *Menninger Quart., XV:*16, 1961.
17. Johnson, Samuel: *Works of Samuel Johnson.* VI, p. 2751.
18. Sorenson, Arthur A.: Research in Educational Therapy. *Amer. Arch. Rehabil. Ther., XI:*2, 1963.
19. *Ibid,* p. 2-7.
20. Arthur A. Sorenson made this statement in the paper which he presented at the Tri-Scientific and Clinical Conference in Memphis, Tennessee, In July, 1963. The Tri-Scientific and Clinical Conference is the annual meeting of the following: The American Association for Rehabilitation Therapy, Inc.; The Association of Medical Rehabilitation Directors and Coordinators, Inc.; and the Association for Physical and Mental Rehabilitation, Inc.

Chapter VIII

VOLUNTEER SERVICES

ALBERT MEULI, M.Ed.

INTRODUCTION

Historical Development

Citizens in our society have been motivated since the beginning of mankind to help those in need. The volunteer movement is deeply rooted in American history. Volunteer work is known in other countries but is particularly an American phenomenon.[1] In the various health and welfare fields, we find that the driving force for reform came originally from the lay volunteer. It was the volunteer who spoke out in behalf of the afflicted and deprived; he was a primary factor in organizing support for change and improved conditions.

A review of the literature reveals the fact that the utilization of volunteers to help the hospitalized patient is not a recent development. It is gratifying, however, to see how the concept of volunteer services has changed during the past thirty years from that of "befuddled activities" of well-meaning do-gooders to that of services performed by the trained and dedicated volunteers of today. Historically, only citizens of the leisure class participated in volunteer services, and their primary contributions were limited to the dispensing of food and gifts to those unfortunates who were hospitalized. This historical record of services given by volunteers in the embryonic years of hospital development was a result of the concept of medical treatment and the role of the hospital and the early American community. The concepts of medical treatment and the role of the hospital in relation to the community have altered in recent years, along with the concept of volunteer services.

The American community has undergone many changes during the first half of this century. One of these has been a gradual shift in the character and organization of welfare and other social services based on alterations in underlying principles. Today the federal government is bearing a large share of the financial responsibility. Emphasis is on broadening and providing more comprehensive programs of assistance to people in need of welfare services, as well as shifting general services from private to public agencies which utilize tax funds. Services to people with demonstrated need have been expanded from a very limited effort to a program comprehensive both in the quantity of services provided and the number of groups and individuals eligible to receive them. The result of government agencies assuming more responsibility for providing various public community services is a changing pattern of acts of charity.

Volunteer services are no longer performed only by members of the leisure class. Citizens with new-found leisure time can now volunteer to assist those who need help. Not only does the average citizen in the modern community have more leisure, but he is also better able to take advantage of new opportunities for volunteer contributions.

The concept of medical care and treatment facilities have also undergone many changes during the first half of this century. Hospitals, nursing homes, outpatient clinics, half-way houses, and rehabilitation centers are becoming a part of community services. The care of patients within these facilities is no longer confined to mere custodial treatment. Treatment of the whole patient or total personality requires many other services. The great majority of the hospitals now have rehabilitation programs, social services, psychological services, recreation, and many other functions not conceived of as part of the hospital responsibility in the early part of the 20th century. The volunteer services program organized as an integral part of the broad medical treatment program is, indeed, a new concept in coordinated medical services.

Only within the past twenty years has the hospital volunteer services been identified separately from the broader all-encompassing volunteer movement. This separate identity has come about even more recently in the psychiatric field. One of the first national meetings devoted exclusively to the subject of hospital volunteer service programs was held in June 1958, in Chicago, Illinois. It was sponsored by the American Hospital Association, the American Psychiatric Association, the American Red Cross, the National Association for Mental Health, and the Veterans Administration. The report of this conference, *The Volunteer and the Psychiatric Patient*,[2] emphasized the importance of volunteer services in mental hospitals. It was the consensus of those present at the conference that growth and success of hospital volunteer service programs depend upon two things: administrative approval and support, and full-time employment of a well qualified director of volunteers. Less than two years later a nationwide Institute for Directors of Volunteer Services was held in Topeka, Kansas. The Institute was sponsored by the National Association for Mental Health and The Menninger Foundation in February of 1960. The report from this workshop, *Volunteer Services in Mental Hospitals*,[3] is considered a basic reference for directors of volunteers in psychiatric hospitals.

With the growth and development of volunteer programs in hospitals came the question of who was responsible for the administration of these programs. The pioneer volunteer coordinators became concerned with program standards and professional preparation. The result of this concern was the development in 1961 of a professional group called the American Association of Volunteer Services Coordinators.[4] The Association is currently developing standards for certification, curriculum development, and preceptorships. It is anticipated that the future leadership of the health-related volunteer programs will emanate from this professional association.

ORGANIZATION FOR A VOLUNTEER SERVICES PROGRAM

Historically, volunteer services have originated in various ways. In some cases, individual volunteers were present in the hospital for some time, and they virtually forced the administration to accept the expanding services of their organizations. In other cases, citizen groups, such as the mental health associations, have organized specifically to help the mentally ill both in the community and in the psychiatric hospital. In a few instances we find that newly established hospitals have been besieged by volunteers even before the administration was sufficiently organized to put them to work. In still other cases, volunteer programs have been developed and organized by an administration that realized the need and wanted an organized volunteer program.

Many volunteer programs have grown out of the work of women's auxiliaries. There are still volunteer programs in existence in which the leader of the women's auxiliary serves as the director of the program on a voluntary basis. These auxiliaries serve as the sole sponsoring agency.

While the concept of the organized volunteer services program in a hospital setting is relatively young, there has been sufficient experience with these programs to analyze their strengths and weaknesses. In the various evaluation studies which have been conducted, we find that much of the dissatisfaction with volunteer services stems from poor organization and administration. Whatever the relation between the hospital and the sponsoring group or agency, it is imperative that the program be the responsibility of the hospital. Careful planning and organization for volunteer services must take place if the program is going to realize its basic objective—improved services for patients.

Administrative Support

Most superintendents and hospital administrators agree that a hospital must be accepted by the community citizens if it is going to provide optimal service. They would probably also agree that the citizens should have first-hand knowledge of the hospital in order to be most effective in interpreting it to the community. What is all too often overlooked, however, is the fact that the community citizen's impression of the hospital is based on his experiences while at the hospital. If the chief administrator of the hospital is anxious to have the citizen's experiences result in a positive attitude toward the hospital, he must provide a sound administrative structure which will effectively utilize the various community resources.

It is practically impossible to find a hospital staff which universally accepts the value of volunteer services. Many of the staff, including medical staff and department heads, will be somewhat reluctant to utilize volunteers in their services. Usually this reluctance is due to a lack of experience and knowledge in working with volunteers. The prime responsibility for setting the proper climate for volunteer services in the hospital rests with the chief administrator. He must reassure the staff that volunteer services has a specific contribution to make and define the ways in which it can contribute. The various department heads must be drawn into the early planning stages of the program. General policies regarding staff responsibility and lines of authority must be clarified at the outset.

It was mentioned earlier that sooner or later the volunteer services program will have to be taken over and administered by the hospital. Proper and effective administration of the program will require the establishment of a volunteer services office. Budgetary provisions will of necessity include the salaries of a full-time volunteer coordinator and a secretary, plus expenses for office equipment and supplies. A volunteer program cannot be viewed as a free or cheap service. It will cost money to staff the volunteer office. Staff time must be invested in recruiting, screening, and orienting the volunteers; considerable staff time will be devoted to the supervision of these volunteers. The hospital administration must be aware of the investment that is necessary to develop an effective volunteer services program, and it must be committed to the idea that the values to be derived are worth the investment. If these facts are not accepted, experience has proven that the program will flounder and eventually destroy itself.

Selection of Volunteer Services Coordinator

The single most important factor in the development of a volunteer services program is the employment of a professional volunteer services coordinator. This person should be experienced in community organization and possess a working knowledge of the hospital's basic objectives and goals. It will be impossible to select a person who has had specific college or university preparation in volunteer services administration since the development of training programs has not been accomplished at this time. It is important, however, that the volunteer services coordinator position be set forth in a job description like any other staff position. The job description can serve as a guide for both the volunteer services coordinator and hospital management. The following is a sample job description:

VOLUNTEER SERVICES COORDINATOR

Definition. This is professional administrative work in planning, organizing, and directing all volunteer services in a hospital.

Typical Work:

Acts as a liaison between community organizations and the hospital in matters pertaining to volunteer services.

Confers with hospital staff to determine needs which can be met by volunteer services in accordance with hospital policy and volunteer resources.

Interprets to the community hospital needs which can be met by volunteers and arranges for services and supplies which will meet the needs.

Establishes volunteer recruitment procedures; interviews, screens, orients, and assigns volunteers to the utilizing service.

Confers with departments on performance, promotion, reassignments and resignation of volunteers.

Keeps volunteers informed on pertinent hospital policies and procedures.

Prepares reports; keeps appropriate records.

Knowledge and Abilities:

Knowledge of hospital structure, function and treatment goals; group leadership principles and techniques; functions of community organizations; methods used to develop a coordinated program of volunteer services in a hospital setting; principles of supervision and inservice training.

Ability to plan, organize and direct a volunteer program as an integral part of the hospital treatment program; create and maintain harmonious relationships with hospital staff and volunteers; speak and write clearly and effectively; establish and maintain effective public relations between the hospital and community.

Minimum Experience and Educational Qualifications:

Graduation from an accredited college or university with a major in sociology, psychology, recreation, occupational therapy, social group work or public administration. (Since there are no specific degree curriculums as such, educational requirements must be, of necessity, flexible.)

Full-time paid experience in the organization of volunteer services or supervision of volunteers in a hospital setting.

There is considerable difference of opinion as to whether primary emphasis should be on experience in community organization or experience in one of the hospital clinical areas. Ideally, the candidate should have both types of experience; but, this combination is rarely seen. It is this writer's observation that those individuals who have a keen working knowledge of the various clinical departments, as well as the basic philosophy and goals of treatment, are most successful in developing a volunteer program which is, indeed, an integral part of the total treatment program. The volunteer coordinator must have genuine understanding of and appreciation for the goals and objectives of each clinical department. Hospital management should give this matter of experience considerable attention when employing a volunteer services coordinator.

Program Coordination

The "nerve center" for program coordination is the volunteer coordinator's office. Generally, aside from the office of the superintendent or hospital administrator, the one office in the hospital which will have the most contact with the community is that of the volunteer services coordinator. The major function of the volunteer services office is that of developing and coordinating relationships between the community and the hospital relative to the volunteer program. It is necessary therefore that adequate secretarial assistance be provided to insure continuity of office coverage and effective public relations with the community and hospital staff.

In an average size program, the employment of one full-time

secretary is adequate office assistance. If the volunteer program develops into one involving several-hundred regularly-assigned volunteers, plus considerable responsibility for community relations and public education, it will then be necessary to employ a professional assistant to the volunteer coordinator.

Several factors must be considered in the function of program coordination. One factor is the matter of discussing the volunteer program with staff. It is of vital importance that the staff understand that volunteers supplement staff services. At no time should volunteer service take the place of staff work. Hospital staff should understand the demands the program will make on them as well as its value to patients. The primary justification is better service to the patients served by the hospital. It takes a hospital staff who can recognize and appreciate the true contributions that volunteers make in the care, treatment, and rehabilitation of patients to train and use volunteers effectively. Services of volunteers, if planned for and integrated into the treatment program, can enhance patient treatment. It is now an established fact that when soundly organized, the contribution of volunteers effects not only patients but also the staff of the hospital and the citizens of the local community as well.

A second factor is that of coordinating the program with both the hospital staff and the various community organizations. Two commonly-used methods of achieving coordination are the volunteer services staff advisory committee and the hospital-community volunteer services council.

The establishment of a staff advisory committee for volunteer services is an essential aspect of the initial organization of this program. The committee can be of tremendous assistance to the volunteer services coordinator in evaluating the needs for volunteer services and the effectiveness of the various programs, and in screening and approving donation requests. This committee will serve to make certain that the volunteer program is hospital oriented. Such a committee should be composed of a representative from each department which will be utilizing volunteers, plus a representative from the business management section and the chief engineer. The need for representation from departments using volunteers is rather obvious; however, the need for representatives from the business office and the chief engineer's office may not be so clear. The latter two representatives are very important as the committee determines needs and priorities for material donations requested by the various departments. It is essential, for example, to know whether or not certain requests for material donations can be purchased from existing hospital appropriations before asking community organizations to donate them. Likewise, it is important to know whether the electric distribution system, water system, etc., are adequate to accommodate the installation of television sets, washers, and dryers before the volunteer coordinator makes official contact with the community outlining the need for such equipment. These are only a couple of examples of how the chief engineer and business office are involved in the staff advisory committee.

Many volunteer projects require interdepartmental planning if they are to be successfully implemented. Examples of such projects are the planning of hospital orientation courses for volunteers, planning of recognition ceremonies, establishing policies for general operation of the program and, as mentioned above, determining needs and priorities for material donations.

The volunteer services staff advisory committee represents the users of volunteer services. The volunteer services coordinator working together with this committee and the heads of departments represented on the committee should determine the specific needs for volunteers and volunteer programs. It will be necessary to work individually with the various departments and with all levels of departmental staff in order to determine the specific volunteer needs as well as the readiness to utilize volunteers. Volunteers should never be placed in a department that is not ready to utilize their services. There must be a specific task to be performed and adequate supervision available. It is essential that the departments to which volunteers are going to be assigned accept the responsibility for on-the-job training and on-going supervision.

Once the volunteer program has been organized within the hospital in terms of identifying basic objectives and determining needs, one can transfer his attention from the users and receivers of volunteer services to the providers and doers. The establish-

ment of a hospital-community volunteer services council to coordinate the requests and services of the community is an important program coordination and communication tool. The exact
organizational structure for such a council will depend on the
local administration. In general the organizational structure takes
on one of two administrative patterns. In one the hospital provides direction and leadership for the council's activities in great
detail. In the other the council acts on its own within general,
hospital-approved policies. In either instance, there must be a
close working relationship, with the volunteer services coordinator
serving as the liaison between the hospital and the council.

Membership on the council may be restricted to those national, state and local organizations which provide volunteer services, or it may be open to all volunteers who are working for the
hospital. Again, this is a decision that the local administration
must make. It is important that during the early phase of the
council's organization the superintendent participate actively to
demonstrate the hospital's interest and support, as well as to
make clear the need for the service which the council can provide.

The hospital-community volunteer services council will be
only as effective as it is supported and it is utilized by the hospital.
It can be used to recruit regular and occasional volunteers, procure material donations, and assist with special hospital projects,
such as the all—hospital carnival, fourth of July celebration, etc.
It can also serve as an excellent communcation tool for interpretation to and education of community and hospital staff. This
form of communication will save many hours for the volunteer
coordinator which he can devote to other aspects of his multi-
farious position.

Physical Facilities

In organizing a volunteer-services program, the development
of proper facilities and location for the volunteer services office is
very important. The volunteer services office should be located
so as to insure easy access for volunteers, and adequate parking
space close to the volunteer services office should be provided.
This office will be the hub for volunteer traffic, they will be going

to this office to apply for volunteer job assignments, to sign on duty, and to unload donations.

Adequate space should be provided for a separate office for the volunteer services coordinator and for his secretary. It is essential that the office be equipped with a telephone service that provides for easy access both inside and outside the hospital. There should be adequate office equipment, such as filing cabinets, clerical equipment and supplies. In addition to the basic office for the volunteer services coordinator and his secretary, there should be another room close by where the volunteers can safely store their personal effects. This room should be so designed that it can serve as a place to hold various meetings involving volunteers and also serve as a "home base" from which they can operate. In a large hospital where volunteers report directly to their specific geographical unit, this type of room may not be as essential as in the smaller hospital where the volunteer office area is the focal point when the volunteer is not actually with patients. Still a third room is needed for the temporary storage and safe keeping of volunteer donations.

It will be necessary to store material donations until they can be processed to the requesting departments. This may be a matter of only a few hours or, in some instances, a couple of days; but regardless, the safe-keeping of such donations is of vital importance. The close proximity of this storage room to the parking area is important. The need for adequate and attractive physical facilities for the volunteer services office cannot be stressed too much. This office is usually the first contact the volunteer has with the hospital. Consequently, he gains his first general impression of the hospital at this time.

Operating Budget

Reference has been made earlier in this chapter to the fact that volunteer services is not free. An operating budget is needed to provide for this service. The budget for volunteer services should include such items as salaries, equipment and supplies, travel, telephone, postage and printing. A miscellaneous expense fund should be set up to cover expenses incurred in connection with the orientation and recognition of volunteers. In general, the operating budget for volunteer services will be very small; but, it is important to recognize that a specific budget is indicated for the on-going success of the program operation.

ADMINISTRATION OF VOLUNTEER SERVICES

Once the framework for volunteer services has been set up, the volunteer services coordinator is in a position to really start working at the actual implementation of the program. Just as there are rather specific criteria used in organizing a volunteer services program, there is a basic sequence followed in the administration of the program. Before discussing this administrative sequence, we should first consider briefly the various types of volunteer services. In general, volunteer services can be classified into two broad areas: (1) direct services, and (2) indirect services. Both areas of service are beneficial, but the real focus of the volunteer program should be on direct services to patients. The emerging role of volunteers in the hospital programs of today means that volunteer services is no longer a peripheral activity but rather is an integral part of the total treatment environment.

Direct services are provided by both regular and occasional volunteers. Regular volunteers are those individuals who have been recruited to serve in a specifically-defined job situation. The primary emphasis is placed on direct patient contact assignments. All regular volunteers have completed a prescribed orientation and training course; they are usually scheduled weekly and are sent directly to the department which has requested their specific service. These volunteers will be working directly with patients on a continuous basis. Supervision and direction necessary for the volunteer to function effectively are provided by the departmental staff. Selected examples of areas in which volunteers may give direct service are: (1) social work—assist with finding employment and housing; (2) recreation—assist in conducting dance classes, individual and group music sessions, physical and social activities; (3) library—conduct book clubs and discussion groups, and (4) nursing—assist with feeding, grooming, and general socialization.

Occasional volunteers who provide direct services come to the hospital periodically, monthly or seasonally, depending on the needs and plans of the hospital. Their type of service does not have the same continuity or amount of direct contact with patients. They receive a brief orientation but seldom become involved in the on-the-job training sessions. Services provided by occasional volunteers might be in the form of entertainment, birthday parties, ward parties, and assistance with seasonal events such as Christmas, fourth of July, and Labor Day. Even though the occasional volunteers do not provide a continuous service, it is very important that adequate supervision be provided for them. No matter how brief or superficial their contacts with the hospital and patients might be, they still gain positive or negative impressions based on their experiences while at the hospital. It is essential that they understand the significance of their contribution and that staff be available to deal with any questions or problems they might have as a result of their visit at the hospital.

Indirect services which involve little or no contact with patients are also provided by both regular and occasional volunteers. Although the primary emphasis of the volunteer program is toward direct service to patients, it should be recognized that certain individuals want to assist in the welfare of patients but for various personal reasons do not want to or cannot serve them directly. Individuals and groups who are located too distant from the hospital or who do not have the time to provide direct service can serve through contributions of material and funds for the welfare of patients. It is imperative that regular volunteers providing indirect service complete the orientation and training session before starting on their assignment. The regular volunteer providing indirect service should have the same working knowledge of the total hospital operation as does his counterpart who is providing direct services. Selected examples of indirect services are: (1) receptionists—assist in social service, volunteer service, or at the information desk; (2) psychology—provide technical assistance in scoring tests, gathering test data, etc., and (3) clerical assistants—help with clerical duties in the various departments, wards, and clinic areas.

Superintendents, hospital administrators, and department

heads are cautioned against the idea that the first priority for volunteer services is that of providing free indirect services as described above. This belief is a definite potential pitfall which must be avoided lest they lose sight of the true mission; namely, providing better services for the patients.

Determining Needs for Volunteers and Material Donations

It has already been pointed out in our consideration of program coordination functions that the volunteer services coordinator working together with the volunteer services staff advisory committee and the heads of departments represented on the committee should determine the specific needs for volunteers. Once the specific needs have been mutually agreed upon it is desirable to develop a job description or assignment guide for each assignment. Responsibility for the development of the assignment guide should rest with the department requesting the volunteer services. The volunteer coordinator should be able to assist, if necessary, with the preparation of the assignment guide. The guide should include at least the following basic information: title of the job; description of the duties; days and hours of work; amount of supervision available and name of supervisor; location; skills and abilities needed; and any special characteristics of the assignment.

The assignment guide serves many useful purposes for both the volunteer coordinator and the department supervisor. On the basis of the assignment analysis and description, the volunteer coordinator can begin looking for suitable volunteer candidates. It can be used to interpret job opportunities to volunteer applicants; to clarify the specific responsibilities of the services to be rendered with both volunteers and staff; to place volunteers in specific assignments; and to interpret to the hospital staff the role of volunteers within the hospital.

Another consideration which should be discussed when determining the needs for volunteers is the specific amount and type of on-the-job training that will be necessary and available. Usually one of the more difficult tasks confronting the volunteer coordinator is that of getting the staff to accept the idea that on-the-job training is an essential aspect of using volunteers in the treatment program. Many times the staff will express the opinion that if on-the-job training is required as well as supervision, they would just as soon do the job themselves. The volunteer coordinator must be sure that adequate training and supervision will be available before making an assignment to any department. It is better to start slowly in making assignments than to rush ahead only to have many volunteers dissatisfied with their work. This will result only in poor volunteer morale and strained public relations.

The matter of material donations is still another consideration in determining the volunteer program needs. A department requesting volunteers must make up an assignment analysis and description; the same principle should be followed when the department requests a material donation. The request-for-donation form should include a detailed description of the requested donation; an explanation or justification of the need; name of staff member making request; and department head's approval. All requests for donations should be considered by either the volunteer services staff advisory committee or a separate donations request committee. The former committee can usually incorporate this function, thereby eliminating the need for the creation of still another hospital committee. It is essential that these requests be approved or disapproved by the committee rather than the volunteer coordinator. The committee should also assign a priority rating to all approved requests; this rating system can then serve as a guide for the volunteer coordinator as he works with the community in obtaining the items requested.

Recruitment Functions

Recruitment of volunteers is one of the key factors in the development of the total program. The recruitment functions involve giving talks to groups regarding recruitment; preparing recruitment literature; preparing publicity for the news media; contacting individuals and groups for service; and contacting individuals and groups for donations.

The volunteer coordinator must make a thorough analysis of the community resources in terms of service and material. This community resource survey should be taking place simultaneously with the process of determining needs for service in the hospital. It is important that the volunteer coordinator not only know about the existence of the various community organizations but also understand their basic objectives and goals. Further, he should develop a working acquaintance with the leadership group of these organizations.

Recruitment efforts must be carefully planned and coordinated to avoid the development of an attitude that all applicants will be accepted. Such an attitude results in poor public relations and a poor volunteer program. All recruitment efforts must be coordinated and approved by the volunteer services office in order to avoid confusion among staff and in the community. This statement does not mean that the only person permitted to recruit is the volunteer coordinator. Other hospital staff certainly can and should be involved in volunteer recruitment. However, their recruitment efforts must be in harmony with the total hospital needs and priorities. Usually, the best recruitment source is the volunteer already serving the hospital. Another excellent recruitment tool is the hospital-community volunteer council.

Generally it is best to use the aforementioned personal contacts for recruitment rather than the mass news media. There is a risk of creating the improper image of volunteer services in the hospital if the mass media are used. Another disadvantage of the mass appeal is that it may result in a number of volunteers who are responding to an emotional impulse, whose interest is only transient, and who are not qualified for the specific assignments requested. It is also possible that the mass appeal will recruit many more volunteers than the hospital can effectively use at the given time, and strained relationships will result if the volunteers must be turned away.

Volunteer Direction

A considerable amount of the volunteer service coordinator's time will be devoted to the general function of directing volunteers. In many ways the role of the volunteer coordinator in this area of volunteer direction is like that of the hospital personnel officer. It has often been said that the volunteer coordinator is a "personnel officer for volunteers." He is responsible for interviewing and screening applicants, orientation and training, assignment and reassignment, and recognition of volunteers. His is a staff function involving the users of volunteer services (departments), providers of volunteer services (organizations), doers of volunteer work (volunteers), and receivers of volunteer services (patients).[3]

Interviewing and Screening. The amount of skill and sound judgment involved in interviewing and screening volunteer candidates relates directly to the overall quality of the program. The volunteer coordinator should develop the special skills involved in interviewing. This process of interviewing and selecting volunteers is based on the requests for volunteer services and the assignment guides. The same techniques used in the selection of employees can be used for volunteers.

Specific criteria and policy to be used in the selection of volunteers are necessary to guide the volunteer coordinator in screening out those candidates not suited to the program. These should be worked out by the volunteer services coordinator and the volunteer services staff advisory committee. Policy should be established to cover minimum and maximum age, if any, for volunteers; employees of the hospital; former psychiatric patients; husbands or wives of staff members; and professional workers serving in their own area of specialization.

All applicants should be interviewed personally rather than depending on a telephone or written acceptance. The initial interview should be viewed as an opportunity for the volunteer coordinator to answer certain questions about the candidate and for the candidate to ask questions and learn more about the work to be done. It is generally desirable for the volunteer's application form to be filled out before the initial interview so that it can be used as a guide for the interview, as well as a partial screening device. The application should be kept on file as a source of information for the departments and for future reference. If the applicant seems to be particularly suited to one of the services requested, he should then be interviewed by the department requesting such services. This procedure is particularly important when special skills, knowledge or personality characteristics are required. In some instances there may be an agreement with the requesting department that they need not interview the candidate. However, the latter procedure should not be encouraged.

In most instances, it will be impossible to accept the applicant during the initial interview, but rather the applicant should be notified after everyone concerned has reached a decision. The rejection of an applicant is undoubtedly one of the most difficult tasks for the volunteer coordinator. However, he should realize that the patient's welfare comes first. Rejection of candidates is rather infrequent; but, when indicated, the issue must be faced and solved. The acceptance of an unqualified volunteer will result in effects worse than the possible poor public relations that might accompany the rejection of this person. A written summary of all interviews should be prepared and placed in the applicant's file.

Orientation and Training. The orientation session is the direct responsibility of the volunteer coordinator and on-the-job training is the direct responsibility of the department in which volunteers work. The coordinator of volunteer services must, however, see to it that the training is provided by the departments. It is standard operating procedure for all regular volunteers to attend an orientation course prior to service in the hospital.

Generally, the orientation course is offered quarterly or at least twice a year. Those individuals who begin service between orientation sessions are usually given an informal orientation by the volunteer services coordinator and assigned with one of the veteran volunteers. Ideally, this procedure should not be used; but, practically, it becomes necessary in order to sustain the volunteer's interest in the program. This session usually contains an introduction to the hospital philosophy, objectives, goals and administrative structure. Specific content, frequency, length and method of presentation should be developed and approved by the volunteer services staff advisory committee. Once the course has been developed the volunteer coordinator is responsible for its guidance and coordination. It will probably be necessary to offer the course both during the daytime and evening hours in order to accommodate those persons who will be serving evenings and who cannot get away from work during the day to attend.

Orientation for groups and individuals who serve on an occasional basis can best be handled individually by the volunteer coordinator along with the staff supervisor from the specific department in which the service is being rendered. Included in this abbreviated orientation is general information about the hospital; administrative policies, if any, that will affect their service; and specific information relative to their participation.

One should guard against the orientation and training sessions becoming sterile in both content and method of presentation. It is this writer's opinion that the sessions should be kept as informal as possible. Less emphasis should be placed on rules, regulations, keys, etc., and more emphasis placed on philosophy of treatment, hospital objectives and interpersonal relationships. It has been my experience that the best time to interpret most hospital policies is at the regular supervisory sessions held by the staff of the department in which the volunteer is giving service. Time spent in orientation and on-the-job training sessions for volunteers is time well spent in terms of quality of service to patients and community relations. These sessions are a vital aspect of the volunteer program and must be actively supported by the hospital staff. It is a well known and accepted fact that a well informed volunteer is the best ambassador the hospital can have in the community.

Assignment and Reassignment. The matter of properly assigning volunteers is one of the prime responsibilities of the coordinator of volunteer services. Matching the right volunteer with the right service requested is of utmost importance. Basic factors to be taken into consideration are the assignment guide, data from the application, applicant's preference, personality characteristics of the immediate staff supervisor, and the amount of supervision available. It should be clearly understood by both the volunteer and staff that if, for some reason, the initial assignment does not work out satisfactorily, reassignment can and will be encouraged. As a matter of fact, assignments should be reviewed periodically by the utilizing department and the volunteer coordinator to determine if a transfer, promotion, or continuance in the same job is indicated.

A sound volunteer program, functioning as an integral part of the total treatment program, must be based on the realistic needs of the various clinical departments. Assignments and reassignments will necessarily have to be based on the indicated needs for service rather than on the desires of the individual or group of volunteers.

Recognition. The final phase in the organization and administration of a volunteer services program is that of recognition. As human beings, we all have a need for our services to be recognized, be we staff or volunteers. Actually, recognition cannot be confined to a specific event such as the yearly volunteer recognition ceremony but rather it should be a continuous process.

Generally, recognition for volunteer services falls into two broad areas: direct and indirect. In many instances, the indirect recognition is the most important. One of the indirect forms of recognition is to make certain that the volunteer is working in a meaningful way. He should share responsibility for decision making in those areas which affect him. Approval by his peers for service performed is still another form of indirect recognition and reward. Indirect methods of recognition must be an inherent aspect of the volunteer's experience as he functions in the program. However, recognition derived from satisfaction with his job and approval from his colleagues and the professional staff with whom he works is not entirely adequate. The more tangible forms of reward must be provided too.

Awards in the form of certificates, pins, chevrons, or other symbols should also be given on a regularly scheduled basis at a public recognition ceremony. It is very important that the key supervisory and administrative staff be present at these recognition ceremonies. Public recognition ceremonies have been held both at the hospital and in the community with equal success.

Standards for the direct forms of reward should be kept high enough that they, indeed, have meaning to the recipients. Policies regarding the standards and nature of direct awards should be reviewed and recommended by the volunteer services staff advisory committee.

Administrative Functions

Organization of the volunteer services program and the general administration of volunteer services are both a part of the total administrative process. However, there are certain detailed administrative functions which should be identified as a part of the volunteer coordinator's responsibilities. Examples of such functions are: preparing reports; keeping records; supervising office staff; preparing specific forms to be used in the program; scheduling; developing a policy manual, and attending meetings.

The number and types of individual reports, records and forms used in the volunteer program must be determined at each hospital. It is customary to submit a report at least monthly to hospital management. A combination statistical and narrative report is usually the most satisfactory. The statistical aspect of this monthly report should list the departments where volunteers are serving; the number of both regular and occasional volunteers serving in each department; the number of hours served in each department by regular and occasional volunteers; the number of recruitment speeches given by the volunteer coordinator; the number of regular volunteers added and dropped; and the number of new volunteers oriented during the reporting period. The narrative aspect should focus on major problems, needs, accomplishments, etc., encountered during the reporting period.

Records are extremely important to the daily operation of the volunteer program as well as for evaluation purposes. Accurate records of hours served for each volunteer are a must as a basis for decisions regarding the type of annual awards the individual is entitled to receive. Although the volunteer many times will minimize the importance of keeping records on hours served, you will realize only too well how important the hours are to him if a public recognition ceremony is held and he is not given an award which he is entitled to or he is given credit for less hours than he actually served. There should be individual files kept for all regular individual volunteers. Files should also be kept on individuals and groups which donate materials. It is from these records that the volunteer coordinator can develop a resource file that can be used when recruiting for volunteers and donation requests.

Communication is a problem in any administrative process, including the administration of volunteer services. The development of operational forms can help to alleviate the communications problem. Several basic forms which should be used are: request for individual volunteer assignment; volunteer application; donation request; request for volunteer entertainment or party; volunteer information card (includes record of service hours and general data), and donation receipts.

The development of a policies and procedures manual for volunteer services is mandatory. The manual should include policies covering the areas of recruitment, selection, orientation, assignment, supervision, and recognition of volunteers. Other areas of operation which should be included in the manual are policies related to volunteer dress, attendance, insurance coverage, minimum and maximum age for volunteers, forms, records, and reports that are to be used.

Community Relations

Community relations and public education are natural by-products of the volunteer program. The volunteer services coordinator is normally involved in conducting tours for prospective volunteers; speaking to community groups and organizations to explain the volunteer program; preparing literature relative to the volunteer program; preparing news releases on volunteer activities; and arranging for publicity concerning this program.

There is a growing trend toward combining the public information and education functions with the functions of the volunteer services office. The volunteer services coordinator will many times be the single hospital staff person most uniquely qualified to carry out the duties of the public information and education officer. In the event that hospital management decides to assign these functions to the volunteer services coordinator, serious consideration should be given to the hiring of an assistant volunteer coordinator.

In order to insure continuity in the public relations and public education program, it is imperative that one office be responsible for the following functions; planning tours for high school, college, and general public groups; developing a speakers bureau; developing special educational programs for both professional and lay groups; and preparing fact sheets, house organ, news releases, and all publicity for the hospital.

Hospital management must not underestimate the need for a well planned and structured community relations program. Community acceptance of the hospital and its treatment program is a most important factor in the realization of the hospital's basic objectives.

TRENDS IN VOLUNTEER SERVICES

The future is nothing more than an extension of the present; therefore, it seems that we can view some of the trends based on the ever-changing medical care and treatment practices.

Medical treatment for both the physically and the mentally ill emphasizes emergency care in the hospital with follow-up services being provided in the community. It is also true that the treatment team now includes several non-medical professions and services not present in past years. As volunteer services is gradually added to this team in the true sense, the role of the volunteer will change. We are already seeing the volunteer image change from the "Lady Bountiful" to one who has a definite role in the total treatment program.

It follows that as more of the follow-up care, treatment and rehabilitation takes place outside of the hospital facilities as such, the future volunteers will be working in a closer relationship with the hospital and the community. The hospital volunteer program will concern itself more with assisting in the follow-up services for discharged patients.

A trend which has already started is the utilization of teen-agers and college students in the volunteer programs. These young people represent not only a vast army of volunteers but also potential health science professionals so desperately needed. The possibility of using senior citizens as volunteers is still relatively unexplored. Herein lies a vast amount of valuable experience and skill which should be used in our mission to assist the physically and the mentally ill.

There is growing concern regarding the volunteer service co-ordinator's training and experience necessary to perform optimally as a professional staff member in the medical setting.[5] Concepts of educational requirements, experience, innate abilities, and personality characteristics necessary for this position will be crystalized in the future. So far, no generally accepted course of formal training or professional standards have been established for this relatively new position. These too will come about in the future as will the continued growth and development of the American Association of Volunteer Services Coordinators.

* * * *

In conclusion, it is reiterated that the volunteer services program cannot function effectively until the administration of the hospital is willing to give it full support and until there is adequate departmental supervision for the individual volunteer. The treatment team must decide where services which can be performed by volunteers are needed. Once these factors have been established, the hospital is in a position to utilize community services to assist in the total treatment program for its patient population. This type of organization and administration will result in more benefit to the patient and in better community understanding, support, and public relations.

REFERENCES

1. Bolstad, Glenna L., and Ginsberg, S. T.: Volunteer workers in state mental hospitals. *State Government, XXXV:1*, 53-56, 1962.
2. *The Volunteer and the Psychiatric Patient.* Washington, D. C., American Psychiatric Association, 1959.
3. *Volunteer Services in Mental Hospitals.* New York, National Association for Mental Health, 1961.
4. *Brief History and Informational Data of the American Association of Volunteer Services Coordinators.* Washington, D. C., American Association of Volunteer Services Coordinators and American Psychiatric Association, 1964.
5. *Job Activity-Time Survey.* Washington, D. C., American Association of Volunteer Services Coordinators and American Psychiatric Association, 1964.

Part II
Elements of the Activity Therapy Service

Chapter IX

PATTERNS OF ORGANIZATION*

A T THE PRESENT TIME, most hospitals are classified according to their relationship with the community, as either clinical, the type of patients they treat, or ownership and control according to MacEachern.[1] The two types of hospital classifications are listed below:

Clinical	*Ownership and Control*
General	Governmental
Special	Federal
Medicine	Army
Internal medicine	Navy
Nervous and mental	Air Force
Tuberculosis	Veterans
Children	Administration
Communicable diseases	U.S. Public
Venereal diseases	Health Service
Surgery	State
Eye, ear, nose, and throat	County
Orthopedic	City
Diseases of women	Nongovernmental
Cancer	Church
Industrial	Fraternal order
Maternity	Community
Chronic diseases	Private-not for profit
Convalescent	Private-for profit

HOSPITAL ORGANIZATIONAL STRUCTURES**

All hospitals, regardless of size and type, have some sort of an organizational structure dealing with the arrangement of the

*The Hoover Commission recommended the following hierarchy of titles for organizational units with Federal agencies; departments, services, bureaus, divisions, branches, sections, and units.

**For a discussion of the structures of hospitals as they relate to patient care, see Brown, Ester: *Newer Dimensions of Patient Care, Part I, 1961,* and *Part II,* 1962, Russell Sage Foundation, New York. For discussion concerning psychiatric facilities, see Emerging Patterns of Administration in Psychiatric Facilities, *Psychiatric Studies and Projects,* 2, No. 9, Published by American Psychiatric Association, June, 1964.

operating departments and facilitating divisions. MacEachern[2] states that "of all modern enterprises, none is more complex than the hospital . . . (and) only by organization in the hospital, can efficiency be produced."

Nearly all hospitals have at their head a board of directors or trustees who act as a governing board and whose responsibility it is to see that adequate service is rendered by the particular hospital. In recent years, within state mental hospitals, the board of trustees is primarily an honorary position to act in an advisory position to the particular hospital. Many state departments of mental health or mental hygiene have a similar advisory board. The reader may draw the conclusion that the public may at times be very weakly represented because the board only advises or makes recommendations which may be accepted or not. But the public within the institutions are also represented through the democratic process; namely, the legislative, judicial, and executive branches which ultimately affect the operation of the hospital. On the other hand, the governing board within general hospitals "must always be regarded as the supreme authority in the hospital, the body to which the director, the medical staff, the personnel and all auxiliary organizations are directly or indirectly responsible."[3]

The governing board delegates their authority of administration to an administrator who may either be a physician or a lay administrator and who, in turn, is responsible to the governing board. Specifically, the duties of the governing board which are performed through the administrative officer, may be divided into three groups: "(1) responsibility for selection of competent personnel; (2) control of hospital funds and (3) supervision of the physical plant."[4] The administrator may, in large hospitals, appoint one or more assistants to relieve him of part of his duties.

Each general hospital is made up of a medical staff who has been appointed by the governing board, and who, in turn, is responsible to the governing board and the administrator of the hospital. In many instances, the medical staff is organized and operates largely outside hospital administration. This, at times, presents difficulties, as Brown[5] comments, "The very fact that there are two competing hierarchies frequently results in the weakening of the social structure of the (organizational) chart and in causing great confusion." The medical staff is usually divided into honorary, consulting, active, associate, and courtesy groups. The active medical staff are those selected to attend the "indigent sick" and are most actively interested in the hospital. The medical staff function is as follows: "providing professional care of the sick and injured in the hospital; maintaining its own efficiency; self-government; participating in education; auditing the professional work; and furnishing advice and assistance to the administrator."[6]

Every physician who has been appointed, has made application in writing, his credentials reviewed by the credentials committee who have made a report to the medical staff, and has been recommended by the medical staff with final approval by the governing body.[7]

A distinction should be made here between the "closed" and "open" types of general hospitals.

> "A 'closed hospital' is one in which all professional services, private and charitable, are provided and controlled entirely by the attending or active medical staff. No other physicians are permitted to treat patients in the hospital except under consulting agreement with members of the medical staff and approval of the governing board.
>
> An 'open hospital' is one in which there is an attending or active medical staff responsible for the *treatment of charity cases,* but in which other physicians—generally known as the courtesy medical staff—are permitted to utilize the private room facilities, provided there is full compliance with the rules and regulations of the institution and such standard technical procedures as may be formulated by the attending or active medical staff and adopted by the hospital."[8]

The hospital departments group themselves into two divisions, one concerned with the professional care of the patient, and the other with business management. The various departments that make up a large general medical and surgical hospital include the clinical departments or divisions of medicine (internal medicine, pediatrics, dermatology, etc.), surgery (general, obstetrics and gynecology, orthopedic, etc.), general practice and physical medicine and rehabilitation. Smaller hospitals will usually have only departments of medicine and surgery. Other departments and facilities include nursing (including nursing education, if the program is affiliated with the hospital and central supply service), adjunct diagnostic and therapeutic facilities (laboratory, radiology, anesthesiology, physical and occupational therapy, electrocardiography, pharmacy, and dental service), dietary, medical records, outpatient, admitting, business, and service, (mechanical maintenance, housekeeping, and laundry).[9] It is possible that some hospitals will also include, in addition to the above, a medical social service department and a medical library (including nursing and patient libraries). Small hospitals or specialty hospitals may combine one or more of the above mentioned departments. Each of these departments will have a department head who will be responsible to the hospital director or administrator.

Although there is a trend away from specialty hospitals, these hospitals or special units of general medical and surgical hospitals will usually follow basic principles of organization. These hospitals usually restrict their treatment to the following: pediatrics; orthopedics; geriatrics; poliomyelitis; chronically ill; physically and mentally handicapped (adults and children); alcoholic; drug addict; epileptic; tuberculosis; and communicable diseases.

If any of the above are affiliated units with a general hospital, they may have an administrator who is an assistant to the hospital administrator. In special hospitals, the medical staff (resident physician or physicians) will be under the supervision of a board of directors or where outside physicians and surgeons are used exclusively, they will be members of the staff of local general hospitals. The various department arrangements in specialty hospitals will be similar to those found in general hospitals although their size will be determined by the size of the particular hospital.

State hospitals for treatment of the mentally ill or retarded will follow an organizational pattern similar to what is found in general medical hospitals. But a major difference between the general hospital and state mental hospital is that the director is usually referred to as the superintendent and is a physician who has specialized in neurology, psychiatry, or both. In most instances, the superintendent has also been certified by the American Board of Psychiatry and Neurology with two or more years of mental hospital administration experience and may or may not be certified as a hospital administrator by the American Psychiatric Association. There have been instances where lay administrators have been appointed as superintendent. One major reason given for this type of appointment is that the specialized training of the psychiatrist or neurologist can be better utilized in contact with patients.

The superintendent of state hospitals are usually appointed to their position by the Governor and/or Commissioner or Director of Mental Health or Director of Welfare of the particular state. In addition to the superintendent, there may be an assistant superintendent and a clinical director or just an assistant superintendent-medical who is responsible for the overall supervision of all clinical areas. An example of the latter is found in Indiana. Also, there will be a business administrator or assistant superintendent-business (Indiana) who has the responsibility for the business affairs of the hospital. While the superintendent is appointed, the other positions within the hospital, including physicians, are usually filled through civil service examinations.

The various departments that make up an average state hospital include social services; psychology, nursing, including central supply and nursing education; activity therapy service; volunteer services; dental; laboratory; and chaplaincy in the clinical services, and medical records; personnel; housekeeping; storeroom; dietary; canteen; maintenance; and farming responsible in the business services. Staffings in hospitals for the retarded are essentially the same as mental hospitals except for the addition of school departments. More and more hospitals treating the mentally ill are employing and developing educational therapy departments.

Since patients in state mental hospitals have similar physical problems as those in general hospitals, facilities are provided for the aged patient, tubercular, and acute medical and surgical patient. In some states, because of the location and size of various hospitals, one hospital within the state will be designed to handle all tubercular patients or other physical problems. Medical and surgical units within the state hospitals will staff this unit similar to those general hospitals in the community. Usually one state hospital handles those patients judged "criminally insane." These hospitals may be a unit of the state prison, a unit of the state mental hospitals, or a separate hospital completely. The staffings patterns and administration will be similar to what is found in other types of state hospitals except for the addition of security personnel.

The Veterans Administration* hospitals have similar organizational structures except there is a change in job titles—Hospital Director or Manager, Assistant Hospital Director (Business) ; and Director of Professional Services (Chief of Staff). The manager may be a physician but not always, and his duties entail running the hospital as a hospital within the community. Depending upon the size and type of hospital the following are the services responsible to the Director of Professional Services; medical; surgical; psychiatry-neurology; tuberculosis; dental; nursing; physical medicine and rehabilitation; radiology; laboratroy; dietetics; social services; pharmacy; and chaplaincy. The business side includes the canteen officer; registrar; fiscal; personnel; supply; engineering; and housekeeping.[10]

ACTIVITY THERAPY ORGANIZATIONAL STRUCTURES

Activity therapy service is a department service within the total hospital organization resulting from a reorganization required by expansion of the various services during the last twenty years. This organization has been necessary for reasons of formal communication; but it has also been necessary to establish executive administration, that is, those specializing in the administrative function—superintendent, (administrator) ; chief of staff, (clinical director or assistant superintendent) ; business admini-

*In 1930, laws were pasesd by Congress which consolidated all federal government agencies and bureaus concerned with veterans under one agency head and established this agency as the Veterans Administration.

strator; coordinator of activity therapy service, (rehabilitation services) ; nursing director etc. Within any organization, there are several organized areas, usually with one director, and these form the executive administration. In a hospital, as in business, one department often functions in or contributes services to several different departments.

The coordinator should, from time to time, consider the departmentation of activities under his direction, the focus of operating responsibilities, and the general structural arrangements. There are questions of structure even within the various specialties that make up the activity therapy service although this may be somewhat limited due to the number of therapists, and program of activities. Nevertheless, the ability to think of organization as an integrated whole instead of a series of semi-independent parts is a distinct asset.

It is desirable that in developing the organization structure that all positions which report to the coordinator or director be of the same position grade. The advantage in having this even strata is partly a matter of attitude and morale among the service units. In addition, department heads are more likely to have equal education and training, similar degrees of responsibility, as well as similar departmental problems; therefore, a proper balanced perspective is maintained on all levels of operation. Also, supervision is made easier because of results of a service unit can be readily compared and possibly applied to those of other service units.

The best guide in deciding which services should be grouped together is the extent to which the activities of the respective services fit together in the overall programming of the hospital and hospital policies. To this end, the organizational structure will vary according to the size of each service unit, the objectives of each service within the total framework of the activity therapy service and the hospital, the personnel and equipment available, time available for conducting activities, the service heads available, types of delegations, and contacts with other services outside of the activity therapy service.

The organization of any business can be shown graphically in an organizational chart. Basically, such a chart for activity therapy

reveals the various functions of the service and shows the relationship between different department heads and personnel who are
assigned within the various specialties. Although some people may
joke about charts, they do represent what is intended in the interest of the purpose of the enterprise. The reader is cautioned
that an on-going organization is not always identical with an
organizational chart at any one time, any more than a constitution is interpreted the same way all the time.*

There are many varieties of organizational plans, but the one
most frequently used within an Activity Therapy Service is the
"line plan" whereby communications are transmitted from the
coordinator to the department heads without interference. This
plan provides for both control and coordination of activities. Although this plan is the simplest and highly efficient, the writer
prefers the merging of the "line plan" with the "staff plan." The
significant advantage of the combination plan is that no coordinator has complete knowledge of all the specialties; therefore, the
"staff" helps him to overcome his own limitations. He is similar
to a general in the field who benefits from the thinking of others
and gains experience from it. In addition, the plan retains the
principle of directness and the advantage of specialization.[10a]

The activity therapy service in large hospitals may be looked
upon, to some degree, as decentralized according to specialties.
The coordinator delegates authority to each unit; that is, the
assignment of self-government and administration to each specialty
under the authority of that department head. In small hospitals,
this type of decentralization may not be needed. How much decentralization takes place is depended upon the amount of independent authority vested in the decentralization unit.[11] The more
experience the department head attains, the more decentralization
can be. On the other hand, uniformity may be required over
budgetary procedures, classification of personnel, programming,
and interpersonal conflicts. Yet these must be combined with the
difficulties and complexities of the various delegated job. "It has

---

*For a discussion of organizational control in voluntary hospitals, see Perrow,
Charles: The analysis of goals in complex organizations, *American Sociological Review*, 26:857-861, 1961.

been demonstrated that the administrator is not strained merely in direct proportion to the number of people under his direct surveillance but in complex and multiplied proportion, because these very individuals form relationships that pose problems of their own fresh kind: new group individualities with which he must cope from out of twos, threes, and fours, and so forth."[12]

The administrative organizational structure of activity therapy or similar services vary tremendously among the various public and private agencies. Since these structures vary so much, samples of typical organizational charts are hereby employed to give this information.

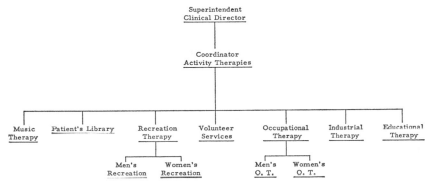

Figure 3. Organizational Chart, Athens State Hospital, Athens, Ohio (courtesy of Athens State Hospital).

Figure 3 shows the organizational structure of the activity therapies within a hospital for the mentally ill in Ohio. Each specialty is a separate department with its own department head who is directly responsible to the coordinator who, in turn, is responsible to the clinical director. The coordinator, in addition to being responsible to the clinical director, may be directly or indirectly responsible to a state consultant in activity therapy.

Gilbert's[13] definition of consultation is interesting to note here. "Consultation takes place in a work-centered, problem-solving situation. A helping relationship is developed through which the consultant gives his knowledge, skills, and experience, and the consultee gives his knowledge skills, and experience in

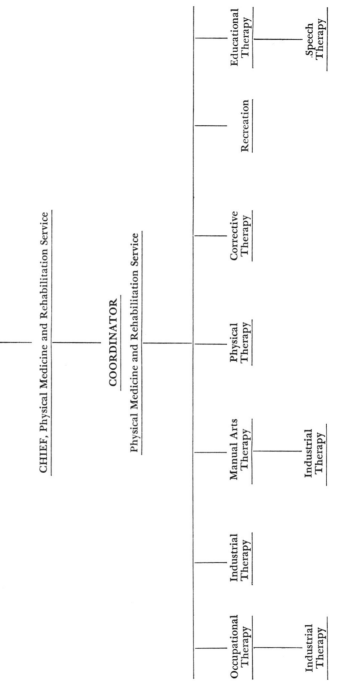

Figure 4. Organizational Chart, Veterans Administration, Washington, D.C. (courtesy of Veterans Administration).

the specific situation to the end that planning can be done and action taken, with the consultee left free to choose and carry out the plan and action." In addition, the consultant usually helps in solving both inter and intradepartment problems, which cannot be solved at the local level, clarifying central office policies, recruiting, conducting workshops, and evaluating programs.

Figure 4 shows a typical physical medicine and rehabilitation service organizational structure in a Veterans Administration hospital.

Figure 5 shows an activities department in a private psychiatric hospital.

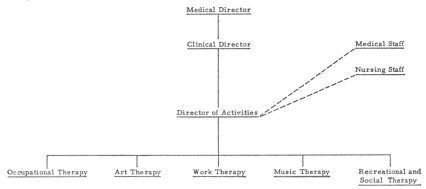

Figure 5. Organizational Chart, Highland Hospital, Ashville, North Carolina (courtesy of Highland Hospital).

Activity Therapy Patterns of Operation

There are to be found a considerable number of different operating patterns within the activity therapy service of the various hospitals. In some services, we still find a traditional pattern of service to be provided by one department and that department only. In others, we find that the various departments will interchange in their personnel and activities if the activities are closely related to their own or if there is a total hospital program such as a special holiday program. Then still, we find services where there is a continual interchange of personnel and activities to the extent that the personnel may lose their professional identification. And finally, we have activities which are conducted by therapist who can do the best job regardless of professional identification. Although the latter would be preferred, it is not always feasible because of professional identification, ethics, personality factors, organizational structure, and hospital policies.

In general medical hospitals, we find the various specialties maintaining their traditional roles although occupational therapy and recreation will interchange or relieve on certain activities. Specialty hospitals, if they have more than one specialty conducting programs, will have more enterchange of personnel and activities than the general medical hospital. The most enterchange of personnel and activities are found in state or private hospitals treating the mentally ill or retarded.

The following exemplifies two operating patterns: one in operation within the state hospitals in California and the other a suggested pattern.

The hospitals in California operate under a program referred to as the "Divisional System." Each hospital has three or more assistant superintendents, each of whom is responsible for one large segment of the hospital, such as acute treatment service, children services, gereatric services, and so forth. Each of the medical and paramedical services have been realigned to work as members of the "divisional team." The various therapists: occupational, recreational, music, industrial, and so forth are assigned to a division where they not only perform services in their own specialty but assist in the motivating and training of other personnel to engage patients in diversified activities. Within the rehabilitation services, there are a number of "Assistant Supervisors of Rehabilitation Services" depending upon the organizational structure of the hospital who may be responsible for the rehabilitation program within a "divisional system," ward services program, centralized services program, or industrial therapy section. It may also be added California has also instituted the use of these rehabilitation services within their day treatment centers.

Another pattern of operating is suggested by Doniger and Dundon.[14] They suggest three divisions designated as: (1) "the unit programmer," (2) "the skill specialist," and (3) "the work specialist." The "unit programmer" would be responsible for planning the patient's day after observing their relationships with each other, and with staff members. He would maintain contact with the medical staff, consult and teach skills to ward personnel, consider the number of patients available for activities in relation to the number of therapists available, and help in the direction of what patients should be involved in the other two divisions. In essence, the "unit programmer" would "attempt to fill the significant gaps in hospital routine which activity programs should fill." The "skill specialist" would develop specific program based upon the needs of the patients, regardless of wards or buildings. The "work specialist" would be concerned with developing a program of work for the patient. The "work specialist" like the "skilled specialist" may either work on the wards with the "unit programmer," or in a centralized place. As Doniger and Dundon[14] point out, the therapist would be assigned by "interest and talents" rather than by training.

Relationship of Activity Therapy Service to Other Departments

It is now advisable to consider the relationship of the departments that make-up the total hospital with that of the activity therapy service. Just as mutual understanding and respect is essential within the activity therapy service, so understanding and cooperation is essential externally. The problems of relationship to a greater degree are unfolded in the character of the duties performed by each of the other hospital departments and the activity therapy service. A wise coordinator will be certain that each of his department heads and their staff members understand the scope of all other departments and services within the hospital, and are aware of the role of each in the total organizational plan.

In the unfolding of patient care, there has been a combination of clinical services and business services that has developed with the hospital. This usually follows: (1) the medical staff; nursing; psychology; social services; physical rehabilitative or activity therapy; pharmacy; dietary, chaplaincy; and various diagnostic departments with the clinical services, and (2) fiscal; personnel; clerical records; housekeeping; laundry, and maintenance within the business service. In addition, there are those individuals who are observed as being with both services—governing boards, hospital and/or business administrators, superintendents or a combination of these.

For an appreciation of the application of these various services to the coordinator and the activity therapy service in general, it is important that we give some consideration as to their administration and duties. The following may be found in all hospitals, institutions, homes, schools, etc.

Hospital Administrator or Superintendent. At the hospital head and in direct charge is the hospital administrator or superintendent depending upon the type of hospital. He may be a doctor or a lay administrator who should meet the standards developed by the American College Administrators, American Academy of Medical Administrators, or the American Psychiatric Association's Committee in Certification of Mental Hospital Administrators. For a general description of the duties of the administrator, we quote from the *Descriptions and Organizational Analysis for Hospitals and Related Health Services:*[15] "Administers, directs, and coordinates all activities of hospital, to carry out its objectives as to care of sick and injured, furtherance of scientific knowledge, and participation in promotion of community health: Carries out program within policies and by general directives from a governing board. Promotes favorable public relations. Negotiates for improvement of hospital buildings and equipment. Coordinates activities of medical staff with those of other departments. Recommends and develops policies and procedures for various hospital activities. Performs related administrative and supervisory duties to insure efficient operation of hospital."

As one can see, the administrator coordinates the activities of the medical staff and other staff personnel. Regarding treatment, the physician is in authority. His orders are given to all concerned with the treatment and care of the patient and the administrator is responsible to seeing that these duties are carried out unless they violate hospital policies.

The coordinator, like all other department or service heads, must acknowledge the authority that is exercised by this individual. Activity therapy service are but a part of the total service and the hospital administrator is responsible for representing the whole; therefore, his authority is to fit together the parts that make the whole. The coordinator's relationship with him varies with the particular type of hospital. In the general medical and surgical hospitals, there may be limited contact except in relation to personnel and fiscal matters while in the state or specialty hospitals there may be considerable contact, especially if the coordinator reports directly to the superintendent. If the latter point is so, then, those duties as outlined in Chapter I are discussed. The various service departments within Activity Therapy usually have little contact with the superintendent since the coordinator represents the activity therapy service.

Assistant Superintendents or Administrators, Chief of Staff, or Clinical Director. Any one hospital may have all three of these positions functioning at one time within the hospital. The assistant superintendent may be a medical or non-medical person while the chief of staff and clinical director are always medical persons. Depending upon the organization and type of hospital, the assistant superintendent or administrator is responsible only for assisting the administrator or, in large hospitals, have assigned duties such as responsibility for the business management or for a particular unit of the hospital. As is the case in many state institutions, the assistant superintendent may be the clinical director or be a separate position whereby he assumes the responsibilities of the clinical director; then he is responsible for the overall development and supervision of the entire clinical services (medical services and staff, psychology, social service, nursing, etc.) In most instances, regardless of the type of hospital, the coordinator will report to this individual and fulfill those duties and responsibilities as discussed in Chapter I. The chief of staff is usually found in the Veterans Administration hospital and has the same duties as the clinical director. Here the coordinator reports to the chief of physical medicine, and rehabilitation services. In the large general medical and surgical hospital, the chief of staff is responsible for the medical staff and has very little contact with the Coordinator.

Business Department. This department embraces certain sections or units which do not have direct contact with the patient but are directly essential to the welfare of the patient. In general medical hospitals and specialty hospitals, these sections or units may be divided into two groups: one concerned with business affairs and the other responsible for maintenance service. In small hospitals, it may be necessary to combine various sections or units, while in large hospitals they may have their own unit head. An example is a state hospital where there are separate units with the business administrator responsible for the overall supervision.

The coordinator usually maintains close contact with the unit or representative concerned with purchasing and supply since he is responsible for the development of the budget for his service and the requisitioning of equipment and supplies. The various services within activity therapy should have only limited contact except for clarification of specific items, since the Coordinator represents again the total service.

Physicians. The physician is responsible for the welfare of the patients. Usually, the various services within activity therapy have more contact with the ward physician than does the coordinator. The coordinator does have the responsibility of interpreting the activity therapy service as a whole to the physicians as well as allowing as much time as possible for all staff members to work with the physician. In the general medical and surgical hospitals, a close professional relationship will be developed between the physician and therapist since much of the program is conducted on a prescription basis.

Nursing Department. Within the nursing department there may be a number of units or sections such as clinical nursing, nursing education, and central supply. The coordinator is usually in direct contact at all times with the director of nursing, especially in the development of a program schedule and resolving interdepartmental difficulties. Staff personnel maintain a close professional relationship with ward nursing personnel since they are in contact with the patient twenty-four hours a day and are fully aware of the patient's condition. The coordinator or department heads may assume a close contact with the nursing education section if student nurses are to receive training in the activity therapies or if activity therapy interns are to receive some training within the education unit.

Personnel Department. This department is responsible for employment procedures, training, and health and safety welfare of the personnel. The relationship between this department, the coordinator, and staff is discussed in Chapter X.

Service Departments. The departments which are included here are maintenance, housekeeping, laundry, and engineering. The coordinator usually maintains the contact with these departments, especially the chief engineer, although other department heads may have contact with the various services from time to time. Least it be forgotten, one of the primary accomplishments achieved by the development of the activity therapy coordinator's position was that much of the communication and working with other departments outside of the activity therapy service could be achieved by the coordinator. Previously the same kind of problems, which were common to all departments in the activity therapy service, were being discussed, for example, with the chief engineer, by each of the activity therapy department heads.

Other Departments. Contact with dietary, social service, psychology, and medical records departments depends upon the nature of the situation. There are times that the social service and psychology departments well be interested in individual patients and, therefore, may contact the activity therapy staff. For example, in the area of contributing to discharge planning, both in terms of describing the patient as the activity therapist sees him at this time, as well as recommending or suggesting various outside resources regarding leisure-time activities. Another area would be the vocational and industrial therapy department working closely with both social service and psychology in terms of their respective operations. Then too, staff members may need to know the background of the patient to provide adequate treatment and assistance.

In summary a wise hospital administrator will learn to develop administrative meeting in which (1) a group of major department heads will meet weekly or perhaps daily, and (2) a group consisting of all department heads or supervisors to meet monthly or occasionally. Regular meetings of both groups are found to have developed a sense of participation in the affairs of the hospital, swift means of communication, and errors and grievances can be cleared up—for example, problems of recruitment.

A word of caution before closing this chapter. Each hospital is a unique institution; therefore, their pattern of organization will vary according to the organizational plan most feasible for that particular hospital.

REFERENCES

1. MacEachern, Malcolm T.: *Hospital Organization and Management.* Rev. 3rd Ed., Chicago, Physicians Record Company, 1957, p. 34-5.
2. *Ibid.,* p. 83.
3. *Ibid.,* p. 90.
4. *Ibid.,* p. 91.
5. Brown, Esther L.: *Newer Dimensions of Patient Care.* New York, Russell Sage Foundation, 1962, Part 2, p. 65.
6. MacEachern, *op. cit.* p. 159.
7. *Ibid.,* p. 161-62.
8. *Ibid.,* p. 169-70.
9. *Ibid.*
10. Organization Chart, Veterans Administration, Washington, D. C. Form V-9.
10a. Terry, George R.: *Principles of Management.* Rev. Ed. Homewood, Illinois, Richard D. Irwin, Inc., 1956, p. 290-292.
11. Truman, David: *Administration Decentralization.* Chicago, Illinois, 1938.
12. Finer, Herman: *Administration and The Nursing Services.* New York, MacMillan Company, 1952, p. 227-8.
13. Gilbert, Ruth: Functions of the consultant, *Teachers College Record, 61* (4) :179, 1960.
14. Doniger, Joan, and Dundon, H. Dwyer: Administrative planning of patient activity programs in mental hospitals, *A.J.O.T., XIV* (5) , 1960.
15. *Job Descriptions and Organizational Analysis for Hospitals and Related Health Services.* U. S. Government Printing Office, Washington, D. C., 1952, p. 21.

Chapter X

ADMINISTRATIVE MANAGEMENT

Management results from the properly mixing of all the elements of the foregoing chapters — program planning (to include facilities, equipment, and supplies), education, evaluation, research, and the previous chapter on organizing, to achieve a desired end — meeting the objectives. It is a tool for achieving objectives. As Klicka[1] comments: "Given a clearly defined objective, with proper short-range and long-range planning available to guide the organization toward that objective, plus practical and functional organizational structure with a well trained executive at its head, good management should be expected." Unfortunately, very few coordinators or directors of an activity therapy service have had executive training. Terry[2] states that management "is a process of basic functions . . . (it) provides effectiveness to human efforts . . . (it) brings order to endeavors . . . it helps achieve better equipment . . . services, and human relations. It keeps abreast of changing conditions, and it supplies foresight and imagination."

Directly related to the activity therapy service, the Veterans Administration states that the Physical Medicine and Rehabilitation Service mission is to insure that rehabilitation services are provided. These services are accomplished through "the media of recruitment of personnel, establishment of standards, promoting educational programs for staff, residents, and affiliate trainee; encouraging and implementing research studies (basic or applied); establishing program designs which reflect changing trends in emphasis and treatment, and the dissemination of information. . ."[3]

This chapter will be concerned with three aspects of management not covered in other chapters of this book: (1) personnel management to include planning for personnel and supervisory structure; (2) business management, including records and reports, finances, standards, and inventory, and (3) ethics.

247

PERSONNEL MANAGEMENT*

Planning for Personnel

It is well, before getting into the specifics of planning for personnel within an activity therapy service or any type of rehabilitation service, to review personnel planning for the total agency. Therefore, the author would like to prevail upon the reader again to quote from a reference he has had occasion to use in his administrative practices. Many of these references can be applied to the specific service of which we are discussing.

"First, the agency must determine and classify the total work required to carry out the program within the framework of designated objectives and policies.

"Second, the agency must classify the total work into primary constituent kinds of work; that is, program, business management, administration, and so forth.

"Third, the agency must divide the work as so classified into manageable components, positions, or jobs.

"Fourth, the agency must group like jobs together into an orderly pattern of organization or structure.

"Fifth, the agency must define salary and wage policies for all positions.

"Sixth, the agency must define responsibility and accountability lines and relationships for each position, and must spell out the relationships between positions.

"Seventh, the agency must establish supervisory controls and relationships and develop a program of supervision.

"Eighth, the agency must organize time schedules for all workers on weekly, monthly, and annual basis.

"Ninth, the agency must develop a system of intercommunication and cooperation so that all workers will engage themselves as team members.

"Tenth, the agency must develop a plan for appraising, measuring and readjusting work loads in relation to evolving standards and changing circumstances."[4]

*An interesting pamphlet concerned with appraisal of personnel programs is "Evaluating . . . Your Personnel Management." U. S. Government Printing Office, Washington, D. C., 1954.

Planning for the number and types of therapists needed can be handled in any of several ways. Therapists may be added as needs arise, according to previously determined quotes, or by staffing ratios where the types and numbers to be treated are adequately predictable. The latter approach has been met with varying opinions. Whichever method is used depends upon the arrangement that has been worked out between the hospital administrator, personnel director, and coordinator. The major consideration here is only that the coordinator, with the assistance of his department heads, has the authority to plan and budget for personnel, to pass upon their qualifications, and directly or indirectly supervise their work.

*Job Analysis and Description.** The job analysis is a means to describe in detail the precise duties and factors involved for efficient performance of the job. On the other hand, the job description comes from the job analysis and includes the duties, responsibilities, work performed, and the equipment, if any, used. Positions within various medical and paramedical settings have pretty much been analyzed - based upon tradition. As new special areas develop and responsibilities increase within professional specialties, new job analysis and descriptions will be necessary. Both the job analysis and description form the basis for the selection and placement of personnel, their training and education, their salary, their promotions, and the handling of their grievances.

Types of Positions. It is impossible to discuss all the job titles and descriptions of the various disciplines within the framework of a single chapter. The present brief discussion will therefore be limited to four general classifications of titles and descriptions each of which has been fairly well accepted.

1. Director or supervisor. This position is primarily of an administrative and supervisory nature concerned with the directing and supervision of personnel and program activities as well as development of an in-service training program, supervision of facilities, and assisting in the coordinating of the departments' activities, with the activities of other departments within the hospital. The scope and em-

---

*See Appendix C for job description of coordinator.

phasis of the program, policies, and budgeting are discussed with the Coordinator. Requirements for the position are graduation from an accredited four-year college in a particular specialty major, with two or more years of supervisory experience or a master's degree with one or more years of supervisory experience.

2. Supervisory. This is primarily a supervisory position concerned with staff supervision and other personnel assigned to the program. Responsibility may include supervising a particular treatment area of the hospital as well as assisting in the planning and direction of overall program. Although work is performed independently it is subject to review and approval by the department head. Requirements usually consist of graduation from an accredited four-year college in a particular specialty major, plus one or more years of experience.

   The title of supervisor may be applied or utilized in various settings to distinguish between the director and staff therapist.

3. Staff, leader, or specialist. This is primarily a beginning staff position responsible for the directing and conducting of activities for the patients. Work is usually performed under the supervision of the next higher occupational level. Requirement usually is graduation from an accredited four-year college in the particular specialty major.

4. Assistant or aide. This is usually a sub-professional classification responsible *within limits* for the directing and conducting of activities. Supervision is by the next higher occupational level. Requirements are usually graduation from high school, special interest in a particular area related to the work classification, and/or previous work experience in the area. An approved in-service training program may be substituted in some instances for yearly experience.

Recruitment. The success of the treatment program depends largely upon the ability to recruit personnel within availability of money budgeted. Employing authorities, whether the personnel director or coordinator, utilizes different methods (formal, informal, direct, or indirect) and sources in recruiting applicants for the various positions within the hospital or clinic.[5]

Regardless of the methods used, the procedure should be a shared responsibility. Although the author feels that the coordinator should answer all inquiries from professionals whether written or personal concerning the status and availability of positions. If nothing else, it gives the coordinator an opportunity to discuss items of mutual interest, develop good relations for the hospital for possible future use, and possibly assist in making referrals to other agencies. If he has doubts about salary, employment starting dates, housing, if it is included, or sufficient monies he should consult beforehand with the Personnel Director.

Unfortunately, there exists a lack of trained therapists within all specialties. For example, the number of registered occupational therapists as of January, 1964, was 6,798 while projected needs to 1966, is 15,000 more. This is compared to only 404 graduates in 1963, while during the period 1963-64 only 2454 were enrolled.[6] In a survey conducted in 1963, by Chapman and Allbresch,[7] only 14.9 per cent of 703 graduates in recreation entered the medical recreation field.

Salaries. Any statement relating to specific salary scales in any one agency or group of agencies has only limited value here because of the wide range paid by the various agencies and the constant adjustments made by federal and state agencies. Most agencies pay salaries commensurating with the training and qualifications required for continuous service. In any event, the salary scale of a music therapist, for an example, within the activity therapy service, should be the same paid a recreation or occupational therapist providing there is comparable equal training and graduation from an accredited college or university with a major in the specialty.

The major consideration when developing a salary structure for the activity therapist in any agency is to provide a reasonable balance between the salaries of one professional group and the next and the salaries paid by other agencies for the same service. Unfortunately, many salary structures within some agencies are determined at such a top level of administration or by legislative action that those who are primarily concerned with this particular services are not always consulted. The present scarcity of activity personnel within the various professional disciplines will continue unless individuals in any one of the professions are given a reasonable financial return for their services.

Listed below is a representative sample of the salaries paid by the state of Indiana for professional positions within the various departments that make up the activity therapy service.*

$5340 - $6300	Occupational, recreational, music, industrial, and vocational rehabilitation therapist.
6600 - 8700	Supervisor of the above positions plus vocational placement supervisor.
7500 - 9300	Director of occupational, recreation, music, and vocational and industrial therapy.

All agencies have some systematic plan determined by a law, act, or policy for annual increments and promotion of their employees to avoid problems of morale and turnover. When promotion is to occur, the coordinator and the department head are to be consulted. This is also true for merit raises, annual increments, or salary adjustments.

Interviewing. The interview is used to obtain information about the applicant, his previous work experience, his ability to express himself, his personal traits and characteristics, and his general attitude. On the other hand, it also provides an opportunity for the applicant to learn about the details of the position for which he is applying. In essence, it is a two-way form of communication; both should ask and answer questions.

The procedure to be used when future applicants are applying for positions within the service should again be one of shared responsibility between the personnel officer and coordinator, in addition to the department head of the specialty. What this shared responsibility will be is dependent upon the agency policy, but is essential that it be a cooperative one for the betterment of the agency.

---

*Permission granted Indiana Department of Administration

Since the coordinator is responsible for the total service, but at the same time, he is not a specialist in every discipline, he should incorporate the assistance of his department heads. Both should plan the manner in which the interview is to take place, including the achievement of specific objectives.

The interview may be handled by having the department head present during the initial interview or referring the applicant to the department head after the coordinator has completed his part of the interview. The author prefers the latter since it does not, in his opinion, cause the applicant to develop further emotional tension than he is already under. Not only should the coordinator be concerned with reviewing the application form, but whether the applicant meets the job classification standards. In addition, he should explain the organization of the services, its structure, the salary range of the position, promotional possibilities, and in-service training program. He will also be concerned with the applicant's strength and weakness as well as attempting to determine whether the individual's personality is of such a nature that he will or will not fit in with other staff personnel. The department head will be concerned with specific skills and how the individual might fit into the total department's operation. It is also wise to take the potential applicant on a tour of the facilities.

Some readers may say that many of the factors that the coordinator is concerned with is also the responsibility of the personnel officer. This may be true, but since the coordinator is responsible for the total services, through budgeting of personnel and program planning, he has the prerogative to ask any questions he so desires. It does no harm to ask similar questions asked by someone else.

Following the interview, the department head and coordinator should analyze the interview with the coordinator reporting the results to the personnel director. Both the department head and the coordinator should be objective in their appraisal of the applicant. If anything, the decision should rest with the department head since he or she will be responsible for the direct supervision of the individual, except in those situations where the applicant is applying for the department head position.

Supervisory Structure

The organizational structure of the activity therapy service must be such as to facilitate two-way communication and delegation, at the same time that there are clarification of duties, responsibilities, and authority, and a span of supervision that permits effective direction and evaluation of performance.

Span of Supervision. Usually the line of authority is through the coordinator to the department head, to staff, and in turn, the staff is responsible directly to the department head and the department head to the coordinator. However, there should also be direct contact between the staff and the coordinator at the request of either.

Since the coordinator is administratively responsible for the total treatment program, he holds the department heads responsible for the quality of work and the carrying out of the program within the framework of the hospital and activity therapy service policies. In addition, the coordinator expects each of the department heads to make a contribution to the institution by continuing to improve his department's administration, activities, making suggestions for the good of the service, improving self professionally, and contributing to the growth and development of the department. The department heads keep the coordinator informed of the quality of the activities, of program problems, and of inadequacies in staffing, facilities, and supplies. It is this combination of working together that desired objectives are achieved. The emphasis is not on the arbitrary control of the department heads through authoritarian methods, but on the development of teamwork, on soliciting ideas, on participation, on considering each department head and for that matter each staff therapist as a member of the total service rather than as being used by it. The importance of this is that good staff personnel in subordinate positions are exposed to a quality of experiences that tend to foster their growth. Growth not only comes from within but from the outside.

Because of the position the coordinator holds, he is always in a position which requires the making of decisions. The literature reveals that decision making is not based upon intuition or experience, but a systematic process of defining the problem, analyzing the problem, developing alternative solutions, selecting the best solution, and effectively implementing the decision.[8] Unless the coordinator can make decisions, he will never attain the status of an administrator. And he will not make decisions unless he has the courage of his convictions. This is a particularly difficult task. As Moore and Poage comment: "All too often, the doctor's long white coat or the nurses' caps will rally and decide on a course of action that is determined by the group alone. Rationality in administration becomes impossible when a superintendent or administrator must evaluate the decision in terms of group loyalties and interest."[9]

Delegating Responsibility. Delegation of responsibility is indispensable wherever an individual is responsible for the direction and action of others. Delegation of responsibility requires delegation of authority to do the work and it is impossible to hold anyone responsible for the results when such authority is not forthcoming. Limits of responsibility and authority are clearly defined in the organizational structure of the activity therapy service, in the written job analysis and description, and in a policy manual if the service has one.

Responsibility gives a sense of security and goes far in maintaining interest in work and developing good morale. Just as the coordinator should know his own functions, the extent of his responsibility, and relationship to his supervisor and hospital, so should the department head know clearly the extent of his responsibilities.

The following are examples of limitations which may be placed upon the department head's authority.

1. New activities cannot be initiated without approval of coordinator.
2. Request for time off, leaves, vacation, repair of equipment must have final approval of the coordinator.
3. Orders for all supplies and equipment must be discussed, approved, and cleared through the coordinator's office.
4. Utilization of facilities of another department within the service may not be made without consulting with the coordinator.

5. All correspondence on the part of a particular activity department which may directly effect the whole hospital must be reviewed by the coordinator.

It is quite in keeping with the principles of good management to delegate authority to department heads for specific activities which affect the whole hospital. All hospitals have some type of special programs for the patients such as July 4, Carnival Day, etc. Although these activities may be the responsibility of the activity therapy service to conduct, it seems perfectly satisfactory to delegate these aspects to some department head. When duties are specifically delegated to certain individuals, opportunity is provided to place responsibility for the quality of results.

Under any circumstances, good judgement on the part of the coordinator needs to be exercised when placing responsibility and authority. No amount of observation or verbal instruction will serve to qualify a therapist fully for a supervisor. Only through the actual performance of management of activities and participation in the formulation of management decisions can the necessary attributes be acquired. Unfortunately, tradition has determined that new supervisors be promoted on the strength of competence rather than on demonstrative ability.

Policy and Procedures Manual. Time will be saved and better treatment will result if policies and procedures concerning the operation of the activity service and each of its departments are outlined in detail, read, and placed in each department. Such a manual is a necessity as well as part of the planning process. But, at the same time, to be effective, it must be used and revised as new policies and procedures are adapted. A policy is usually a plan of action concerned with basic or specific issues, whereas procedures concern themselves with the way policies are carried out. Although there are many different items which could be incorporated into such a manual, it is important that all policies form a framework around the operation of the service and support each other. It should always be remembered that there are already in existence certain hospital policies and procedures which directly or indirectly affect the activity therapy service; therefore, these cannot be changed to suit the individual service, but should be integrated into the activity therapy service manual.[10]

In the policy and procedures manual, there should be included such items as formal organizational structure of the service, lines of authority, personnel policies and regulations (hours of service, vacations, special leaves, promotions evaluations, attire, absence from duty, etc.) , rules and regulations concerning general and specific activities (work schedules, movement of patients to and from activities, rainy day procedures, etc.) , volunteers, records and reports, budgeting, inventory control, program planning procedures, in-service training, and function of individual departments with description of activities. This latter item, a part of the author's manual at Logansport State Hospital, has been sent to all ward physicians to assist them in the assignment of their patients through prescription to specific activities. It also is used as a tool in educating the hospital personnel to the Activity Therapy Service.

Figure 6 shows a typical policy and procedure.

POLICY MEMORANDUM
A T — 4
ACTIVITY THERAPY SUPPLY REQUEST

1. . . . . all request for services and/or supplies, equipment, facilities from other departments and wards are to be acknowledged only on an "Activity Therapy Supply Request" form unless otherwise designated by the coordinator or his appointed designate

POLICY PROCEDURE

1. Request
    a. All request for services and/or supplies are to be filled out in duplicate by the ward or department and forwarded to the Activity Therapy Coordinator for action, distribution, and approval or disapproval.
    b. All request from the ward must be signed by the head nurse and approved by the nursing area supervisor before any action can be taken. Request made by various departments must have the signature of the person making the request and the department head who is approving the request.

2. Action
    a. The coordinator or his designate upon receiving the request will forward to the particular department for its action.
    b. If the request requires a substitution, the particular department head,

except dietary, may take the liberty of contacting the nursing area supervisor or department head to work out an appropriate substitution. When the substitution is made and the request requires no further action, the form will be returned to the Coordinator. It is suggested that the Activity Therapy Department Head make note of the request and return the form immediately.

c. If the request cannot be filled for any reason, it shall be returned immediately to the Coordinator with the reason stated for disapproval.

d. Dietary substitutions will be made at their discretion and the form returned to the Coordinator. The Coordinator will then notify the area supervisor of the substitution.

e. If action on the request is required by more than one department, the Coordinator will route to the department that requires the most time in filling the request. It then will be returned to the Coordinator for re-routing to the next department for its action.

f. The department head or his designate will initial his approval of the particular request before returning the request.

3. Return Communications

a. When action is taken by the department head of any of the therapies or by dietary the request form will be returned to the Coordinator, who in turn will notify by telephone or in person the nursing area supervisor or department head of the action taken.

b. One copy of the Activity Therapy Supply Request form will be circulated back to the head nurse through the nursing area supervisor or to the department after dietary and therapies have completed their action. The other copy of the form will remain in the Coordinator's office for one month following the request and then will be destroyed.

c. The Coordinator's office will notify the ward or department when and where services and/or supplies and refreshments can be obtained when action is approved.

d. The Coordinator's office will notify nursing area supervisor or the department head if services and/or supplies are disapproved by dietary or therapies.

e. The nursing area supervisor or department head will relate all pertinent information to the head nurse or ward attendant and to the p.m. shift supervisor concerning action taken.

Figure 6.

Although the manual is of assistance to the regular employee, it is especially helpful to the new employee. Louise[11] comments that "the supervisor should endeavor to teach from the manual and refer to it frequently. In this way, reference to it will become a spontaneous act in time of need on the part of new personnel."

Two excellent manuals in use within an activity service at the present time is the one utilized at The Menninger Foundation and the other at Jamestown State Hospital, Jamestown, North Dakota.

Supervisory Conferences. Conferences and group discussions should be as frequent as possible in order to solve problems, resolve differences, obtain new ideas, and supervise work done. Conferences may be of two types: informal and formal. Informal conferences are those which are held during the day with staff personnel as needs arise. The coordinator and a department head, for example, may confer together on how a piece of equipment is working out or discuss patient participation in a particular activity. On the other hand, those conferences which are conducted for a specific purpose to discuss specifics about the overall work of the department head or problems relating to the functions of the department are usually referred to as formal or supervisory conferences.

Supervisory conferences should be held on a regular basis. The author prefers to conduct such conferences on a weekly basis with each of his department heads. These conferences are conducted on Monday; thereby giving the author and his department heads an opportunity to project plans for the whole week as well as posible review, if need be, or problems that may have occurred over the past week-end. Since the activity therapy service department head meeting is held on Friday, it also provides an opportunity to follow up with specifics as they relate to an individuals department at the first of the week. Additional conferences may also be held at either the request of the department head or the coordinator. In turn, the department head should have similar conferences with his supervisors and staff personnel.

It is assumed that the reader is well aware that the success of such conferences depends largely upon the preparation made by both the coordinator and department head. It should also be noted that the time for the conference is extremely important since fatigue according to research psychologist is an important deterrent to objectivity. Therefore, conferences should be held early in the day, if at all possible. And finally, the conference should be free of interruptions.

Items discussed might include department budgeting, staff relationships, activities, and information the coordinator or department head may want to pass on to each other which was gathered from other meetings or discussions inside or outside of the activity therapy service. But regardless of what is discussed, the discussion should be kept on an objective level with the department head being encouraged to express himself. As many times occurs, the department head may provide solutions to his own problems just by talking the particular problems over or by having a better clarification of specific matters.

On the other side of the desk, the coordinator needs to be a good listener. He needs also to guide the discussion and keep it on the subject. If there is need for criticism, it should be directed at the way a particular problem was handled and not at the individual. No two individuals are exactly alike. Only by recognizing individual differences can human resources be fully utilized. The conference should end with a summary of what decisions were reached and the future plans or goals.

Following the conference the coordinator should write down the highlights of the conference especially those points in which decisions were mutually agreed upon or decisions made by the coordinator affecting the department. A copy of the written conference should be sent to the department head. This information is used as a review for both before the next conference and serves as a guide as well as a measurement of progress. It goes without saying that the writing up of such conferences is extremely helpful if a time comes when discipline action is necessary. The conference helps also to improve the technique of the coordinator in conducting conferences by reviewing and evaluating his methods.

While conferences with department heads are held on a regular basis, additional conferences or special conferences with all department heads are necessary, at times. These conferences would undoubtedly be concerned with budgeting, development of master schedule, important information that needs to be dispensed immediately, or policy development to name a few items. The author does not necessarily classify weekly department head meetings as a special conference since he looks upon such meetings as a method of providing general information concerning the service and departments or the exchange of the same type of information. It also provides an opportunity to review the forth-coming week's program.

The coordinator may wish to have conferences with staff personnel at times, but it is preferable for the department head to hold those which relate specifically to the individual's work since the department head is in a better position to know than the coordinator. There are times, especially if there is a major grievance between the department head and a staff member concerning a specific problem, that the department head or staff person may request a meeting with the coordinator. In such cases, it is important that the conference be written up and if it involves a disciplinary action, that a carbon of the conference be forwarded to the personnel officer.

Personnel Evaluation. At least once a year, regardless of agency, there is some kind of an evaluation of personnel's performance. The evaluation may be required after so many months of employment for new employees, a basis for promotion,* for salary increases or adjustments, for annual ratings, working satisfaction, separations, and demotion or layoff when necessary. Staff personnel are usually evaluated by the department head, the department head by the coordinator, and the coordinator by whoever is his supervisor.

By any system that has been developed to date, the evaluation of personnel's performance is more or less subjective. The effectiveness and value of performance ratings depend largely upon the rater, and how well they use the goal devised for evaluating the personnel for whom they are responsible. The performance rating is only a tool.

The primary function of evaluation is to serve as a guide for the individual in determining his adjustment, competence, and attitude. The aggregation of the written supervisory conference serves as the basis for the evaluation or assists where agencies provide some kind of performance rating forms. The supervisory conference record serves the useful purpose in that it gives the rater a tangible source of material upon which to base his rating, thus freeing himself from making a rating that might be influ-

---

*For an interesting promotion check sheet, see Fair, Ernest A.: She's ready for promotion when . . . . . *Hospital Management,* December 1959, p. 93-94.

enced by his "feelings of the moment." Where such is the case, a guide sheet usually accompanies the form. Unfortunately, many forms used for performance ratings are worthless and do not measure what they are intended to.

When evaluating the performance of the department head, the coordinator should be fair; the tendency for one or two characteristics to color the judgement in relation to other characteristics is unfair to the individual. Evaluation should show progress whether slow or rapid; if not, then it is quite possible that poor judgement was made some place. But is should be remembered that it takes some individuals longer to "find themselves" if they have been recently promoted or are new to the agency. The evaluation should be based upon how well the individual has succeeded in relation to his own ability and quality of his work in relation to his ability. Compare the employee with what you expect of him, do not compare him with others. The evaluation should summarize the strengths, needs, and progress into a composite whole which reflects the elements that make up the individual.

When the evaluation is completed, the individual on which the evaluation is about, should be called in for a discussion about the report. Supervisory conferences based on the written records keep both the coordinator and department head aware of the latter's development. If the department head has been helped to evaluate his own work and follows his progress, nothing in the evaluation will come as a surprise. If there is rejection or severe criticism of the evaluation, it should be noted. In most agencies, the supervisor of the coordinator is usually the reviewer of his department heads evaluation; therefore, the individual who rejects his evaluation may want to discuss it with the coordinator's supervisor.

Although there are a number of reasons for having the evaluation reviewed by another person, the primary one is to keep the rating objective and free of personal bias, favoritism, or subjective feelings. In addition, it is a guard against the "halo" effect by the rater in which the rater tends to rate his employees usually high in each area.

Relationship With Others. The coordinator is in a key position for establishing and maintaining morale. Good relationships between all departments within and outside of the activity therapy service are enhanced when individuals know one another and understand each other's problems. The coordinator, as coordinator of the service, takes the initiative for getting acquainted with other therapists and department heads before a clash of interests brings them together.

BUSINESS MANAGEMENT

Records. Records not only provide an enduring record for the activity therapy service, but a source for future program planning as well as a reflection of past expressed needs. The kind of records required for the successful operation are many and varied. Records may take the form of personnel records, program and service records, daily, weekly, monthly, and annual reports, property records, financial and business records, etc. Only as they are available can the administrator determine the cost of the various services, justify budget request, demonstrate special needs, evaluate new methods, or interpret effectively the services. Patients may go, but the hospital and services must remain. On the other hand, they should not be kept unless they contribute to the effectiveness of the service and are essential to its efficient operation.

An example of an all inclusive form concerned with the Activity Therapy Service at Logansport State Hospital is shown below. This form is not only utilized for patient programs, but for any programs directly or indirectly involving hospital departments or personnel. As you will note, the form is primarily a request for supplies or for assistance to be provided by any one of the various disciplines of the Service. The form is used by the wards when they are in need of various types of equipment, by various hospital departments, for example, if they want photographs taken of something or want to use a specific facility utilized by a particular department. Since the Recreation Department is responsible for all ward parties or picnics sponsored by either the hospital or by volunteers, no food for these activities can be ordered directly through the Dietary Department before clearing first with recreation; therefore, the reason for having dietary listed, as well as recreation being able to control the scheduling and assignment of staff therapists to the activity.

LSH-A-35 (3-61)

ACTIVITY THERAPY SUPPLY REQUEST

TO: ACTIVITY THERAPY COORDINATOR   Date:....................

FROM: Ward or Department...

                                                     Area

            Approved: .... (Head Nurse) .... (Supervisor)

            Event: ....

            Date: .... Time: .... Sponsored by: ....

            Number to be Present: .... Place: ....

ITEMS NEEDED:
  1. Equipment:
  2. Supplies:
  3. Facilities:
  4. Food (See other side)
  5. Other:

TO BE FILLED OUT BY COORDINATOR:

                                              Music

Route to: Recration.... Dietary.... Art Therapy.... Photo.... Therapy....

                 Occupational....

                 Comments: (Action, Approved, or Disapproved) ....

RETURN TO ACTIVITY THERAPY COORDINATOR

Area notified as to action taken on ....

Figure 7.

Reports. Probably no other single factor is more vital to good administrative management than oral and written reports. Good reports save duplication of effort and often save embarrassment due to ignorance of a situation. The coordinator depends upon accurate reports from his department heads for efficient management.

Reports should be made promptly if they are to serve their purpose well. A good report is clear, concise, and complete. If it is written, all pertinent facts are clearly stated and well organized for easy understanding. No extraneous material is included. Oral reports are likewise well organized.

Oral reports are given when information is for immediate use. Frequently, reports are supplemented by written reports or by observation. Although oral reports are often time-consuming, they offer an opportunity for further objective explanation and interruption. It is well to set aside a block of time to be kept for oral report purposes. It should be an unbroken rule that oral reports are not interrupted except in an emergency, for if continuity is broken, important points may easily be forgotten.

Written reports not only provide information of a permanent value on performance for present or future evaluation, but are adaptable and utilized for statistical purposes. Also included in this category are administrative interdepartmental, interagency, and accident reports, reports on policy changes, and reports about unusual conditions which may reflect the quality of care the patient has received.

An example of an administrative report used by the author for a number of years is given below. In essence, it is a guide for the department heads to utilize when developing their monthly report. In turn, the author utilized the same guide in preparing his monthly report for the hospital administration. In addition to the written phase of the report, all departments turn in a statistical report concerned with the number of patients seen, activities conducted, and hours spent with the patient in conducting activities.

1. Basic plans, policy goals: This to be concerned with any changes concerning these items or desired changes as they would apply to the particular department submitting the reports or the total Activity Therapy Service.

2. Administration: Here we are concerned with any particular changes and procedures for direction and cooperation within the individual department. Also, any new procedures that the particular department might be effecting, such as utilization of work schedules, organizational charts, statistical reports, etc.

3. Supervision: To be concerned with any new techniques of supervision, any particular problems in this area that may have developed, any solution of problems and techniques which should be relayed on.

4. In-service training: Here is noted any changes in in-service training, the content of such and any future plans.

5. Volunteers: Comments regarding the use of them, future use, and any other pertinent information concerning the volunteer program.
6. Program coverage: Any changes in programming (old or new) or any re-evaluation.
7. Department needs: To be concerned with personnel needs, supplies, and equipment, as well as any other pertinent information as projected into future needs of the particular department.

It is well to remember that a report to be of greatest use, and to save time and duplication of effort must be prompt, complete, accurate, and objective.

Finances. Money is needed to acquire, equip, and operate the activity therapy service. The financing of this service has not always been an easy operation. Administrators of hospitals, as well as budget committees, commissioners, and state legislatures have not always looked upon the services provided by these disciplines as having therapeutic value. In many instances, the service has had to depend upon the sale of occupational therapy items, the contribution of individuals, and/or donations to support themselves. Only in general medical and surgical hospitals and Veterans Administration hospitals has there been a consistency in support of the various forms of adjunctive treatments. Most service within state systems, however, no longer depend upon these methods for securing supplies and equipment. Nearly all public and private psychiatric hospitals now receive appropriated funds in addition to the use of profits from their hospital canteen.

The acquisition of finances is through the development of a budget. A budget may be looked upon from two aspects - its formulation and its execution.

1. *Formulation.* A budget is an expression of financial needs based upon total planning to include both personnel and program requirements. The preparation of the budget is based upon past experiences, present conditions and their influences, and projected future conditions along with provisions for special situations.

The budget is usually developed on an annual basis, although many state agencies may use a biennial system whereby expenditures are projected over a two year period because of legislative arrangement. Also, within the annuality of a budget there may be monthly or quarterly stages. The length of time that the budget is for depends upon the purpose of the budget. Although the extent to which reasonable forecasts can be made should be considered in determining the budget period.

There are usually two types of budgets which can be applied to the operation of the activity therapy service. One, an operating budget from appropriated funds used for personnel, supplies, equipment, facilities, renovations, etc., and secondly, a supplementary budget from the profits of the hospital canteen, sometimes called a Patients Recreation Fund used for supplies and equipment which are of a recreation nature and which cannot be provided through appropriated monies for some reason or another.

The first step taken by the coordinator in preparing the budget is meeting with the hospital administrator responsible for the total over-all hospital budget. What usually occurs is that the hospital administrator will call a meeting of the various department heads within the hospital to outline the operation of the hospital's forthcoming year. This type of meeting usually includes projected programs, expansion or curtailment of present services, new or renovation of existing facilities, salary revisions, policy changes and so forth.

After the initial conference, the coordinator disseminates the information to his various department heads. Since the coordinator is responsible for the total service, he relies heavily upon continuing conferences with his various department heads to counsel and provide information for him in the actual development of the proposed tentative budget. It is not easy at times to forecast the services to be rendered in the projected year (s) ; however, records of past years will shed light for program planning, personnel, facilities, supplies, and equipment.

The budgeting of personnel is probably the largest item by the activity therapy service, if not for the whole hospital. Ewalt[12] estimates 70 per cent of a hospital's operating funds go for salaries. Consideration must be given to the hospital location, patients served, type and extensiveness of the activity therapy service treatment programs, supplies, equipment, and facilities and number and qualifications of employees needed, including salary adjustments, and how well the services have sold themselves to the hospital administration. Although the activity therapy service, in most hospitals, is an accepted service, it still is an adjunctive service. Whether it is truly accepted depends upon its treatment program and the professionalism of its staff.

Supplies and equipment, unfortunately, are difficult to budget and are often unintelligently planned. Records of purchases in previous years should be studied to determine adjustments desirable to meet the succeeding years needs. In addition, most budgets for supplies and equipment include separate columns to list whether the item is new, addition to that already on inventory, or replacement.

Within due time, the tentative budget for the total service is completed with attached cost data and justifications and is ready to be forwarded to the hospital administrator or financial officer. A series of meetings involving the budget committee then follows at which time the various departmental budgets are discussed and adjustments made to represent the total budget for the hospital. It may occur that the coordinator will be involved in further meetings with the hospital administrator to justify particular items or to discuss minor adjustments.

It sometimes happens that it may be necessary to increase certain department's request while the request of others will be decreased. Experience has shown that it is proper and right to submit a realistic budget.

2. *Execution.* After the budget has been adopted, it becomes the financial blueprint for the ensuing year. This does not mean that adjustments cannot be made because revisions and adjustments will take place due to some new development or information. Therefore, it is well for the coordinator to have a periodical review. As so many times occurs, especially in federal and state agencies, will the total hospital budget be accepted due to legislative action. Therefore, when the activity therapy service budget is returned, it may require a further adjustment. A good procedure to follow in such instances is to deduct in percentage from each department what was deducted from the total activity therapy service budget. In this way, all departments are treated in a fair

way. It may happen that because of projected plans, it would not be advisable to utilize the procedure just mentioned. In such instances a conference should be held with the various department heads to reconsider the whole budget and agree to the necessary changes.

It is the duty of the coordinator to make comparisons between the budget and actual performance. Having records in such form as to ascertain quickly whether or not expenditures are being kept within the appropriated budget is a must. It may be necessary, as well as good administrative practices, as the occasion requires, to have meetings with the specific department heads to discuss irregularities in their spending, if such is occurring or appropriate praise if it is warranted.

Not only does comparison assist in planning and control but also aids in coordination by promoting a balance in activities, disclosing weaknesses in program planning, encouraging an interchange of ideas between department heads regarding program planning, assisting department heads and staff to know the goals of the hospital and services and revealing personnel weaknesses, whereby possible means of correction can be instituted.

Standards. It is basic to any program to have established quantities which are required to meet the needs of departments and program objectives. These standards are determined by the type, age, and sex of the patients, program content, cost of items, durability and the period of time between orders.

To establish standards for a department or activity, its basic needs should be analyzed by the department head and coordinator together. The aim is to establish the needs of the department for good service and efficient management without waste. Standards need to be flexible. As activities change, standards should increase or decrease. Where supplies and equipment are no longer used or smaller quantities required, there should be some provision for removal and consequent change in the standards.

Standards prevent an oversupply and serve as a guide in preparing the budget and program planning. An oversupply can be wasteful. There is less economy in the use of supplies when there appears to be no limit to the amount available.

Inventory. Inventory is basic to an adequate program of control and record. An inventory is a detailed list of all supplies and equipment, their specifications, and standard number of quantity. This serves as a basic instrument for keeping an up-to-date record of all property to facilitate the program of activities. Not only does the taking of inventory give an opportunity to determine whether standards are being maintained but it provides an excellent chance to dispose of excess and obsolete material, to recommend changes in the standards, to determine the condition of articles of equipment, to order repair or replacement if necessary, and to provide information which reflects the need for supplies and equipment for the forthcoming year, with anticipated cost. It also is an ideal time to return items to their proper place. It might be added that they justify additional space as well as having special significance in case of loss through stealing, fire, or other destruction.

The only way to insure efficient management of supplies and equipment is to establish a definite routine and develop specific directions for its accomplishment. This material should be placed in writing, preferably a policy manual and used for teaching the persons responsible for inventory. Most departments within the activity therapy service have their own central storage area or a combination of such in addition to keeping a minimum of supplies and equipment within their own department.

Items drawn out of a central supply area should be recorded on what is usually referred to as a "perpetual inventory form." This form furnishes an up-to-date daily record and entries are made each time a transaction or withdrawal takes place with the signature of the person who took the item.

Finally, it should be the function of every individual to report breakage, equipment which is in need of repair and low stock of material. Along with this goes the education of staff therapists in the proper use and care of supplies and equipment.

In summary of management, the coordinator need not master every function that is essential to administration but he must be able to coordinate all activities into a unified whole which will provide a smooth-running service. This not only includes the establishment of an organized system for accomplishing the day's program which fits in with the programs of the other groups throughout the hospital, but the responsibility for making decisions about it and for the supervision of it.

ETHICS

To this point in the chapter we have been discussing the concept of administration of the activity therapy service to meet the objectives of the particular hospital in which the concept is now operating or its projected operation. The objectives of the activity therapy service and all of its efforts to attain these objectives should be governed by ethical practices. Every professional occupation working within the hospital, including the hospital itself, finds policies and decisions many times directly and indirectly based upon the Medical Code of Ethics and the Hospital Code of Ethics. Within the activity therapy service, we find again policies and decisions based on still another facet, the individual profession's ethics to which he belongs. To be professional, a man must act within an ethical framework, defined by a professional code. But in addition, he must apply the knowledge he has acquired to himself. "He is his most important professional tool. Therefore, his professional preparation cannot be considered adequate unless it includes learning to reconcile what he has always thought and believed about himself with the knowledge about other people that he is acquiring and using in his practice."[13]

It may be said that hospital occupations, in contrast to a business or industrial enterprise is very far from being motivated by insistence on monetary profits: the chief mark of its ethics is providing a service. Ethics in a hospital is characterized by a continuous and conscious self-abnegation for the well being of the patient, a dedication thereto beyond the crisp call of the dollar proportionate to the effort.

According to Webster, ethics is defined as "the science of moral duty, broadly, the service of ideal human character." In other words, ethics is concerned with the problems of man's adjustment to the actual conditions in the midst of which he lives. Ethical refers to "conforming to professional standards of conduct." Combining the two, ethics and ethical, professional ethics gives attention to certain ideals and practices which grow out of man's professional privileges and responsibilities. To be of service is of little or no value unless it is administered with tact and insight. The stimulation one receives from serving is the dividing line between a profession and a job.

The need for professional ethics is very apparent, since the more specialized the knowledge, the higher the skill, and the less the public knows about the quality and the technical aspects of the work, the greater is the opportunity for abuse to arise. Consequently, the need for developing and maintaining higher standards of conduct is greater.

How urgent it is to keep fast the characteristic ethics of a profession may be learned of course, from the oaths that must be taken — "The Hippocrates Oath" by the doctors, the "Florence Nightingale" pledge by nurses, and the "codes of ethics," "rules of professional conduct," "standards of practice," principles of conduct," "canons of ethics" established by legal, business and other paramedical professions. One of the most important roles that professional organizations play, according to Finer,[14] is that they "are the keepers of the conscience of the profession. They can raise and sustain the individual because though it is not possible to convince others of spiritual values by any objective demonstration to the point of requiring their sacrifices of time and energy over the years, the visions of others, one's colleagues, acting under a sincere conviction, is itself a demonstration that seems to produce imitation and acceptance."

An example of ethical obligation is that the coordinator and his department heads have an obligation to assist their staff to advance either within the hospital or encourage them to find new opportunities outside the hospital, if they so desire.

Professional Ethics. One of the factors that has influenced the development of the activity therapy service, as we have said before, is the increase of professionalization in the various services. Training is becoming more standardized, credentials more formal, and admission to professional societies more stringent. What recognizes a profession? According to the McGlothlin[15] conception, a profession: " (1) Deals with matters of great urgency and significance; (2) is directed to human benefit and is guided by ethical standards; (3) is learned, and (4) undertakes tasks which require the exercise of judgment in applying knowledge to the solution of problems and accepts responsibilities for the results." He continues by saying that "Each profession exhibits these characteristics in varying degrees at different points in time. The more advanced professions exhibit them all." Codes, whether written or unwritten, are very essential to the growth of professions. "They are moralized in the sense that they go beyond the mere administrative obligations in a particular situation but affect standards and norms of conduct."[16]

In summary, the coordinator's position provides the opportunity to channel into one office those administrative functions which are common to all of the various activity therapy specialties, thereby increasing efficiency, both in the administrative sense and by giving the department heads more time to work in the area of supervision and leadership within their particular discipline. This prevention of duplication of administrative matters is one of the major reasons for the grouping of the various specialties.

There must be a spirit within the activity therapy service which makes possible the pooling of experiences, the sharing of new ideas, the dedication of accomplishment, the readiness to continue monotonous tasks, the feeling that it is a privilege to serve in every possible way, and a sense of pride in the achievements of the hospital and one's own services, and the members of which are working together.

REFERENCES

1. Klicka, Karl S.: It's hospital's business to be a business. *Modern Hospital, 97* (3) :120, 1961.
2. Terry, George R.: *Principles of Management*. Rev. Ed., Homewood, Illinois, Richard D. Irwin, Inc., 1956, p. 4.
3. Personal letter with enclosures. Richard A. Silver, Director, Personnel Service, Veterans Administration, Washington, D. C. April, 1963.
4. Trecker, Harleigh B.: *New Understanding of Administration*. New York, Association Press, 1961, p. 190.
5. Caplow, Theodore: *The Sociology Of Work*. Minneapolis, University of Minnesota Press, 1954.
6. *Facts . . . About Occupational Therapy*. American Occupational Therapy Association, 250 W. 57th Street, New York, New York, January, 1964.
7. Chapman, Frederick M., and Abresch, William J.: Placement of recreation graduates. *American Recreation Journal, 5* (3) :73, 1964.

8. Moore, E. Calvin, and Poage, Edwin F.: The art of decision making. *Mental Hospitals*, June, 1964.

9. *Ibid.*, p. 307.

10. Smith, George A., and Roland, Christensen C.: *Policy Formulation and Administration*. Rev. Ed., Homewood, Illinois, Richard D. Irwin, Inc., 1953.

11. Louise, Sister Mary: The internal planning committee. *Hosp. Prog.*, April 1961, p. 64.

12. Ewalt, Jack: *Mental Health Administration*. Springfield, Thomas, 1956, p. 64.

13. Henry, Charlotte S.: Criteria for determining readiness of staff to function without supervision. In *Administration, Supervision, and Consultation*, New York, Family Service Association of America, 1955, p. 43.

14. Finer, Herman: *Administration and The Nursing Services*. New York, The MacMillan Company, 1952, p. 190.

15. McGlothlin, William J.: The place of nursing among the professions. *Nursing Outlook, 9* (4) :214-15, 1961.

16. Taeusch, Carl F.: *Professional and Business Ethics*. New York, Henry Holt and Company, 1926, p. 99.

Chapter XI

PLANNING THE ACTIVITY THERAPY PROGRAM

THE DEVELOPMENT of the activity program is the function of the entire activity staff. While the responsibility and duties may fall more heavily on the coordinator and department heads, the participation of all staff is essential to the success of the program. Though the task of administering and supervising the activities of the program may be shared by the coordinator and department heads, its total effectiveness depends to an immeasurable degree upon the performance of every staff member. Activity programs are inseparably related to many other programs in the hospital and the quality of one is almost certain to affect the quality of the others. Moreover, the activities usually identified with all of the activity departments are inseparably bound together by purpose and ineffective achievement in one aspect of the program affects the entire program.

MEETING OBJECTIVES

The principles governing program planning should be based primarily upon a clarification of the objectives, both short and long range, as outlined by the administrator and the obligations necessary for their fulfillment. Short range objectives will not help achieve long range objectives unless the administrator works with long range goals in mind. The decision as to the responsibilities, personnel required, necessary assignments and scope of activities is established after careful analysis of the situation. It should be understood that special adaptations must be made at times to fit the specific needs and interest of the patients and the hospital, and to the facilities in which programs will take place.

Objectives stated in vague and double-meaning terms have minimum administrative value. It is pertinent that the objectives and functions be defined and responsibilities be delimited to assure satisfactory coverage of necessary activities and avoid duplication of efforts. Furthermore, a clear conception of the essential objectives and needs must be formulated before any planning of programs can take place since policies, procedures, and other plans are a direct outgrowth of the explicit recognition of the objectives.

To develop good planning requires a realistic recognition of the primary and secondary objectives by the various services. Therefore, following the clarification of the objectives between the clinical director and the coordinator, the coordinator must clarify these same objectives with his own staff as well as the unique goals as they relate to the objectives of each service. This is a particularly difficult assignment because of the highly specialized groups with whom he works. Patience and knowledge must be combined if this work is to be carried out with skill. From these, we develop the objectives for each service including ordering of time, material resources, personnel skills, and character, and institutional arrangements to secure an end. It is, of course, easier to define the objectives of some services than that of others but, in every situation, a clear understanding of the objectives is of great assistance to each service. The staff therapist who has the direct responsibility for conducting the activities must have an understanding as to the reasons for the specific activities and realize the importance of knowing how to best conduct such activities.

While each department may be distinctive in its function and responsibilities it is impossible for any one department to stand alone since its embodiment is dependent upon the aggregate contribution of the other departments. It is the completeness and individuality of the various elements which enhance the total program and makes it valuable, since each department is an aid to each other for a common purpose. Therefore, inter-relationship must be recognized and ways of working together for the benefit of all concerned is necessary.

The relationship of the program to the objectives involves all the departments of the activity therapy service with the leadership of the coordinator. This fact should be paramount in program planning within the psychiatric hospital. In general medical and surgical hospitals, this relationship is not always apparent since, in most instances, the physician is usually in direct contact with the therapist. At the same time, the size of the hospital and the volume of business must also be considered as a primary difference.

It is quite possible that the particular objectives as outlined by the clinical director in a psychiatric hospital may not always coincide with the objectives which are felt by the activity therapy service who are in constant contact with the felt needs of the patient. In such situations, the information should be relayed to the clinical director. This can be accomplished through frequent communication and conferences. It may also occur that ward physician may discuss this with the clinical director or make recommendations directly to the individual therapist serving the ward or to the coordinator.

A program in which activities are planned and conducted so the whole patient receives benefit will do most to assist the medical staff. The program cannot be routine; it must be adapted to the conditions and needs of the patient. Patients not only differ from one to another in their needs, but also have a varying interest from age to age, day to day. Unless the program provides activities that appeal to the patient's different taste and varying moods, they will present problems when it comes to attending activities. In any event, the program plans should not be sacred. They should be looked upon as tentative outlines to be modified when needs arise. It is important that the department heads and coordinator consider as many alternatives to the program as possible.

For successful operation of the program, information must flow two ways. The ward physician and patients must be informed about what activities are available and what is going on in the program. This includes the utilization of medical referral or prescription slips. Activities must be designed to motivate the patient to voluntarily contribute to the management of their own time, acquire new skills and interests, adoption of previously learned skills, and attain a feeling of security through recognized achievement.

FACTORS IN PLANNING

Five factors must be taken into account in planning the activity therapy service program—the patients to be served, the staff personnel, the facilities, finances, and activities that will assist in the treatment process. Since all of these items differ according to the various medical and paramedical settings, no standardized program can be presented; however, several guiding principles and procedures can be followed. Therefore, let us look at these five factors which influence the scope of the program planning process.

1. The Patients to be Served. The needs, interest, and capabilities of the patients should be the factor underlying all program planning while the primary objective is to provide more and better therapeutic programs within the limits of the personnel and facilities available. As Tillock[1] comments: "The areas of patient need encompasses all contacts and experiences that the patient is conscious of from the time it is decided (if elective) that it will be necessary for him to undergo hospitalization until such time as he may be discharged or transferred from the hospital." Success in the performance of this necessarily implies a clear understanding on the part of the therapist of the problems involved and, also, a knowledge of the patient as an individual.

To know a patient requires a study of him as a whole. Such a study necessitates careful scrutiny of the patient's personality traits, emotional reactions, intellectual status, and his behavior under various conditions. It also involves analysis of the whole environment to which he has been exposed; his social background, occupation, conditions in the home, and his place in the community. It is the analysis of the individual in a most inclusive sense and it provides the basis for therapist's relationship with the patient.

Regardless of the setting, the patient's understanding, interest, and cooperation are of greatest importance in both planning and carrying out the program of care. While the patient is hospitalized, he may be forced into a certain treatment regime, but usually even in the hospital, this cooperation is essential to successful therapy; and ultimately the health of the individual will depend upon his interest in recognizing and maintaining his health and his ability to take care of himself.

2. *Leadership.* While the coordinator takes a large part in coordinating the total program, he leaves the execution of the program to the various departments and staff therapist. The success of the program is in large measure the quality of leadership provided by the therapist. Each therapist "must have leadership qualities commensurate with his position. Each person must be encouraged to exert his maximum initiative for the good of the group and be respected for his work in terms of his methods, value systems, and goals."[2]

The therapist serves an important function as intermediary between doctor and patient. The physician's explanation, instruction, or admonitions often require interpretation; it is the staff therapist who, in his discussion with the patient, can best clarify these pronouncements, lending them more effective emphasis.

In the development of any program plans, consideration must be given to the personnel required to conduct the program and their attitude so as to assure its success. A uniformity of attitudes among all therapist is necessary if a consistent "milieu" is to be maintained in the total treatment program for the patient. Key,[3] in discussing attitudes of ancillary therapists, states that "personality differences between the activity therapists is of major importance in determining the perceptions of the patients about patient-activity therapist relationships." He continues by saying that "it appears from this finding that differences between activity therapist personalities are major determiners of patient's perceptions of activity therapist. Efforts on the part of the activity therapist to adopt different roles with different patients are apparently ineffective and are overshadowed by the personality of the activity therapist." In conclusion, he recommends that the coordinator "have a thorough knowledge of his staff in order that he can recommend particular people to work with a particular patient. He would be responsible for maintaining a staff of therapists who are specialist in creating different desired relationships with patients." Whether Dr. Key's recommendations can be incorporated into an organizational complexity such as being discussed within this book is difficult to say, but with the rapid changes that are being made within hospitals and the large number of different kinds of specialists, the coordinator, as well as the professionals in the various specialties, must give consideration and thought to these comments.

The therapist is responsible for the quality of treatment which the patient receives from the time of admission to his discharge. Therefore, the therapist must possess certain attributes which are essential for good leadership. The following list of traits are probably representative of the qualities that should be present at least to some degree in all therapists.

"1. Energy. A capacity for performing a wide field of activities . . . (and) stamina to see things through. . . .

2. Emotional stability. The effective leader is relatively free from bias; is consistent in his actions, . . . respects authority, . . . is well adjusted, . . . (and) is self confident. . . .

3. Knowledge of human relations. A leader needs to know as much as possible about human behavior. . . .

4. Personal motivation. The desire for leadership must come from within the individual.

5. Communication skills. A leader is able to talk and to write clearly. . . .

6. Teaching ability. . . . teaching is one of the best ways to develop people, to inspire them, and to make them aware of particular objectives. A teacher is employing his teaching skills when he asks questions and offers suggestions in place of issuing orders. Demonstrating how to accomplish a particular task. . . . and preparing followers for advancement. . . .

7. Social skills. A leader understands people and knows their strength and their weaknesses. He has the ability to work with people. . . . (and) gain their confidence and loyalty.

8. Technical competence. . . . The ability to plan, organize, delegate, analyze, seek advise, make decisions, control, and win cooperation requires the use of important abilities which constitute technical mastery of leadership. . . ."[4]

No therapist will ever agree wholly on a list of traits, but this is of little importance if all recognize that the therapist should be intelligent, cultured, and well grounded in the science and art of his particular specialty and that he should have a keen insight into human personality and a love and respect for people that comes from the conviction that each individual is of infinite worth.

3. Areas, Facilities and Supplies. To provide good treatment not only requires good staffing with intelligent and technically competent therapist, but there must be sufficient activity areas, facilities, and supplies, indoor and outdoor, in proportion to the patients for whose treatment the activity therapy service are responsible. These items are highly important contributing factors to a smooth running program which, in turn, reflects directly on the quality of patient care and treatment.

Planning an activity therapy program for a whole hospital requires an understanding of the nature and function of the various departments need of supplies and equipment to insure a diversified program. If the supply of materials is inadequate, the treatment of the patient may be jeopardized. Equipment which is not in good repair or ready for use is often more troublesome than if it were missing altogether. The situation is not only embarrassing but is wasteful of time and wearing on the nerves of all concerned. A deeper discussion of this whole area may be found in Chapter XII.

4. Finances. Programs cannot be carried on successfully or continuously without sufficient funds being provided through appropriated or contributed funds or directly by the patients for their care. The cost of providing personnel, equipment, supplies, and other essential items are high by todays standards, but they are necessary for total treatment.

5. Activities. Activities are the media through which the patient is assisted in his recovery; in essence, they are a constructive tool used as a means to an end, the end being that the activities help bring about desired changes in behavior so that the patient may be enabled to improve himself and the social order to which he belongs. The activity should be structured in such a way that self-development through achieving, creating, improvising desirable kinds of recognition, socialization, overcoming difficulties, and respecting the rights of others is as important for the patient as it is for the normal individual. Program planning, therefore, requires a knowledge of the needs, interest, and capabilities of the patient so as to provide the best programming for the patient since medias must be chosen according to the stages in which the patient is found. Such a program to fulfill the purpose for which it is intended and to take advantage of the full benefits inherent in the activities requires that the content be selected for the contribution therein. Although many inherent values of an activity remain within the activity, unrealized and undiscovered by the therapist.

In many hospitals in the past, especially in large public mental hospitals, the guiding principle of the activities program was to keep as many people active as much as possible, almost without regard for the kind of activity the individual needed. That this total effort has certain merit has been demonstrated, but more important than the activity is the emotional atmosphere in which the activity is carried on, and the relationships created between the patient and the therapist who guides the activity.

Another factor to be considered which was not commented upon above, but one which is receiving more and more attention is community program planning for the recently discharged patient. Although there is a correlation between the hospital and various community agencies regarding referral of patients with impairment of function or physical deformities to rehabilitation centers or sheltered workshops, there seems to be a lacking of the same correlation when it comes to the mentally ill or retarded. More patients, according to recent surveys and the literature, are being released and discharged from psychiatric hospitals and more psychiatric patients are remaining within the community.

The importance of this to the activity therapy service according to Meuli[5] is that ". . . it has become imperative that the activity therapy service plan for and coordinate their hospital programs with other community agencies offering similar services. Community planning of this nature must be started first in the hospital and then a referral system must be developed to insure proper communication with other agencies, both public and private, in the community." In addition, the author would like to add that such programs should not be isolated ones only for discharged patients.

The development of such programs for patients in the community is a cooperative undertaking, not a task for the hospital alone. Community leaders, patient families, employers, ordinary citizens of the community, including the patients themselves, must accept common responsibility through individual and group effort for assisting patients to function as members of our society.

Perhaps this need for more effective cooperation among community groups has been more clearly recognized by hospitals than it has by the community and its agencies. The hospital has long felt a need for community cooperation in its attempt to assist the patient in his return. In an attempt to educate the community about this problem, the Indiana State Department of Mental Health in 1962, made available funds to the Indiana University, Department of Recreation and School of Medicine to conduct an Institute "aimed at effecting among those whose responsibility it is to serve recreation needs in local communities. . . ."[6] The participants were from municipal recreation departments, YMCA and YWCA agencies sponsoring community recreation programs, and recreation directors from the state hospitals for the mentally ill and retarded in Indiana. If the gains made by the patient are to be continued, it is necessary for community cooperation.

PLANNING ELEMENTS

Experience has indicated several elements that influence the attainments of the hospital objectives in addition to the factors listed above, in program planning, whether for a larger psychiatric hospital or the small specialty hospital. In addition to the goals of an activity therapy service as listed in Chapter I, opportunities are provided for structured normal activities of daily living, assist in diagnostic and personality evaluation, augment psychotherapy and other therapeutic efforts, and assist the patient to bridge the gap between the hospital and the community the following elements should be considered.

Organization Methods

First and foremost is that program planning is a cooperative venture, its organization necessarily intricate because of the great variety of activities entailed and the numerous responsibilities borne in connection with these activities. As the number of patients and their needs increase in any one hospital, then the scope of the program becomes larger and more diversified. The importance of getting together for the planning of the program with the various department heads cannot be underestimated. There must be mutual understanding as to the underlying philosophy of the program, as well as the ability to give and take.

It must be recognized that program planning is not a mere matter of dividing up the patients among the various departments and delegating treatment. As Ridgway[7] comments, "Program division should be based on their functions for patients." In a large hospital which is necessarily highly organized, the planning of program becomes a painstaking process which requires a detailed program and full records. Programming for the sake of programming has no place in the hospital. All pre-planning must provide for an atmosphere in which the various departments can set goals and continually modify these goals as new patient needs are seen in the process of group treatment. Treatment, balance and variety, flexibility and continual evaluation within the program notes of successful planning.

The efficiency of any organization is largely dependent upon the personnel and advantage should be taken of the various skills of the various therapists in the development of program since the department and therapists will be challenged to greater effort and anxious to demonstrate their ability. "Staff therapists with specific talents, skills, and abilities should be utilized regardless of their primary professional specialty. For example, an occupational therapist may be adept at drama, and in turn, be responsible for the drama program, which is normally provided by the recreation department."[8]

As a means of determining duties and responsibilities within the activity therapy service, the coordinator must survey the needs and decide upon the most efficient means for attaining the objectives within his jurisdiction. Through the procedure of analysis each major aspect is clarified and it then becomes possible to carry through the sequential step of each phase. With such a foundation, a program may be very narrow or exceedingly broad, but nevertheless it must have the elements of flexibility and progression for effective action. The ability to move in new directions and apply theoretical principles to a practical situation, makes possible a more dynamic, expanding, and yet integrative program.

Program Scheduling

No attempt will be made to define the priority of program for each department since this area is still very much clouded by philosophical and theoretical issues of each specialty, by the educational and professional background of the particular coordinator and/or clinical director or superintendent of the hospital, and by the petty jealousies that still exist between the various departments. All that can be said is that it is the mutually acceped and understood inter-relationship of their functions that makes for adequate programming. Therefore, the role of the various disciplines must be defined on the basis of their specific objectives and methods rather than the media used. Only the future may bring actual mutations in the character of the services rendered and the professions rendering them. It is therefore necessary that all specialties clearly define its scope, limits, and basic objectives as they relate to an integrated program of activity therapies.

The development of a master schedule is nothing more than making a list of the type of activities that are to be conducted by each of the departments, where they are to take place, the ward(s) involved, time, and day of the week. In addition, the schedule should include the general policies of the activity therapy service as they relate to patients going and coming from activities, a listing of the activity therapy service department heads with their office phone numbers, the ward arrangements (active intensive treatment service, intermediate treatment service, etc.), a listing of staff personnel who may be assigned to specific wards to counseling the wards on parties, obtaining supplies for the ward, etc., and a listing of the vocational and industrial therapy counselors and their ward assignments, who are responsible for assisting the medical personnel in the assignment of patients to work placement positions. If the educational therapy department is responsible to the coordinator, the class period can be an integrated part of the regular schedule or can be separate. The master schedule, in essence, gives a complete breakdown of all activities conducted by the activity therapy service for the patients. In addition to the master schedule, there is usually needed a supplementary schedule which gives similar information as the master schedule, but relates only to activities which are conducted only for that particular week as well as making announcements concerning ward sponsored volunteer parties, name of movies, special programs, etc. Examples of both of these schedules are given below:

ACTIVITY THERAPY MASTER SCHEDULE

DAY AND TIME	WARDS	TYPE OF ACTIVITY	LOCATION
TUESDAY (Cont.)			
9:00 a.m.	14	Recreation (Physical Fitness)	Gym—A. T. Bldg.
9:00 a.m.	10	Recreation	Ward 10
9:00 a.m.	All	Recreation	Game Room
9:00 a.m.		Staff Reporters Meeting (Hilltop)	A. T. Bldg.
9:00 a.m.	6	Industrial Arts (Assigned Patients)	Vocational shop
10:30 a.m.	L	Art Therapy	Ward L
10:30 a.m.		Art Therapy (Assigned Patients)	Art Department
10:30 a.m.	Teen-agers (Boys)	Art Therapy	Art Department
10:30 a.m.	14	Music Therapy	A. T. Bldg.
10:30 a.m.	15	Music Therapy	A. T. Bldg.
10:30 a.m.	16/17	Music Therapy	Ward 16/17
10:30 a.m.	11	Recreation	Ward 11
10:30 a.m.	2F/2M	Recreation	Ward 2F/2M
10:30 a.m.	All	Recreation	Game Room
10:30 a.m.	M	Recreation (Physical Fitness)	Gym—A. T. Bldg.
10:30 a.m.	I	Recreation (Physical Fitness)	Gym—A. T. Bldg.
10:30 a.m.	4	Recreation (Physical Fitness)	Gym - A. T. Bldg.
10:30 a.m.	All	Library (Cont.)	A. T. Bldg.
10:30 a.m.		Staff Reporters Meeting (Cont.)	A. T. Bldg.
10:30 a.m.	W. Inf.	Occupational Therapy	A. T. Bldg.
10:30 a.m.	L	Occupational Therapy	A. T. Bldg.

Figure 8.

WEEKLY PATIENT'S ACTIVITY SCHEDULE
November 16—November 22

Monday, November 16 OD for the day—Dr. Cheng
1:30 p.m. I.T. & C.T. Disposition Staff Room
1:30 p.m. Miami Co. Pts. Party—Volunteer Game Room

Tuesday, November 17 OD for the day—Dr. Mackey
9:00 a.m. Clinical Ward Conference Ward O
1:00 p.m. Clinical Ward Conference Ward 5
1:00 p.m. Disposition Staff Staff Room
7:00 p.m. Ward C Party (Volunteer) Ward C
7:00 p.m. Ward 6 Party (Volunteer) Ward 6
7:00 p.m. Veterans Party (Volunteer) Game Room

Wednesday, November 18 OD for the day—Dr. Matheu
7:00 a.m. Catholic Mass Auditorium
1:30 p.m. Ward L Party (Volunteer) Ward L
1:30 p.m. Ward 14 Party (Volunteer) Ward 14
7:00 p.m. All Dance Auditorium
7:00 p.m. Ward I Party (Volunteer) Ward I

Thursday, November 19 OD for the day—Dr. Shallow
9:00 a.m. Diagnostic Staff Staff Room
1:00 p.m. A.I.T. Disposition Staff Room

Friday, November 20 OD for the day—Dr. Phipps
9:30 a.m. Ward Rep. Inter-Ward Council Ward C
9:30 a.m. Clinical Ward Conference Ward D
3:00 p.m. Catholic Devotional Hour Auditorium
3:30 p.m. Adolescent Meeting Adm. Conf. Rm.
7:00 p.m. Benton Co. Pts. Party (Volunteer) Game Room

Saturday, November 21 OD for the day—Dr. Burnett
 Nurses on duty—T. Huddleston, M. Kandler, D. Klink
9:45 a.m. Protestant Bible Class Auditorium
2:00 p.m Closed Wards Movie—Never Steal Anything Small Auditorium
2:30 pm. Teenagers and Children Protestant Bible Class R. C. Classroom
7:00 p.m. Open Wards Movie—Never Steal Anything Small Auditorium

Sunday, November 22 OD for the day—Dr. Maschmeyer
 Nurses on duty—T. Huddleston, M. Kandler, D. Klink
8:45 a.m. Protestant Church Services Auditorium
9:45 a.m. Catholic Church Services Auditorium
2:00 p.m. All Entertainment by Putnam Co. Auditorium

Signed . . . .
       Coordinator of Activity Therapy

Figure 9.

Referrals, Reporting, and Recording

Adequate information about patients is necessary as a basis for the activity program. In order that all activities may become more effective, the ward physician should furnish information about patients, and in turn, the therapist should provide information, in order that the treatment may be carried on. Through no other means can the effectiveness of the program be accurately appraised. The referral of patients to activities may be handled in one of two ways. One, through written prescription whereby the patients are referred directly to specific activities for specific treatment at the request of the doctor; and secondly, by clearance or approval in which a whole ward or a group of patients are given approval to participate in various activities. The former method can be found in all types of hospitals while the latter is usually found only in public or private psychiatric hospitals, although this form may be applicable in the general medical and surgical hospital when patients are being taken out of the hospital to a recreation activity. The master schedule discussed above is another example of a clearance or approval.

The written prescription should contain the patient's name and age, diagnosis, ward or room, chart number, date of referral, precautions, treatment recommended or results desired, and signature of the referring physician. Besides the data that bear directly on the medical problem, there may be a varying amount of sociological information that may indirectly affect diagnosis and treatment and that is necessary for identification of the patient.

Probably no other single factor is more vital to a good treatment program than reports and records. So too is the management of the hospital dependent upon these same reports and records. As patients leave the hospital they need counseling service. This need may extend over a period of months or years. But aside from their use to the total hospital, they offer a means by which the effectiveness of the program can be accurately appraised and possibly give suggestions with respect to additional activities needed. Without this follow-up, no objective data concerning the program can be formulated and periodic evaluation and analysis cannot be conducted.

Patients receive better care when reports are thorough and give all pertinent information. Reporting of observations should

LSH-K-46 (6-58)

Logansport State Hospital

Referral to Activity Therapy Department

Patient's Name: .... Ward: ...... Age: ....
Type of Therapy Requested:
C.T. Individual...: Rec. Individual...: M.T. Individual...: Art Individual...:
    Group....   Group....   Group....   Group....
I.T. Individual...: V.R. Individual...:
    Group....   Group....

Specific Activity: ....

Objective:
    Pre-Vocational ....
    Outlets for Aggression ....
    Socialiaztion ....
    Muscular Coordination ....
    Means of Expression ....
    Development of Special Interest ....
    Training in Special Skills ....

Suggested Attitudes Permissive.... Restrictive.... Other....................

Ground Privileges: Yes.... No....

Mental Status: Alert.... Retarded.... Confused....

Precautions: Depressed....... Suicidal or Homicidal....... Assultive.......
           Seizures....... Hyperactive....... Elopment Tendencies.......
           Others (specify) ....

Special Instructions: (contraindications, etc.) ....
....
....
Comments: ....
....
....

Referred by .... Date ....
                Disapproved
                Approved by ....
                    Ward Physician

Figure 10.

be as specific and as objective as possible since reports give the therapist a sense of security which comes from knowing all factors in a given situation. On the other hand, it is essential that records be exact and correct since a number of professional workers are usually coordinating their efforts in their respective service to the patient. Insofar as it is possible, the record should consist of facts rather than opinions since it is important that each therapist knows what the other plans to do, are doing, and have done for the patient.

In summary, the activity program should contribute materially to the improvement of the hospital's entire program. It should provide to the administrator, physician, psychologist, and other members of the staff information about patients that will make them better able to perform their duties related to the adjustment and improvement of patients. Since the activity program is patient centered, it introduces purposes and techniques adapted to assist and encourage the individualization of other therapies. The therapist should be prepared to assist other staff personnel and departments to better recognize and meet the needs of the patients. The individualization of the activity program will lead staff members to recognize and observe significant patient attitudes and behavior, and this practice will, in turn, contribute to the total effectiveness of the activity program.

REFERENCES

1. Tillock, Eugene: A mental hygiene program for general hospitals, *Hosp. Prog.,* *42:*110, 1961.
2. Myers, J. Martin, and Smith, Lauren H.: The organization of a mental hospital, *Ment. Hosp., 7:*6, 1956.
3. Key, William: *Coordination of the Ancillary Therapies.* Convention Address, December, 1959, Sheraton-Lincoln Hotel, Indianapolis, Indiana.
4. Terry, George R.: *Principles of Management.* Rev. Ed. Homewood, Illinois, Richard D. Irwin, Inc., 1956, p. 385.
5. Meuli, Albert L.: An organizational complex. In *Recreation in Treatment Centers.* Washington, D. C., American Recreation Society, Vol. II, 1963, p. 15.
6. Therapeutic Recreation in the Community. (Ed.) MacLean, Janet R., Bloomington, Indiana, Department of Recreation, 1962.
7. Ridgway, Elizabeth P.: Personal letter. March, 1963.
8. Meuli, *op. cit.,* p. 15.

Chapter XII

FACILITIES AND EQUIPMENT

Today, a well-developed activity program is considered one of the basic treatment modalities in hospitals treating both the physically and mentally handicapped. At the same time, this increasing emphasis on activities calls for greater emphasis on suitable facilities and equipment for rehabilitation of the patient. These facilities are the means of implementing the diversified but interrelated functions of the various departments, as patterned by the process of planning and organizing. Although facilities and equipment are tools in assisting the therapist to perform his therapeutic function, they cannot be overemphasized. The role of the therapist is directed toward education and/or reeducation of the patient; therefore, adequate facilities and equipment will influence the therapeutic value of his education.

FACILITIES

The requirements for facilities within the various hospitals and rehabilitation centers vary with the type of agency in which the facilities are to be developed and the program designed.* It can be stated that the distribution of facilities for activity therapy programs will have some resemblance to the distribution of other

---

*Presently in progress is a movement toward the accredidation of rehabilitation centers and sheltered workshops. This movement is being studied by an "Ad Hoc Committee on Accreditation of Rehabilitation Facilities" formed by the National Rehabilitation Association, National Association of Sheltered Workshops and Homebound Programs and the Association of Rehabilitation Centers. Consideration is also being given to the involvement of the American Hospital Association on the proposed accreditation program. Further information concerning this whole area can be found in the *Journal of Rehabilitation,* January-February, 1964, "NRA Policy Statement on Rehabilitation Centers" and "Accreditation of the Rehabilitation Facility," *Journal of Rehabilitation,* May-June, 1964. The latter issue also includes a "Directory of Rehabilitation Facilities" in the United States and Canada. The directory includes a listing of admitting conditions, type of ownership, patients served by care and by age, bed capacity, service programs, and type of professional personnel employed.

kinds of hospital facilities while the accessibility to program areas will be of a greater or lesser extent influenced by the type of service in the specific hospital or the rehabilitation center.

State and federal hospitals treating the mentally ill or retarded should locate their activity building in close proximity to the center of the hospital grounds. This location will contribute to a better integrated whole within the total hospital. It should be readily accessible to both "open and closed wards," and patients with "ground privileges" should be able to come and go unaccompanied since it can be estimated that between seventy and eighty percent of the patient population of the hospital will frequent the building during the year. In addition, smaller stations or sub-stations for specific department activities will be located on the wards, especially those wards in which patients need bed care or are limited in their physical or mental ability to move freely around the grounds.

Rehabilitation centers or physical medicine departments in general medical and surgical hospitals may or may not provide facilities which are accessible to both those within the hospital and those being served on an out-patient basis. Specialty hospitals or clinics will determine their location of facilities upon the type of mental or physical handicap involved, although in most instances the location will be similar to those found in the hospitals mentioned above.

Planning new facilities, especially an activity therapy building or a rehabilitation center involves a considerable amount of work and should not be undertaken without a well-conceived plan. No standard plan can be applied to all activity therapy buildings, wings, or rooms since the design and development of each present a specific problem. However, the architectural keynote should be flexible to insure the future changes in concepts and practices. While a new building is not a guarantee in attaining a therapeutic program, the better the building the greater the potential of the treatment program.

The type and philosophy of the hospital for which the facility is being considered must always be kept in mind. In addition, the size of each department will depend upon the extent to which the hospital proposes to furnish the various forms of therapy. And finally, *those who will eventually use the facility should have a major part in its development.*

The most important component of a program is the trained therapist. Therefore, if we expect them to function properly we must provide them with a proper setting in which to work. In many hospitals, the therapist has had to utilize areas designed entirely for different purposes. This puts them at a disadvantage.

At present, there are sixteen of the fifty states planning rehabilitation building during the next five years.[1] It is hoped that in their planning some or all of the basic guide lines listed below will be utilized.

1. The facility should be based upon the needs of the patients in the hospital.
2. Planning should be based upon the regard for existing facilities and the relationship to potential outdoor facilities.
3. Visitation to other facilities of the same nature.
4. The facility should be in close proximity to the rest of the hospital. If possible, centrally located.
5. Functional design with flexibility. In many instances, program areas must serve a dual purpose.
6. Consideration of the possible expansion of the facility at a later date due to patient population growth.
7. Consideration of the equipment needed to operate the facility.
8. Utilization of professional advisory organizations.
9. Selection of a competent architect.
10. The building being free of political and especially personal interest.

It should be noted that where funds are not available for the total structure, construction of the necessary area should be started with the other areas completed as soon as funds are available. It is unfortunate, but as so often occurs, partial completion results in a permanent structure.

The increased demand for facilities has often resulted in the use of buildings originally planned for other departments. Often adaptation of these buildings presents serious problems, but, with some ingenuity, imagination, and effort, remarkable results have been accomplished. In adapting old buildings, care must be taken to make sure that the structure is sound, meeting building codes, and providing adequate exits.

Facilities: Indoor. No two structures are identical in their arrangement and facilities, but there are certain basic facilities which should be provided or included. An ideal building should be functionally designed so as to provide a varied program of recreation, music, and occupational therapy for all types of mentally ill, mentally retarded, and physically handicapped. It is quite possible and desirable that this building provide facilities for education therapy, vocational and industrial therapy, and the patient's library. It is recommended that separate rehabilitation centers and/or physical medicine departments should include facilities for physical, recreation, and occupational therapy respectively, hearing and speech therapy, prothetic and orthesis service, vocational service, library service, and facilities for teaching activities of daily living. Large rehabilitation centers may also contain medical, dental, psychological and social service facilities.[2] All areas should be so designed taking into consideration the handicapped, to allow the patient to feel that he is in normal and natural surroundings. This is no small way encourages patient participation, thereby bringing about socialization. Ideally, the design must put emphasis on features which tend to attract and hold interest.

The following proposed activity therapy structure is designed primarily for a large mental and/or retarded institution although many of the facilities may be adapted to smaller institutions and general medical and surgical hospitals.

The structure should, if at all possible, be of a one-story design thereby providing ease of administration and accessibility to program areas by patients, especially those who are physically handicapped. Multi-floor design may be justifiable in congested areas or general medical and surgical hospitals but construction costs usually are higher. In addition, multi-floor structures may require activities to be conducted on the roof. This presents many problems, such as the installation of proper fencing or railings, provisions for adequate drainage, inadequate space, and supervision. Certainly activities can be provided more economically on the ground floor or by making arrangements for use of community facilities.

The main entrance into the building should open into a central foyer or lobby with the lobby being so located that patients and personnel can readily reach the various activity areas. One entrance or more should be of the ramp-type with handrails or all entrances to be flush with the ground. Adequate corridors of proper width and surface are essential, especially in those hospitals serving the physically handicapped. Experience has indicated that even the smallest activity therapy building need offices and a large conference room if the building is to serve as a central administrative building for all of the activity therapy services. Martin[3] believes that this single factor (of offices) may encourage "team" action because of the "constant informal communication which can be carried out—through personal contact." Adequate office space would include private offices for the directors to have conferences and discussion with their staff. Study areas should also be provided if students are working in the activities. Moreover, it is important to have the administrative offices adjoining the lobby thereby presenting ease of supervision and coordination of patients going and coming from activities. Another factor to consider is that in many hospitals, it may be an advantage to locate the canteen or snack-bar, with an outdoor patio, adjacent to the building, through the lobby.

The recreation unit of the building should include a gymnasium which serves a dual role as an auditorium. This arrangement has both its advantages and disadvantages, but very seldom will there be two mass activities programmed at the same time which require separate facilities. If activities are to be programmed in that manner, then separate facilities should be provided and consideration be given to having permanent seating with an inclining floor in the auditorium.

The gymnasium-auditorium should not be less than 60 x 90

ft. to a maximum of 100 x 110 ft., with a basketball court 42 x 70 ft. to 50 x 80 ft., ceiling height should be 22 ft. or more. Telescopic folding bleachers are preferable to permanent seating facilities, thus additional space is provided for floor games. If the gymnasium doubles as an auditorium, a portable stage may be used although it is preferable to have an elevated stage at one end which can be used for dramatic and music productions and motion pictures. Stage size will be determined by the over-all gymnasium-auditorium size, patient population, and programming although a desirable stage size should provide a minimum width of 40 ft., a depth of 20 ft., height of 3 ft., above the proscenium opening, which should not be less than 12 x 25 ft.[4]

Adequate storage, dressing rooms and entrances for bringing in and taking out scenery should be provided and be easily accessible to the stage. It is desirable that the gymnasium-auditorium area be equipped with a proper public address system, permanently installed, with electrical outlets for phonographic equipment and microphones, as well as controls of lights and sound from several points, such as the stage, athletic office, and projection booth. Additional switches for lights will be needed at various entrances. Where the gymnasium-auditorium is used for motion pictures, an adequate size projection booth, completely fireproofed in itself, is essential.

Conveniently located storage, dressing, locker, and shower rooms can not be over emphasized where facilities are being used for different activities. The gymnasium-auditorium storage room should be of a large size so as to accommodate both small and large pieces of equipment such as folding chairs, combination standards, exercise mats and apparatus. Special attention needs to be taken when planning toilets, locker, and shower rooms for both sexes. Gang showers are recommended for men while individual showers and dressing booths are recommended for women. Control of water and water temperature should be by a mixing chamber located near the men and women shower areas. When the building is serving outdoor facilities, separate entrances to toilet and shower rooms should be provided as well as exits from the area into the lobby without having to pass through the gymnasium-auditorium. Some hospitals may desire to have an exercise room adjacent to, and opening into the gymnasium although exercise activities can be conducted in the gymnasium proper. Attention should also be given to providing a small room with a serving counter opening into the gymnasium-auditorium area for the preparation of food. If possible, a kitchen should be provided within easy access to the area.

Recreation game or activity rooms are an essential part of the activity therapy building and should be provided and designed for multiple use. It is feasible, to provide folding partitions, so rooms may be divided as well as making all of the rooms soundproof. Sufficient storage space for equipment and supplies within the rooms as well as adjacent to these rooms can not be overstressed.

The music therapy unit will be in need of several activity rooms, practice rooms, listening rooms, and library room, of which all should be provided with accoustical tile and sound insulated. The actual number of rooms needed will be based upon the present and anticipated staff available for giving lessons, supervision, and patient population. A useful guide in multipurpose rooms to be used by music therapy is to allow 20 sq. ft. for each participant. Again, it can not be stressed enough for adequate storage room with specific storage cabinets for instruments, phonograph records, choir robes and uniforms. The storage room should be well ventilated and protected against excessive moisture or heat or extreme changes in temperature, since many instruments are made of wood with glued joints. If a separate auditorium is planned, music therapy is usually responsible for the area and can utilize some facilities adjacent to the stage and the stage proper for their programs.

Some hospitals have developed facilities when working with individual patients whereby it is possible from a master station to switch on any or all of the music practice rooms to hear how the patient is progressing. Other hospitals, working through the music therapy department, have a wired music distribution system throughout the hospital or to particular wards. This can also be accomplished if the hospital has a closed circuit TV station with music traveling over the same coaxial cable. Before entering into the development of such a program in an already existing facility, serious consideration must be given the project because of the extensive cost.

Two approaches may be utilized when developing the occupational therapy department; one, separate rooms for specific medias, i.e., wood, ceramics, etc.; and two, a multi-craft clinic where all varieties of medias are provided. An exception here would be in kitchen facilities, large woodworking equipment, etc., which should be in separate rooms. Regardless of the developmental approach the area should have adequate cabinet storage space for supplies, equipment, and unfinished craft articles. In addition, separate storage space is needed for the storage of large quantities of material and supplies, and for double duty as a preparation room. West[5] recommends that the occupational therapy department be planned on a "U" or the "H-shaped" design, with the office being located at the base of the "U" or on the crossbar of the "H". She further recommended that the walls of the activity rooms be glass thereby providing exposure to all rooms and easy supervision of the area. Minimum space of 26 sq. ft. is recommended for each patient, while in large hospitals it is suggested that the clinic facility be based upon the "unit system, allocating 100-200 square feet per unit . . ."[6] A kitchen, if possible, should be provided for a home economics program which would also serve a dual purpose for the preparing of food in connection with special programs. Easy accessibility from the kitchen to one or more of the multi-purpose rooms or auditorium should be provided.

It is desirable to have the patient's library within the building and easily accessible to the lobby or an outside entrance. A patient's newspaper which may be sponsored by any one of the departments should also be located within the building, and if possible, adjacent to the library. Serious consideration should be given to providing a bookbinding and utility room adjoining the library.

Optional facilities within the building may include space for bowling lanes, swimming pool, handball courts, indoor driving range, etc. If plans are to include the educational therapy and vocational and industrial therapy departments then additional classrooms, training and testing units, located so that distraction would be at a minimum, and offices must be provided. If a children's unit is included within the hospital, consideration should be given as to whether to have a separate activity area within the unit or to use existing facilities. Regardless of the type of facilities used, some of the furniture and equipment will need to be scaled down. A volunteer lounge is another consideration that must be given serious thought, as well as a facility for speech and hearing units. Speech and hearing laboratories should be removed as far as possible from sources of extraneous noise but still conveniently located for both in and out patients. If the hospital is involved in research and/or teaching, one-way observation windows may be indicated in one or two rooms of the activity room.

An inter-communication system between main areas and offices as well as a central sound system with conduits large enough to provide future television installations are well worth the money spent. Anticipated use of television should include a master television antenna from the roof to various installation points within the building and should be carefully studied and designed by specialists. However, it should be pointed out that television can be a dangerous anti-social instrument at times—replacing social interaction.

Provisions should be made within the building for adequate custodial storage and a transformer room. The heating of the building should be adequate and provisions for air-conditioning, especially in the gymnasium-auditorium, as well as adequate lighting for all rooms should be made. Safety precautions, such as a master switch for power tools should be built in. The physical environment within the building is established not only by the shape of the spaces, but by the lighting, color, acoustics, ventilation, heating, and durability of materials which are easily cleaned and require low maintenance.

The prime consideration of locating the activity therapies in general medical and surgical hospitals should be easily accessibility to all parts of the hospital, near to the elevators, for patients who will be brought to the treatment clinic and in order to bring service apparatus to the wards and rooms. The various departments need not be large, but should include some of the basic items mentioned previously such as one or two multi-purpose rooms for recreation and music programs, an additional room or two for occupational therapy with adequate space for storage and offices.

More hospitals, including specialty hospitals, are now providing swimming pools for their patients as well as exercise or corrective therapy rooms. Besides treatment rooms, there must be a waiting room or space for patients, an examination room for physician, rest rooms, as well as sufficient storage space for supplies.

Those interested in pursuing the development of a large rehabilitation facility or facilities just discussed, are recommended to read *Planning Multiple Disability Rehabilitation Facilities* published by the U. S. Department of Health, Education, and Welfare, Public Health Service, Washington, D. C. Another excellent source is *Planning Facilities for Health, Physical Education, and Recreation* published by the Athletic Institute, Chicago, Illinois. This particular publication gives an excellent description of suggested floor lay-outs, lighting intensities, furniture arrangements and equipment which can be used by all specialties working in a rehabilitation center.

The following pages give a graphic design of activity therapy areas within various types of hospitals. It is emphasized that these following designs are presented only as a guide for planning similar units.

Figure 11 is an activity therapy building designed along the lines described in this chapter. Particular attention has been paid to functional departmental units, office units, and flow of traffic.

The Rehabilitation Center of McLean Hospital presently under construction (Figure 12) is a day-care center for both in and out patients. "McLean Hospital, a division of Massachusetts General Hospital, is a 276-bed, voluntary, non-profit teaching hospital,

—————————————————→

Figure 11. Activity Therapy Building designed from Contents of this Chapter.

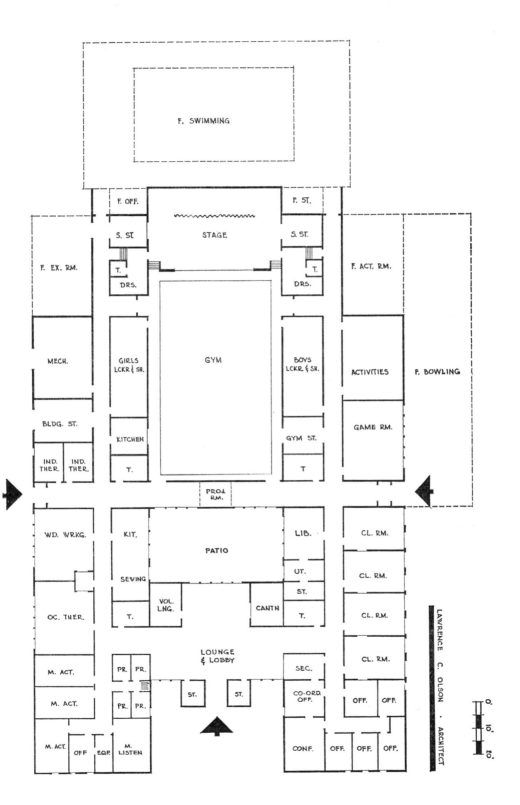

F. SWIMMING

F. OFF. F. ST.

STAGE

S. ST. S. ST.

F. EX. RM. F. ACT. RM.

T. T.
DRS. DRS.

MECH. GIRLS LCKR & SH. GYM BOYS LCKR & SH. ACTIVITIES F. BOWLING

BLDG. ST. KITCHEN GYM ST. GAME RM.

IND. THER. IND. THER. T. T

PROJ. RM.

WD. WRKG. KIT. PATIO LIB. CL. RM.

UT. CL. RM.

SEVING ST.

OC. THER. T. VOL. LNG. CANT'N T. CL. RM.

M. ACT. PR. PR. LOUNGE & LOBBY SEC. CL. RM.

M. ACT. PR. PR. ST. ST. CO-ORD. OFF. OFF. OFF.

M. ACT. OFF EQP. M. LISTEN CONF. OFF. OFF. OFF.

LAWRENCE C. OLSON · ARCHITECT

0' 10' 20'

caring for and treating all types of psychiatric illness . . . Except for a "Village Green" area, the structure will be a single-story, slab-on grade unit, plus a partial basement. The main floor will consist of a series of modular structural units 33 feet square, arranged in series to create landscaped courts in addition to providing for the functions described below. Total floor space will be about 20,000 square feet. The basement, under the occupational therapy wing only, will provide another 4100 square feet.

In the O. T. wing, patients will engage in painting, sculpturing, pottery and ceramics, fine woodwork and weaving. There will be a kitchen, sewing room, and some office space. The basement, accessible both from upstairs and directly from outside, will have a darkroom, and machinery for heavy woodworking. The present printing, typing, and dancing facilities will be transferred to the basement."[7]

Figure 13. Represents a plan for multiple disability rehabilitation facility based upon information which has been developed by the Joint Committee of the American Hospital Association, American Physical Therapy Association, and American Occupational Therapy Association, and other . . . operating centers. . . ."[8]

Figure 14. Is the Activity Therapy Building at Faribault State School and Hospital; a hospital for the mentally retarded. Emphasis is put upon educational and recreational activities in design.

Facilities: Out-doors. Again, as with the activity therapy building, no two outdoor recreation areas are identical in their arrangement and facilities. Out-door facilities are needed in quantity and variety to serve the mentally ill, mentally retarded, and the physically ill and handicapped. The development, selection, and design of out-door facilities will consist of a combination of specific uses as are appropriate to the area available. The site should be located within a short walking distance of the activity therapy building or as centrally located as possible to the rest of the hospital, thereby providing access to lockers and shower facilities. Multiple use of the area and facilities can extend service and

⸻⸻⸻⸻⸻⸻⸻⸻⸻⸻⸻⸻⸻⸻⸻⟶

Figure 12. Rehabilitation Center, McLean Hospital, Boston, Massachusetts (permission to reprint courtesy of *Mental Hospitals*).

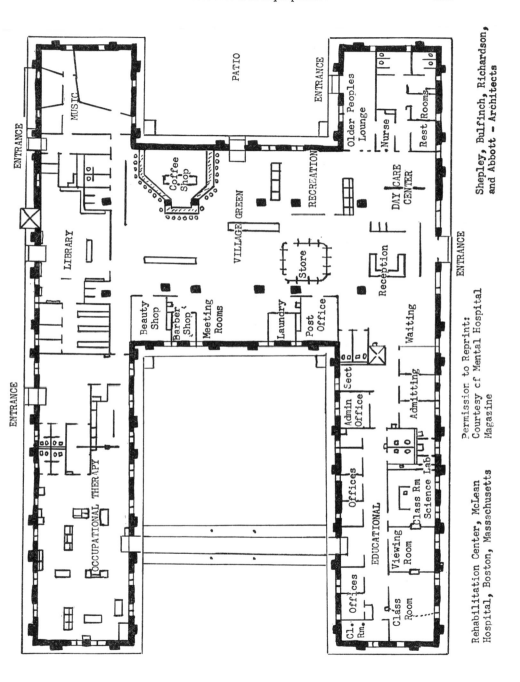

Rehabilitation Center, McLean
Hospital, Boston, Massachusetts

Permission to Reprint:
Courtesy of Mental Hospital
Magazine

Shepley, Bulfinch, Richardson,
and Abbott – Architects

partially off-set the cost of developing the facilities such as utilization of the basketball court for dances or the varied uses of a cement tennis court for badminton, volleyball, etc. Careful planning facilitates a maximum variety of uses.

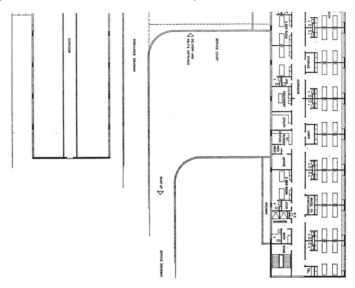

Figure 13. Plan of a Multiple Disability Rehabilitation Facility. Developed by Joint Committee of the American Hospital Association (permission to reprint courtesy of Department of Health, Education, and Welfare, Washington, D.C.) .

Butler[9] suggests the following factors and objectives should be considered when planning outside facilities "regardless of the type of recreation area:

1. Effective use of the entire area.
2. Location and arrangements of the areas and facilities.
3. Adequate space for the facilities.
4. Ease of supervision or operation.
5. Accessibility and relationship of various features.
6. Utilization of natural features.
7. Safety.
8. Economy in construction.
9. Economy in maintenance.

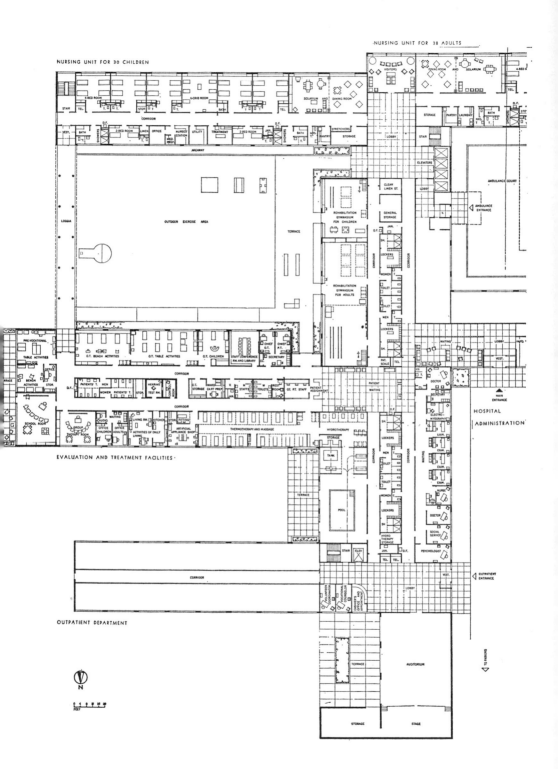

10. Convenience of people using area.
11. Appearance."

Facilities for the mentally ill, retarded, and physically handi-capped children should include an area for playground apparatus apart from the play area for older children and adults. Opinions differ as to the value of apparatus for the mentally ill although some pieces are justified only if it provides an outlet for past known interest. Other facilities for all types of patients should include baseball and softball diamonds with effective illumina-tion, sandboxes, open turf areas for field sports, tennis courts, paved areas of nonabrasive material for multiple use, shuffle-board, and horseshoe pits. Shelters, picnic areas, camp sites, and pitch and putt golf courses are other outdoor facilities which can be provided.

Swimming pools are now being provided in many hospitals. Location of such should be adjacent to the activity therapy build-ing where locker and shower facilities are available. If it is away from the building, then proper bathhouse facilities must be built. A heated pool is desirable and will receive more use and the length of time of its use will be extended. Provisions should be made in hospitals which work with children to provide a wading pool. Consideration of types of pool facilities: indoor and out-door, cost of construction, size, and equipment; the author recom-mends the references listed at the end of this section. (See refer-ences 10 and 11.)

Few hospitals have golf facilities due to the expense involved but it is quite possible to have a "Pitch and Putt Course" or a driving range. Those interested in developing driving ranges should refer to "Golf Operators Handbook" published by the National Golf Foundation. The "Pitch and Putt Courses" can be developed on as little as five acres for a nine hole course with a par 3 and a range anywhere from 40 yards to 250 yards. Approxi-mate cost is $1000.00 per hole.[10] Miniature golf courses also enjoy a considerable amount of popularity within the hospital.

Shelter buildings may be of the open or closed type. A build-ing of this type provides many opportunities for informal par-

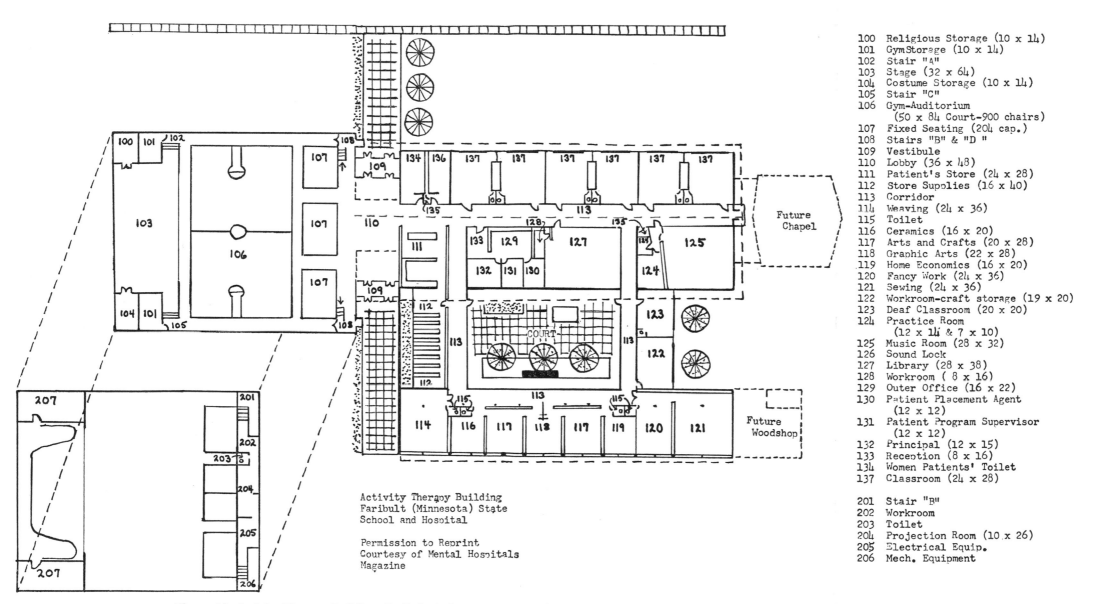

100	Religious Storage (10 x 14)
101	Gym Storage (10 x 14)
102	Stair "A"
103	Stage (32 x 64)
104	Costume Storage (10 x 14)
105	Stair "C"
106	Gym-Auditorium
	(50 x 84 Court-900 chairs)
107	Fixed Seating (204 cap.)
108	Stairs "B" & "D "
109	Vestibule
110	Lobby (36 x 48)
111	Patient's Store (24 x 28)
112	Store Supplies (16 x 40)
113	Corridor
114	Weaving (24 x 36)
115	Toilet
116	Ceramics (16 x 20)
117	Arts and Crafts (20 x 28)
118	Graphic Arts (22 x 28)
119	Home Economics (16 x 20)
120	Fancy Work (24 x 36)
121	Sewing (24 x 36)
122	Workroom-craft storage (19 x 20)
123	Deaf Classroom (20 x 20)
124	Practice Room
	(12 x 14 & 7 x 10)
125	Music Room (28 x 32)
126	Sound Lock
127	Library (28 x 38)
128	Workroom (8 x 16)
129	Outer Office (16 x 22)
130	Patient Placement Agent
	(12 x 12)
131	Patient Program Supervisor
	(12 x 12)
132	Principal (12 x 15)
133	Reception (8 x 16)
134	Women Patients' Toilet
137	Classroom (24 x 28)
201	Stair "B"
202	Workroom
203	Toilet
204	Projection Room (10 x 26)
205	Electrical Equip.
206	Mech. Equipment

Activity Therapy Building
Faribult (Minnesota) State
School and Hospital

Permission to Reprint
Courtesy of Mental Hospitals
Magazine

Figure 14. Activity Therapy Building, Faribult (Minnesota) State School and Hospital (permission to reprint courtesy of *Mental Hospitals*).

ticipation and supervised activities as dances, table games, music, and crafts. The building itself should contain a kitchenette, rest rooms, storage rooms, drinking fountains, and base and wall outlets. Size of such buildings vary depending on whether it shall be of the closed type or open type. The open type is a small compact unit with a covered porch approximately 400 to 600 sq. ft. A common size of the closed type is 1500 sq. ft.[11] Lighting should be provided so evening activities may be conducted. It is an advantage to have a multipurpose paved surface area adjoining the building.

Camp sites are being developed more and more for utilization by the handicapped so as to teach skills, knowledge, and attitudes about outdoor living. Camps call for special planning and should be available for several months of the year. The site should include attractively designed buildings for living, a central building for offices, a spacious dining room-recreational hall with a modern kitchen attached and an outdoor patio. Also facilities including outdoor recreational areas, hiking trails, fishing holes, and swimming areas should be included. The geographical location of the site should be determined by the type of program, frequency and duration of the camping visit (day camp, overnight camp, resident camp).

One of the most difficult decisions to make in developing outdoor play areas is the selection of the type of surface to be used for various play and sport areas. When selecting a surface material, there are certain factors that must be studied carefully before a decision can be reached. Gabrielsen[12] lists the following factors which should be considered:

Level of performance (general play, tournament play, professional play).
Seasonal use (summer only, year-around use).
Multiple use or single purpose (surface to be used for more than one activity).
Durability (for quality of use).
Resilience (the spring or bounce).
Traction (footable).

Appearance (esthetic value, or harmony with surroundings).
Cost (money available for initial construction and maintenance).
Maintenance (availability of funds and personnel for maintenance).
Local climatic Conditions (amount of precipitation and range of temperature).

Discussion of the three major types of surfaces; turf, asphalt, and concrete would take a considerable amount of time; therefore, the reader is recommended to refer to the references at the end of this section. (See reference 12.)

The quality of illumination requires uniformity over the play area. Illumination levels recommended for play areas whether indoor or outdoor depend upon the purpose for which the area is used. The Illumination Engineering Society[13] states that the "Correct choice among the various design factors depends upon a balancing of economic cost against such factors as appearance, relative safety and reliability. . . . A true comparison (of lighting systems) should involve systems proving comparable quality and quantity of illumination."

Additional features essential to a well-developed play area are: tables and benches for participants in quiet games or for use by visitors, bleachers for softball and baseball diamonds, drinking fountains strategically placed at various points, attractive and well landscaped grounds, and fireplaces for outdoor grilling and picnics.

Facilities: On-wards. Facilities for conducting activities on the ward may, at times, present difficulty due to the lack of adequate space and storage rooms. The question of space is quite a problem in old hospitals where space is at a premium; hence, one often sees activities being conducted in poorly lighted and ventilated rooms. Newly developed psychiatric units in general medical and surgical hospitals usually provide a large enough dayroom whereby table games, social gatherings, and small activities can be conducted. Wards in state and federal hospitals usually have day rooms which can be utilized for activities as well as other building areas within the hospital. The location of these rooms on the ward should be centrally located although even the basement of the ward building is not undesirable, providing the rooms are high and there is adequate light and ventilation. It is desirable to have a gardening area adjunct to geriatric wards. Specialty hospitals, especially children's hospitals, have similar arrangements. Hunt's[14] *Recreation for the Handicapped* gives a good description of facilities and equipment needed for orthopedically and cerebral palsied incapacitated children or adults.* Active programs can not be very well presented in general medical and surgical hospitals due to the physical arrangement of the ward and the physical incapabilities of the patients. Therefore, consideration must be given to the development of multi-purpose rooms in another area of the hospital.

All departments which do conduct activities on wards should have access to a storage room or cabinet. If this arrangement is impossible, then some type of a cart should be developed which could be utilized for the transportation of supplies from the department to the ward. Occupational therapy should have a small sub-station or stations located in various treatment areas of the hospital since their activities are not always conducive to day-rooms. Recreation and music can usually requisition two or more large rooms for their activities. Vocational and industrial therapy and educational therapy departments can utilize various offices or rooms within the hospital to conduct their business.

EQUIPMENT AND SUPPLIES

No activity can be conducted without equipment and supplies. In turn, the activity wil largely determine the type of equipment and supplies needed. For the procurement of adequate equipment and supplies of various amounts for different purposes and the justification; the coordinator or director must lean heavily on the counsel and information of his department heads. Other factors

---

*Also see *Making Buildings and Facilities Accessible to, and Usable by the Physically Handicapped and Design of Buildings to Permit Their Use by the Physically Handicapped*. National Society for Crippled Children and Adults, Inc., 2023 W. Ogden Avenue, Chicago, Illinois 1961.

which must be considered in determining the type of supplies and equipment needed are the age, sex, mental and physical ability, and skills of the participants, space and facilities presently available, and cost and seasonal use.[15] Martin[16] observes that "destruction is at a minimum when even the most disturbed patients are presented with an attractive area pleasantly and comfortably furnished. On the other hand, loss by destruction and misuse is high when patients are surrounded by unattractive, worn-out equipment." The Athletic Institute[17] states that "the investment in facilities will not yield the return expected unless sufficient quantities and varieties of equipment and supplies are provided." All apparatus should be of a standard type and purchased from manufacturers of good repute who will agree to furnish adequate service of periodic inspection and adjustments. It may be well for the coordinator or department heads, when furnishing a completely new building, to ask for a blanket appropriation for equipment, thereby facilitating matters more quickly.

It is not possible to give a complete standard list of equipment and supplies because the number and types of apparatus, as well as that of the many necessary accessories, will vary according to the predominant type of work, but an attempt will be made to briefly outline basic equipment. The planning for necessary equipment and the mode of its installation should be left to the department head involved and not be planned for them by others.*

The Veterans Administration has developed methods of testing equipment whereby equipment is sent out to various types of hospitals. It is put to use in various types of wards and for various patients. An observation is made over a period of time to ascertain its use to the patients and whether or not the equipment is satisfactory.

The gymnasium-auditorium, acoustically treated, should be equipped with equipment which is essential for its particular use —sound systems, scoreboard, microphones, basketball backstops,

---

*For some assistance in recreation equipment see *Criteria For Judging Recreation Equipment,* American Recreation Society, Inc., 1404 New York Ave. N.W., Washington, D.C., 1962.

portable standards for volleyball, badminton and tennis, bleachers, long tables, if banquets are to be held in the area, various types of lockers, choir risers, stage curtains, and a movie screen to name just a few of the items. Multiple-use areas indoor and outdoor should be provided with the various types of billiard-pool tables, folding table-tennis, tables, lounge chairs, television set, table shuffleboard, and folding card tables. Music listening and practice rooms usually include a piano, a hi-fi or stereo system, and comfortable lounge chairs. Another useful piece of equipment is a piano "dolly" equipped with ball-bearing rubber casters. Such equipment facilitates movement and pays dividends in helping to keep the piano in tune and preventing damage to the piano legs and floor. If there is a separate auditorium, then a decision must be made whether to equip the area with folding chairs or permanent theatre type of seating. Where funds are not available for the regular size stage, then a portable stage should be secured.

The occupational therapy department will need a kiln and potter's wheel for ceramic programs, woodworking machinery, various floor and table size looms, and cutting tables and sewing machines for sewing programs. A pegboard wall facilitates storage of hand tools. A mobile cart for servicing ward patients is essential. The kitchen should include adequate tables and counter space, range, oven, sink, dishwasher, and proper ventilation. The library should not only include book cases but a bulletin board or two to display colorful decorations or items prepared by the patients, a book cart, newspaper stick holders, index card file case, and other related material. The occupational therapy and recreation departments in general medical and surgical hospitals and specialty hospitals should study the numbers and categories of disabilities to be treated before the ordering of equipment and supplies although equipment and supplies seem to be applicable to both general medical and surgical hospitals. If possible, this area should be close or adjunct to the physical therapy department.

Speech and hearing clinics usually include head-phones, amplifier, tape recorders, microphones, wall mirrors, and chalkboard, to name a few items. Classrooms for the mentally retarded and physically handicapped should consider chalkboards and track boards which are mounted on rails to allow them to be raised and lowered to fit the size of the students using them.

The careful selection of supplies and material for the program is essential. What is required depends upon the nature and scope of the program, the number of kinds of facilities, and the personnel available to conduct the programs. Some supplies may be made by the patients themselves as part of a project such as bean bags, table-tennis paddles, checkerboards, etc. Hospitals may also find assistance by appealing through the local newspapers, civic organizations, and philantropic groups. The danger involved here is the receiving of supplies which have reached their life span.

Quality vs. Quantity

The importance of a good quality of merchandise can not be overstressed. Quality is an inherent factor of quantity. The quantity of equipment and supplies should be determined by the nature and number of participants, and fields and courts available. Funds, especially state funds, are not usually adequate to provide all of the supplies needed, but it is essential in hospitals to have durable safe equipment and supplies provided in specific amounts. It is assumed before we close this chapter that adequate methods have been developed for inventory control so that depreciation can be correctly calculated and proper maintenance recured. Date of purchase, original cost, serial numbers, property tax number, and estimated useful life must be recorded. Unit cost and standardization of color, style, and size are other important considerations. In order to secure proper supplies and equipment, to keep an adequate quantity on hand, and to avoid waste, proper systemization and control must be exercised over purchasing, storage, and distribution.

The fact that this chapter dealt primarily with facilities and equipment at the hospital does not preclude the importance of taking full advantage of integrating the patient with the community. Nearly all activities which are provided within the hospital can also be found within the community and it behooves the therapist and the hospital to take full advantage of these facilities.

The patient must be given the opportunity to keep in contact with the ouside world and to experiment with better ways of adjusting to it. One of the general recommendations made by the American Association for Health, Physical Education, and Recreation, at their 1958 national convention and later published in their conferences report, *Recreation for the Mentally Ill* was that ". . . institutions and outpatient treatment centers for the mentally ill should be encouraged to enter into an agreement with schools, parks, and other community agencies for the cooperative planning and joint use of their recreation facilities. Such cooperation would tend to lessen the problems resulting from the isolation of the institution from the community."[18]

REFERENCES

1. *A Marketing Survey of Annual Expenditures and Purchasing Patterns in Public Mental Institutions.* APA, Washington, D. C., January, 1961, pp. 11-14.
2. *Planning Multiple Disability Rehabilitation Facilities.* U. S. Department of Health, Education, and Welfare, Public Health Service, Washington, D. C., 1960.
3. Martin, Harold R.: Architectural planning for activity areas. *Ment. Hosp.,* 9 (4) : 23, 1958.
4. Butler, George D.: *Introduction to Community Recreation.* 3rd Ed., McGraw-Hill Book Company, New York, 1959, p. 211.
5. West, Wilma: Organizations and administration of occupational therapy departments. *Principles of Occupational Therapy,* 2nd ed., (eds.) Wallard, Helen S. and Spackman, Clarence S., Philadelphia, J. B. Lippincott Company, 1954, p. 66.
6. *Manual on the Organization and Administration of Occupational Therapy Departments.* William C. Brown Company, Dubuque, Iowa, 1951, p. 9.
7. The McLean Hospital Rehabilitation Center. *Ment. Hosp.,* August, 1962, p. 411.
8. *Planning Multiple Disability Rehabilitation Facilities. op. cit.,* p. 9.
9. Butler, George D., *op. cit.,* p. 179.
10. Gabrielsen, Alexander: Golf facilities. *Sports and Recreation Facilities for School and Community.* (ed.) Gabrielsen, M. Alexander, and Miles, Caswell M., Englewood Cliffs, New Jersey, Prentice-Hall, Inc., 1958, p. 294.
11. *Planning Facilities for Health, Physical Education and Recreation.* The Athletic Institute, Chicago, Illinois, 1962, p. 93.
12. Gabrielsen, Alexander: Selecting the proper play surface. *op. cit.,* p. 219.
13. Gabrielsen, Alexander: Lighting for sports and recreation facilities. *op cit.,* p. 209.
14. Hunt, Valerie V.: *Recreation for the Handicapped.* Englewood Cliffs, New Jersey, Prentice-Hall, Inc., 1955.
15. *Equipment and Supplies for Athletics, Physical Education, and Recreation.* The Athletic Institute, Chicago, Illinois, 1960, p. 3.

16. Martin, Harold: *Architectural Planning for Activity Programs, in Psychiatric Architecture,* (ed) . Goshen, Charles, American Psychiatric Association, Washington, D. C., 1959, p. 79.
17. *Equipment and Supplies for Athletics, Physical Education, and Recreation. op. cit.,* p. 2.
18. Recreation for the Mentally Ill, Conference Report, (ed.) Phillips, B. E., American Association for Health, Physical Education, and Recreation, New York, New York, 1958, p. 33.

Chapter XIII

STAFF DEVELOPMENT

STAFF EDUCATION is taking place every day and is a part of supervision and administration as well as a group process. It is in no sense considered as a substitute for professional education. It is necessary to instruct all members of the team regarding the character of the activities assigned to them and the relationship these bear to the training of their colleagues in the collective enterprise. All training and education is for improvement and growth. Without these, the job is nothing.

The gaining of knowledge, showing others how to perform a job, and stimulating thinking takes place as a result of a specific training program, of trial or error, or of gradual infiltration. Whether we recognize it or not, training is going on all the time. It is a mistake to look upon training as mere indoctrination to be completed in a short time after a therapist begins his work in a hospital. Experience shows that education must be viewed as a creative process and as a period for development and growth of the whole individual. Any training given to as many as one employee makes its impact on the group and rebounds to the progress of the group.

Training, as observed by Terry,[1] "is in the nature of a development of people and is a continuous requirement in most enterprises; it offers the means of increasing an employee's efficiency on a present job and of qualifying for a better job." The Committee on Employee Training in the Public Service states that "employee training is the process of aiding employees to gain effectiveness in their present or future work through the development of appropriate habits of thought and action, skills, knowledge, and attitudes."[2]

The success of the education and training of any individual depends upon his acceptance and understanding of why this education and training is needed. In addition, it is necessary for both the staff therapist and newly employed therapist and those charged with the training program to have a clear conception of the precise skills to be attained. A basic concept pointed out by Wolfe[3] "is that the content of a staff development program must be related to the goals and objectives of the agency and based upon the specific knowledge and skill needed by each staff member to carry out the purpose of the program."

Education may be provided in four ways within an activity therapy service: (1) In-service education or training, whereby the therapist within each specialty continues to receive training and further his or her professional development. Another form of in-service training which may be a part of the former or separated entirely is a program for new employees and/or for semiprofessional personnel. The American Occupational Therapy Association has developed training programs for assistants in the fields of psychiatry and general practice. The latter may also be looked upon as on-the-job training. (2) Activity therapy staff development, whereby the entire staff of the activity therapy service are involved. (3) Clinical affiliation program, whereby students who have completed their schoolroom education in their specialty affiliate with one or more hospitals. (4) Volunteer training, whereby volunteers who are assigned to the various specialties receive specific training with regards to patients and programs.

In-service Training

A college education is now considered a basic requirement for nearly all professional positions within the activity therapy service while a high school diploma may be the requirement with additional on-the-job training for assistant or semiprofessional personnel. In some situations, persons trained in other fields will continue to fill many of the vacancies that exist in the service. Therefore, an adequate in-service training program is even more essential to further develop the partially trained or untrained therapist as well as to assist the trained therapist in his continuing education and professional development.

In—service training programs are usually conducted by the department head of the specialty, although the department head may delegate a particular program session to another therapist, or each staff member, in rotation, may be responsible for certain topics of interest to the whole staff. The program should be officially announced in advance and carry the approval of the administrative head. The announcement should indicate the nature of the course, its objectives, and the time and frequency of training sessions. Moreover, if the department head is conducting the training program, he should be aware of the supervisory element. This element according to Wolfe[4] "can produce either positive or negative reactions in the group, since each member has a particular relationship with his supervisor. The supervisor should recognize these various reactions and must learn to deal with them in working with the group."

The training sessions should be held on a weekly or by-monthly basis with attendance being *compulsory* and conducted during scheduled working hours. In addition, the training sessions should be conducted in the work area if demonstrations and activities are part of the session, otherwise, meetings can be held in a conveniently located area. The particular day and time of day that the sessions are conducted will have some influence upon the ability to comprehend and retain the material presented. If possible, the sessions should be scheduled when it will least interfere with the regular program and when the therapist find it most convenient to attend. The department head, when developing the patient program, should allocate a period in the program for the conducting of an in-service training program.

If wisely conducted, in-service training programs offer a wonderful opportunity for raising the standard of work, contributing to employee growth, preventing stagnation, and for developing a spirit of cooperation among staff therapist as well as developing a professional attitude. To the summer student, it supplements their schoolroom theory by providing a better understanding of their duties, a practical introduction to activities, and a guide to the solution of activity problems.

It is essential that the department head or whoever is in charge of the program have a definite program for each training session. Active learning requires participation. Material presented should be alive and interesting and meaningful to the learners. He must give the staff therapist every opportunity to share in the session and encourage them to express their opinions on the program under discussion. A worker may not understand situations which are similar to others he has handled unless he has an understanding of the underlying principles. By stimulating them to express their opinions and share in the program, the therapist is kept more alert and watches for new ideas that may be useful to the training sessions. The director may also utilize this time to point out weaknesses and suggest methods of correcting them. Under competent leadership, therapists can help others to realize their own potentialities and to face their problems realistically. In other words, help them to develop a faith in their own resources.

A brief comment should be made about the in-service training program for those who are classified as semiprofessional. This type of program might possibly be looked upon as apprentice training. A number of suggestions are hereby given to improve the quality of the assistant therapist: (1) careful selection of candidates with good selection techniques; (2) on-the-job training supplemented by in-service training; (3) advancement according to demonstrated ability and not according to time expanded and (4) the use of textbooks and manuals showing the levels of skill to be attained at each stage of progress.

A well planned and administrated program for semiprofessional therapist has a number of distinct advantages for both therapist and the department or hospital operating the program. For the department, it insures a steady flow of semi-skilled personnel to replace those who leave and helps make changes in programs less confusing. The therapists themselves learn a specific skill and are less susceptible to unemployment if they leave the hospital. Moreover, the therapist is paid while learning and is motivated to obtain a higher degree of skill, thereby obtaining an increase in position, money, or both. Finally, in such a program there is a maximum opportunity for integrating academic theory with practical problems often leading to improvement in the solution of the latter.

Following are a few suggestions as to content and conduct of in-service training programs within each specialty:

1. Cover the aims and objectives, the function and duties, and the major problems that develop within each of the specialties.
2. Include types of program activities. Each staff member should have special skills in one or more activities.
3. Interspace lectures and discussion periods with periods devoted to participation in activities, demonstrations, and practice leadership.
4. Schedule formal presentations and allow time for questions and discussion.
5. Utilize every opportunity to relate discussions to problems that the therapist will face.
6. Before closing the meeting, inform all therapists of their next assignments and indicate briefly the next meeting's program.
7. Summarize the work covered during the session.

In-service programs for the newly employed therapist who could later be reclassified to a higher position would not only include the above mentioned areas but medical lectures, ward attendant experience, area rotation of programs, field trips, philosophy and theory and tests of the particular department one is working in.

Another form of in-service training conducted within a number of states, primarily in the field of mental health, is the bringing together of personnel of similar specialties for skilled workshops or conferences. These skilled workshops are usually conducted by the state consultant of the specialty, or the association of a particular specialty. These workshops vary in length from two to four days, usually with two or more sessions daily. Although only a few high spots can be reviewed or considered, it does provide a means to discuss mutual problems or ideas, clarification of policies and procedures, and heighten interest in professional repsonsibilities. In addition, there may be quarterly meetings for department heads.

Such conferences should be easily accessible to personnel with time off with pay. The conference area should provide a building with suitable facilities for conducting either lectures or active programs. Faculty may include in or out-of-state personnel. Before the workshop begins, a preliminary announcement outlining the workshop contents and containing any specific directions should be made. It is quite possible and a good idea, at times, to ask the participants what they would like to discuss.

Some states have designated a particular hospital for the training of new employees in a particular specialty or for refresher courses. These courses, of one to three months in duration, often prove a fertile ground for recruiting better qualified individuals.

In the final analysis, the department and hospital that has provided proper educational facilities and has established adequate training programs will develop the rounded specialist and will itself reap a twofold benefit: (1) Improvement in the treatment of the patient, and (2) greater interest of the staff in their patient and in the hospital. Remember, only a rolling stone gathers no moss.

Activity Therapy Staff Development

The author basically looks upon this type of staff development as involving the total staff of the activity therapy service. Many of the thoughts discussed under in-service training can be applied here but the major emphasis is upon the total hospital and related subject matter.

The rapid growth in the number of special techniques and the increasing greater contributions that these specialist make to the hospital have put new and heavier requirements upon the departments and therapist within each of the activity therapy service. Furthermore, a greater appreciation of the value of each of the specialties and the hospital has increased the demand for total staff development. If the therapist is to meet the requirements of today's situations, there must be a better understanding of each other. The staff needs to possess certain information and attitudes if they are to become fully satisfied with these positions. Beyond his effectiveness as a team worker and social human being, the therapist depends on (1) his feeling of security and individual importance; (2) his sense of personal responsibility, and (3) his considerate attitude toward other employees and their rights.

No therapist should ever be satisfied with his present knowledge of his specialty or related fields. Medicine is moving forward so rapidly each year that only by constant reading, observation, association with other specialties, and other educational experiences can the therapist hope to keep abreast of his own specialty.

It is being suggested by the author that staff development programs involve all the specialties within activity therapy. Because these programs require considerable advance preparation and involve the total staff, they should be less frequent than the weekly or semi-monthly in-service training programs. The author has found it satisfactory to conduct one meeting a month. If all in-service training programs are conducted by each specialty on the same day, the staff development program could be conducted in its place on a monthly basis. It is feasible to set up a committee which will be responsible for the activity therapy staff development program. It is suggested that the committee be made up of the coordinator, two department heads, and two experienced staff therapists from departments other than the department heads' departments.

Recognizing the deversity of interest of the various departments, clearly defined programs should be arranged as far in advance as possible. This allows the entire staff to become better acquainted with the subject matter prior to the meeting and so increase the value of the discussion. It is hoped that such total discussion of subjects related to all will serve as an added stimulus to each therapist to use the contributions in solving the problems encountered in the therapist's daily work. It is also expected that these meetings will further enrich the new employee's background by emphasizing in statement and action the importance of other departments to the total hospital operation.

The outline below reveals the philosophy and methods of the Activity Therapy Service Seminar as conducted by the staff at Logansport State Hospital.

ACTIVITY THERAPY STAFF DEVELOPMENT PROGRAM
(An On-Going Process)

A. Philosophy:

Any knowledge or information which will broaden the understanding of the total environment within the hospital with the purpose of expanding culturally and professionally oneself.

B. Method:
1. The staff development program will be conducted on the third Tuesday of each month beginning at 3:00 p.m. in the Activity Therapy Auditorium.
2. Attendance is compulsory for all Activity Therapy staff personnel.
3. All departments within the total hospital setting will be involved at some time.
4. Presentation of material by individuals outside the hospital setting will be encouraged (faculty from nearby universities, consultants from departments of mental and public health, etc.).
5. Topics should have some relativeness to the Activity Therapy.
6. Method of presentation will be at the discretion of the person or persons giving the presentation. Method may include: films, panels, visual aids, formal lectures, role playing, seminars, etc.
7. Personnel presenting the staff development program should have prepared, if possible, a resume of the topic presented to pass out to personnel attending program.
8. All interested personnel outside of Activity Therapy are invited.

Figure 15.

Following is a suggested list of topics for staff development programs:

1. History and development of the various specialties within the activity therapy service. It is surprising how little is known by each of the specialties of the specialties.
2. Group dynamics.
3. Professional qualifications of specialties within activity therapy service.
4. Drugs and the effects on patients.
5. Role of other specialties (psychology, social service, nursing, ward physician) in the treatment of patients.
6. Staffing and diagnosis of patients.
7. Professional ethics.
8. Release planning for patients.
9. The clinical team approach.
10. History and development of the hospital.

In summary, the well-trained therapist becomes a competent member of the hospital staff by his participation in staff development programs. Because of his ability and because of his understanding of hospital problems and procedures and the vital role the hospital plays in medical treatment, he is almost sure to support the administration in its endeavors to improve service.

All these benefits to the hospital can be obtained at a cost of only a few cents per patient day. To the patient this would provide, at almost insignificant cost, the personal attention of the therapist as a member of the clinical team and an improvement in service pervading the entire hospital.

Clinical Affiliation

A clinical affiliation is a part of the total educational process for those interested in specializing in any of the specialties that make up the activity therapy service. It can not be thought of as a separate entity in itself, as it is inevitably related to classroom study, and at the same time, clearly distinguished. The knowledge essential to the practice of a specialty can not be learned solely through books and lectures. Contact with the patient is vital if the student is to gain the proper perspective and discipline and the ability to apply the scientific facts that he has acquired.

"In any discussion of the subject, it seems important to repeat and stress the fact that an internship is concerned with the students' practical experience, as contrasted with his classroom theory. In the internship, the student must translate into activity the knowledge, the thinking, and the emotional response he has acquired in the classroom. . . . In the internship, the student has (the) opportunity to learn facts of a kind and range different from those that can be taught in class, to coordinate all this information into a usable whole and to put the total sum of the information into service. If the maximum value is to be had from the time allotted to an internship, there should be as little duplication of classroom activity as possible and a conscious effort not to cover areas which could better be included in a classroom study."[5]

During the entire internship, stress should be laid upon the patient as an entity rather than exclusively upon his pathologic conditions. His mental as well as his physical condition should be given careful consideration. This recognition will constitute a substantial portion of his internship.

Consideration of the advisable content of an internship will inevitably raise questions as to the processes of teaching in such a situation. There should be periods assigned for certain specific educational pursuits. This establishes a routine that is beneficial to the intern and to the staff alike. Various schedules and allocations of duties and time can be made that will achieve the major objectives. Emphasis should be on standards, not on standardization.

In the development of an internship program, the hospital as well as the total activity therapy service must become aware of its teaching responsibilities. This requires department heads within each specialty that are competent, experienced, and are recognized in their specialty. These department heads should develop the teaching program in cooperation with their professional organization and/or college.

All the schools at the present time that give a degree in any of the specialties that make-up the activity therapy service require an internship of from three to nine months in one or more clinical settings. The most demanding internship is that required to be an occupational therapist. The time devoted to a clinical affiliation in occupational therapy must be approximately nine months of which twelve weeks are spent in a psychiatric setting, eight weeks with physical disabilities, and four to eight weeks in tuberculosis, pediatrics, and general medicine and surgery other than physical disabilities respectively.[6] Further material concerned with an adequate clinical practice in occupational therapy can be found in publications entitled *Standards for Training in Occupational Therapy* prepared by the Educational Committee of the AOTA and the AMA.[7] Another guide is the *Director's Guide for a Clinical Training Program for Occupational Therapy Students* which is concerned with affiliation of the student and the clinical teaching program.[8] A *Manual for Occupational Therapy Students in Clinical Training* has been prepared to orient students to an understanding of what is expected of them during their clinical work.[9] A program recently developed by the AOTA to offset the shortage of registered Occupational Therapists in the

Occupational Therapy Assistants' Training Course[10] whereby individuals who do not have a degree but have certain interests and skills, previously acquired, may train to become an assistant at specific hospitals—general medical and surgical and psychiatric hospitals. It is recommended that the training program be conducted through the resourccs of a single hospital (general medical and surgical, or psychiatric) whereby various agencies would develop a cooperative program by sending their students to a single hospital. Following completion of the course, the student may apply for certification to the AOTA. In addition to the schooling, the student may and should become registered. Admittance to the Registry is by examination conducted by the American Occupational Therapy Association.

The National Association for Music Therapists,[12] in association with the National Association of Schools of Music, have a similar internship (six months), and registration as found in the American Occupational Therapy Association. Affiliation is with approved phychiatric hospitals following a four year academic course leading to a bachelor's degree. Although in recent years, clinical affiliations are being established in several kinds of special schools, hospitals and institutions.

Those working in the area of medical recreation have usually found their internship worked out between the particular school granting the degree and the medical setting. Registration in this specialty is with the "Council for the Advancement of Hospital Recreation."[13] Industrial therapy, physical therapy, education therapy, have similar registrations which will be discussed further in the Appendix.

Because the purpose of the internship is to round out the training received in school, it should be considered as a part of the basic preparation for practice. This is true whether the degree has already been granted or has been withheld until the completion of the internship.

While only one specialty has a rotating type of internship, there is beginning to be felt a need for all specialties to provide a rotating internship in the various medical settings. Emphasis so placed will make the intern more able to assimilate the various branches of medicine and to apply them to whatever medical setting the student will eventually settle in.

The satisfactory internship should include work with specific and general patients, assume some clerical and administrative responsibilities; present case histories and solutions to such with his skill, rotation within the various other specialties that make-up the activity therapy service, observe other departments outside of the activity therapy service, attend various types of staff meetings, utilization of library and maintain a daily record. It should be mandatory that at the time the intern begins his service, he should be given a manual of the standard procedures followed in that hospital.

No matter how excellent the physical equipment or clinical material may be, the first requirement of any hospital offering acceptable internship is that it have a well-organized medical staff with department heads selected on the basis of competence who, in turn, will accept the responsibility for the development of an adequate educational program.

It is advisable that an educational director be appointed, at least on a part-time basis, to see that the work of the student is truly educational. In turn, the educational director should appoint one person from each specialty to act as the student's special advisor and guide during his period of internship. This arrangement should not change the relationship of the intern to the department head if the department head is not the advisor. Naturally, the advisor should have the necessary background. In many instances, the coordinator, in addition to his regular duties, assumes the responsibility of educational director.

Some suggested duties of the educational director would include the following:

1. Carry on all correspondence with each school prior to the appointment of the intern.
2. In cooperation with the department head, should arrange the overall intern's schedule.
3. He should arrange the schedule of conferences, meetings, lectures, etc.

4. He should act as a general advisor.
5. He should assist the department heads in working out uniform procedures and teaching methods.
6. Assist in the development of a manual of procedures for interns.
7. Arrange a series of conferences with other hospital heads—administration, medical, social service, etc.
8. He should keep a permanent record of the accomplishment of the intern during his period of service.

Because schools have an obligation to their students which extends beyond graduation, there should be close cooperation between them and the hospital in the development of a sound educational program for the internship. This relationship should warrant visits to the hospital by the educators to counsel, advise, and encourage the staff in their educational activities and services. Conversely, such visits will help the educator to gain a better understanding of the problems confronting the specialist in actual practice.

In summary, the internship prepares the student to enter his profession and provides a broad base upon which further specific training can be built. It should be developed so that it offers a period of clinical responsibility under supervision which aims to complete the school courses, but also his professional attitude, cooperation, and stability.

Volunteer Training

Volunteers play an important part and are needed in the activity therapy service to extend treatment to a greater number. Since volunteers play a part in the treatment service, this implies, according to Conte,[14] "That the volunteer is a therapist." The increasing demand for more services by everyone concerned delegates this, but for maximum effectiveness, volunteers must receive some training in philosophy, theory, and technic within the specialty they are assigned to. While the volunteer has many strengths to contribute, he also needs to recognize his limitation and accept supervision. For this reason, it is imperative that the volunteer be thoughtfully indoctrinated and thoroughly trained in the techniques of working for and with the patients. We are all aware that it is impossible to prepare a person for leadership in a few days; but an intensive course dealing with objectives, methods, activities, and problems serve a useful purpose.

The training should be conducted in the hospital with formal lectures, personal conferences, and practical experience, by the departments who are going to use the volunteer. The amount and type of training depends upon the nature of the task and the extent to which the volunteer is prepared to perform it, but, to be a success, the training program must be organized and administrated soundly. However, training does not consist merely of preliminary preparations for the position. It is a continuing process throughout the period of service by means of conferences, advice from supervisors, reading, and observation of the work of others. In addition, the volunteer must learn to follow a routine, which, in turn, will make him far more efficient. Further, it is important that the therapists themselves understand the value of the volunteer to the program as well as the limitations involved. Recognize their ability, their training, and experience. Many of them have been leaders within their respective fields. Listen to them. Share with them. They may have something of value to offer. If the therapist does not recognize their abilities, show appreciation for services rendered; no matter how well organized is the hospital effort to recruit qualified volunteers, it will be wasted. Volunteers learn the service rendered at the hospital and appreciate its worth, and become interpreters and effective ambassadors for the hospital in the community.

The volunteer is the carrier of information to the general public and the promulgator of concern among citizens of the state for those who need preventive care or hospital treatment. Many hospitals have annual recognition dinners for their volunteers where certificates are given out. With proper screening and training, most of the volunteer aspects that professional despair of—tardiness, lack of responsibility, unfitness for the job—are eliminated. The weeding out process should be done before the job; not on the job.

Another type of leader which is receiving a considerable

amount of attention recently is the junior leader. The services rendered by these leaders takes a variety of forms. They may issue equipment, work in children's wards, read to older patients, collect game materials, repair small equipment, etc. The training of the junior leader follows much along the lines of the adult volunteer but caution should be exercised as to their specific duties.

The recruitment of volunteers is the responsibility of the director of volunteer services who coordinates all voluntary services for the institution. But he alone cannot be the final judge, for this rests with the department head of the specialty. Persons being considered should have a genuine concern to service others, some knowledge of the activities, personal skills in one or more of them, and the ability to teach and lead groups. Although some volunteers offer their services on their own initiative, it is most common that they are asked to help. Personal contacts with people having specific skills, appeals to interested service organizations and groups have proven the two most successful.

The training program for volunteers should be set-up on a regular time schedule with a specific meeting place, method of teaching, content, and responsibilities. This not only holds true for the volunteers but for those who are conducting the training sessions. The content of the program should be similar to the program developed for training the assistant within the specialty, but modified.

In summary, experience has shown that the training of volunteers is facilitated if sound policies and procedures are adopted and followed:

1. Assign volunteers worthwhile duties which contribute to the program.
2. Define the duties and type of work.
3. Provide for supervision.
4. Maintain and appraise records.
5. Assure good working conditions.
6. Express gratitude and appreciation for services rendered.

Although a person trained at the expense of the hospital may leave the employment of the hospital or institution, his training is not in vain because the community benefits by the ex-employee or volunteer working in another rehabilitation center, clinic, or industry. By training employees who may leave the service of the institution, the hospital is rendering a community service and advances the cause of public and mental health.

Finally, for training to be effective, it must be in a climate conducive to training. Training programs have little effect upon individuals if the work placement is opposed to what he has learned. Where management makes no provision for training or handles it in a shipshod, haphazard fashion, the message to employees is likewise clear and unmistakable and the reaction predictable. In the light of what has been commented on throughout this whole chapter, the Civil Service Commission[15] states that "There must be a climate in the organization characterized by a sense of devotion to the objectives of the organization and a willingness to work cooperatively towards the attainment of these objectives. There must be created or there must exist in the organization on the part of supervisors and employees, a will to improve. Management policies must be so structured and oriented as to encourage this will to improve, and to recognize it, and to reward it.

"The training program must be part of an overall effort directed by the top executive, aimed at the increased effectiveness of the organization within the framework of democratic administration. This climate must be known. A training policy must be established and issued by the executive of the organization, preferably in writing. This policy should indicate management's view of training as a management function, the broad objectives of training, and a clear indication that effective employee training has management's fullhearted support.

"There must be employee understanding and acceptance of what are the supervisor's responsibilities.

"There must be a clear delegations of authority and responsibility for carrying on the training program. . . ."

REFERENCES

1. Terry, George R.: *Principles of Management.* Richard D. Irwin, Inc., 1956, p. 686.

2. *Training the Supervisor.* U. S. Civil Service Commission, Government Printing Office, September, 1956, p. 1.
3. Wolfe, Corinne H.: Group training methods in public assistance agencies. In *Administration, Supervision and Consultation,* Family Service Association of America, New York, 1955, p. 21.
4. *Ibid.,* p. 24.
5. O'Morrow, Gerald: What you should know about internship in hospital recreation. *American Recreation Journal, I* (8) :12, 1961.
6. Fish, Marjorie: Education aims in occupational therapy. In *Principles of Occupational Therapy.* 2nd Ed., (eds.) Wallard, Helen S., and Spackman, Clarence S., Philadelphia, B. J. Lippincott Co., 1954, p. 32-33.
7. The Council on Medical Education and Hospitals of the AMA: *Essentials of an Acceptable School of Occupational Therapy.* Rev. Ed., American Occupational Therapy Association, December, 1949.
8. *Directors Guide for a Clinical Training Program for Occupational Therapy Students.* Rev. Ed., New York, American Occupational Therapy Association, 1950.
9. *Manual for Occupational Therapy Students in Clinical Training,* New York, American Occupational Therapy Association, 1950.
10. *Requirements for an Acceptable Training Program for Occupational Therapy Assistants.* New York, American Occupational Therapy Association, 1962.
11. *Program Outline for Occupational Therapy in General Practice and Psychiatry.* New York, American Occupational Therapy Association, 1962.
12. National Association Music Therapists, Lawrence, Kansas.
13. Standards Approved by the National Professional Organizations of American Recreational Society, American Association Health, Physical Education, and Recreation, and National Association for Recreation Therapists.
14. Conte, William R., and Liebes, Edith: *A Voluntary Partnership.* University of Texas, Hogg Foundation for Mental Health, 1960, p. 6.
15. *Training the Supervisor.* Washington, D. C., U. S. Government Printing Office, 1956, p. 92.

Chapter XIV

EVALUATION AND RESEARCH

EVALUATION

N̲o̲ ̲p̲r̲o̲f̲e̲s̲s̲i̲o̲n̲ ̲c̲a̲n̲ ̲g̲r̲o̲w̲ unless it can give evidence that it is willing and able to evaluate its own particular contribution. Diversity of patients' needs puts a strain on the ingenuity of the activity therapy service and commands a mustering of all its resources to satisfy the conditions of the patients. Many talk more and do less about evaluation than any other phase of the program. Routine, perfunctory attention is impossible; the conditions can not be taken for granted. A continual and exacting alert is necessary. Evaluation is a continual process. The coordinator who is responsible for the planning and organization has the task of follow-through of seeing what is planned for the hospital meets the objectives. The only thing that can be planned beforehand is the basic skills and their scientifically selected variety, and the conditions, philosophy, and techniques of securing cooperation.

Evaluation is based upon planning. All must recognize that evaluation is an important function, that it is not just another routine procedure tacked on to other easily recognized procedures. It is total effort by all affected by the service. Programs and facilities largely determine the kinds of activities which can be carried on, thereby the problems that develop in evaluation is due in a large measure to a lack of interest in the actual planning for it. The serious and often difficult process of examining objectives and of evaluating the activities in the light of goals are seldom engaged in conscientiously, but are somehow passed by as something for the future. Evaluation is rarely scheduled for or time budgeted and less time is spent in studying its techniques than other program areas. A knowledge of the essential factors in program planning is not sufficient to assure success in evaluation. A well-balanced program of activities and the ability to administrate and conduct programs are also essential.

Evaluation Consideration

In consideration of evaluation, let us examine and review a number of important factors which must be taken into consideration when evaluation is to occur, although ways of evaluations are numerous.

1. Clarification of Objectives. Objectives must be clarified and resolved before actual planning can take place. Direction is indicated by the objectives, thereby the course along which the program is to progress is already suggested.

2. Relation of Program to the Objectives. When programs are developed by different services, there is a need to review each of the service programs for consistency. To insure consistency among programs, it is necessary first to check one against the other to see whether they add up to a unified program. No one service has all the skills or energy to aggregate to all the patients within the hospital. When discrepancies are discovered, it is not always easy to correct them. Therefore, it may be necessary to develop a new course of action, compromise, or develop alternatives in order to achieve the objectives. Sufficient flexibility should be provided in order to permit adjustments as needed.

3. Program Scheduling. Scheduling of programs give vitality and practical meaning to the planning. Management is needed to carry out the program, to organize the groups, and to conduct on schedule the activities. Since the master schedule consists of procedures and methods so arranged and designed in order to provide the courses of action to achieve the objectives, it requires advanced planning; otherwise, program planning has little or no value. If experience indicates that certain programs should be omitted or changed or less time be given to them, the schedule must be revised accordingly.

Effective planning, both long and short-range, requires the answering of certain questions; *What* action is necessary? *Where* will it take place? *When* will it take place? *Who* will do it? *How* will it be accomplished? Thus, as we have stated before, the program relationship to the objectives grows out of the objectives and requires advanced planning.

4. Response and Representativeness. If the program has developed out of the objectives, then adequate response and representation in the program should be forthcoming. A program that provides only a limited number of activities or too broad a variety of activities will fail to serve or attract the needs of the patients.

5. Balance. A conscious effort must be made to achieve a well-balanced program; otherwise, some aspects are bound to be over-emphasized. Activities must be scheduled so that there are as few as possible frustrating experiences in which the patient has to choose constantly between several activities. Proper preparation of a master schedule is one way of eliminating such problems.

A common weakness in program planning, in the large mental hospital, is the tendency to offer such a variety of programs that it exerts pressure on the patients to take part continuously and upon the therapist to see that the program is carried out. On the other hand, too few activities or all special interest activities will only attract a small segment of the patients. Daily, weekly, and seasonal programs are among the many kinds needed.

A happy balance is attained when there is sufficient programs, with variety in day-to-day activities, including evenings to meet the needs and interest of each patient and enough special events to challenge the interest and participation of all patients. Quantity of activity must give way to quality.

6. Adequacy of Leadership and Supervision. The key to success of program is leadership and the quality of leadership with proper supervision. It has been said that leadership and program cannot be separated—so consequently evaluation will determine how effective both leaders and programs are. Although quantity of staff does not insure quality of treatment, it is nonetheless true that quality treatment is impossible to achieve without a sufficient number of people to carry out the treatment.

It is an important supervisory responsibility to motivate staff members and stimulate in them an honest desire for appraisal that conceives of evaluations as a positive force seeking for growth and development. Two ways of accomplishing this is through individual conferences and a satisfactory in-service training program.

We might say that with insight as to purpose and understanding of the problems demanding consideration comes interest. The appreciation of the intrinsic worth and importance attached to the work of the activity therapy service motivates the staff to a high degree of efficiency and results in excellent service and cooperative progress.

7. Records. Records are part of the responsibility of every therapist. The written record gives an analysis of the program content in addition to providing the physician with a report concerning the reactions of the patient to the treatment situation. Through this experience, the therapist relives the activities and becomes aware of the whole which seemed only fragmentary as he went through the experience. It provides a source for present and future program planning because it expresses the felt and unfelt needs and interest of the patients as well as an account of what actually happened. And finally, it provides a permanent and continuous record for the activity therapy service—a tool for evaluation and planning the activity therapy program, self study, training, and research.

8. Facilities and Equipment. Objectives can not be met successfully in programming, without adequate facilities and equipment which are the tools to performing a therapeutic program. Here intertwining of clinical knowledge and administrative policy and activity is apparent.

The attainment of these objectives by a variety of methods, and their importance varies with different types of hospitals. The problem of determining the most essential areas and facilities is comparatively simple in the case of the small hospital or general medical and surgical hospital, but complex when a plan for a large hospital is under consideration. Accessibility is less important in selecting the site for a softball diamond than it is in locating a shelter house to serve patients for outdoor activities.

The effective solution of program demand, on the part of the coordinator and his staff calls for an understanding of the needs and interests to be met by the area; a knowledge of the facilities which can meet these needs; their requirements as to space, location, and construction; and the ability to impose these features upon the area in such a way as to produce an effective and attractive plan.

RESEARCH

Research is important in discovering and identifying information and facts helpful in formulating and evaluating plans. Every profession needs its working concepts. These are ideas that add new knowledge or tie together previously isolated facts. Linn[1] defines research as a "process of learning by direct observation, in contrast to learning from books or from teachers." Research is important today because we must replace opinion by fact, guesswork by principles. In some instances, research is concerned with what is commonly termed "pure research." "Pure research" is important because it provides the fundamental principles and knowledge upon which further research can be pursued. In contrast, "applied research" is used to denote research conducted for a definite purpose and which can be applied immediately. In many instances, the two are inter-related.

Unfortunately, many individuals react negatively to the word "research," but, as observed by Gurel,[2] "research is basically nothing more than the application of systematic observation and objective fact-gathering for use in answering some particular question." He continues by stating that "properly utilized, research provides the foundation blocks for a sound evaluative structure and the practical benefits which results from rigorous evaluation."

Research is not difficult if it is pursued in a systematic method. Oken and Grinker[3] comment: "The specific problems which a hospital chooses to study grow naturally out of the clinical questions it faces. There is no dearth of these. The investigator begins by formulating hypothesies, then tries to narrow them down through observation. He develops and tries out techniques appropriate for detailed observing and for measuring the phenomena. Next, he outlines an appropriate research design for a formal but still pilot investigation. Thus, informal observations grow into pilot studies, then into more controlled specific research projects. Eventually a broad program of interrelated studies may evolve."

Extensive research is being conducted by several foundations,* governmental units, private enterprises, and professional organizations. In addition, the federal government through legislative action is providing more and more money for research in all areas of health. Former President Kennedy's request for federal funds and the passage of the Mental Health Act to increase research in mental health has spurred this area. Governors in numerous states have requested state appropriations for mental health expenditures. Private agencies lending a hand in mental health research include The Menninger Foundation, Chestnut Lodge, Austin Riggs and Michael Reese Hospital and Medical Center in Chicago, to name a few. One government unit, the Division of Vocational Rehabilitation Administration,* Department of Health, Education, and Welfare, has done considerable research through grants in the area of rehabilitation and related fields which have value to the activity therapy service. Some of these studies represent the effort of a two or three year research program and have contributed highly significant findings, such as *The Vermont Story,*[4] *Day Hospital,*[5] and *Project 52.*[6]

Another unit of the same department providing research grants in the biomedical sciences and health-oriented disciplines as well as supporting studies in hospitals and other community health services and the application of the results of such studies is the Public Health Service with headquarters at the National Institute of Health, Bethesda, Maryland.**

Need for Research

Another important role of the coordinator is that of research,

*For extensive listing of Foundations providing grants, see *Foundation Directory,* New York, Russell Sage Foundation, published yearly.

*Those interested in obtaining a bibliography of research and demonstration projects provided through the Vocational Rehabilitation Administration, should write U. S. Department of Health, Education, and Welfare, Vocational Rehabilitation, Administration, Division of Research Grants and Demonstrations, Washington, D. C., 20009, asking for their *Reports resulting from Research and Demonstration Projects, A Bibliography, 1962.*

**An information pamphlet about the services of the Institutes is *Public Health Service,* Rev. ed., Publ. #81, Washington, D. C., U. S. Government Printing Office, 1963.

especially in the area of improvement of methods relating to the coordination of the activity therapy service. The coordinator has a vital role to play in collecting data sufficiently inclusive in scope to contribute to the further development of the total activity program of the hospital. Each of the various professional organizations have completed significant research within their own specialty which has been wholeheartedly welcomed by the medical profession, but little has been done in attempting to research the integration of their philosophy, theory, and activities into a whole. Possibly this is limited by the lack of clear statements of existing philosophies and theories of each specialty in forms which will permit the derivation of really critical testable hypotheses. If significant progress is to be made in the integration of these specialties, it will result from break-throughs at the conceptual rather than the operational level. Working concepts are necessary for the development of suitable instruments for evaluating techniques and practices.

The problem of greatest importance in the area of the activity therapy service and one which will continue is the development of a philosophy acceptable to all specialties regarding the content of and elements of coordination or administration of all these specialties within a whole. Possibly this problem results from fear because it means an attempt at progress. Sheffel[7] observes that administrative research findings from other fields are not being applied to hospital administrative systems since the results may threaten individuals or procedures. A philosophy is a system of thought. It is based on some orderly, logical statements of objectives, principles, policies, and general methods of approach. Therefore, the research program for this requires more than agreement between disciplines concerning what are the basic objectives, policies, and functions in the field. It requires some agreement concerning the fundamentals underlying the work of each specialty. It is one thing to do the research, but it is another thing to use the research that has already been done.

If integration is to occur, there must be developed a better liaison and cooperative research effort with research specialists or sub-committees of professional organizations in related professions. In addition, more frequently scheduled conferences in which concrete efforts are made to assess the value of cooperation needed in the development of an activity therapy service and identifying need for future investigation. It should be realized that having a set of concepts of one's own does not isolate a profession from other groups. A good concept, usable to members of one profession, is hardly ever rejected by members of other professions. Unkefer[8] writing about the activity therapies as a whole, comments that "never before have we been so close to working together on joint developments at the treatment level. The wide adoption of hospital staffing plans which place all activtiy therapies in a single department has opened the opportunity for carefully controlled joint work and study." He continues: "Administrative changes and new staff plans do not in themselves cause willing cooperative work. They may open channels of communication which can support cooperative efforts. With more channels open, it is imperative that we join our co-workers at the treatment level, and later at the organization level, to solve our common problems, and to bring better care and treatment to our patients."

The following list of references from selected periodicals and books from time to time have material concerned with the activity therapy service as a whole:

> *American Archives of Rehabilitation Therapy.*
> *American Journal of Occupational Therapy.*
> *American Recreation Journal.*
> *Archives of Physical Medicine and Rehabilitation.*
> *Bulletin of National Association for Music Therapy, Inc.*
> *Hospital Management.*
> *Hospitals.*
> *Journal of The Association for Physical and Mental Rehabilitation.*
> *Journal of Rehabilitation.*
> *Mental Hospitals.*
> *Modern Hospitals.*
> *Music Therapy Yearbooks,* 1951 to present.
> *Nursing Research.*
> *Psychiatric Quarterly.*

Recreation.

Recreation for the Ill and Handicapped.

Recreation in Treatment Centers.

Research Bulletin, Division of Mental Health, State of Washington.

Research Quarterly of the AAHPER.

Social Work.

Listed below are some problems in which exploration and study are needed in relating to the activity therapy service.

1. The role of the coordinator in an activity therapy service.
2. Employment of research specialist within the activity therapy service.
3. Integration of the activity therapy service.
4. Adequacy of existing professional preparation for the position as a coordinator.
5. Consideration of program planning in the activity therapy service.
6. Relative value of all services in program planning.
7. What are the relationship of coordinators to hospital administrators?
8. What is budgetry practice?
9. What is the influence of the size of the hospital on the activity therapy administrative problems—the distribution of work, the grouping of service, etc.?
10. Improved use of activity personnel.
11. Effective teamwork within the service.
12. What administrative skills are especially required?
13. What is the optimum span of control in the service?
14. What personal qualifications are needed by the coordinator?
15. What is the contribution of activity therapy service in the hospital—how do we demonstrate it, how do we interpret it?

Conclusion

Although this book is an attempt to outline administrative procedures for the total activity therapy service, the writers hope that it is not the last. Since there is a limited amount of literature on this subject, the administrator of such a discipline must depend upon administrative works offered by parallel disciplines; public administration, educational administration, and business administration. The advancement of the total services to the giving of better patient treatment is dependent on the gathering of far more information than is available at present. It is urged that the petty and verbal confusion which exists between the various disciplines be dissolved and that a rigorous and continuous effort be made to improve the administrative aspects of the total. The author is well aware that individuals and professions resist changes or adjustments, but changes are an important characteristic of our society. Changes are made necessary by the occurrence of new concepts, new social ideas, and new problems.

REFERENCES

1. Linn, Louis: A philosophy of psychiatric research. *Ment. Hosp.,* January, 1963, p. 21.
2. Gurel, Lee: Evaluation and research. In *Recreation for the Mentally Ill,* Conference Report, 1958, Washington, D. C.: American Association for Health, Physical Education, and Recreation, 1958, p. 38.
3. Oken, Donald, and Grinker, Ray R.: A setting for clinical research. *Ment. Hosp.,* September, 1962, p. 486.
4. Chittick, Rupert A., Brooks, George W., Irons, Francis S., and Deane, William N.: *The Vermont Story,* Vurlington, Vermont, Queen City Printers, Inc., 1961.
5. Kramer, Bernard M.: *Day Hospital.* New York, Grune and Stratton, 1962.
6. *Project 52, A Study In Adjunctive Therapies Coordination.* Topeka, Kansas, Washburn University of Topeka, Kansas, June, 1958.
7. Sheffel, Irving: Financing administrative research. *Ment. Hosp.,* February, 1961, p. 63.
8. Unkefer, Robert F.: Factors Contributing To The Professional Growth of Music Therapy. *Bulletin, National Association for Music Therapy,* May 1961, p. 5.

BIBLIOGRAPHY

A Guide for Executive Selection. Washington, D. C., U. S. Government Printing Office, 1961.

A Guide for the Development and Administration of the Training Program for Occupational Therapy Assistants. AOTA, Rev., October, 1961.

ALA Bulletin. April, 1961 and October, 1964 are both devoted to Hospital and Institution Library Service. (Invaluable in information and inspiration)

A Long Range Plan for Mental Health Services in California. Sacramento, California, Department of Mental Hygiene, 1962.

A school for emotionally disturbed children. *Ment. Hosp.,* April, 1961.

Activity Therapies. *Perspective,* Olympia, Washington, Department of Institutions, Spring, 1963.

Adrian, Daryl B.: Correspondence study proves effective adjunct. *The Alumni News,* a publication of the Kansas State Teachers College, Emporia, XLI, 1963.

Patients go to school. *The Menninger Quart., XV,* Winter, 1961.

Affeldt, Thomas O.: A survey of inpatient programs for adolescents. *Ment. Hosp.,* April, 1963.

Ammon, Gunter K.: *Theoretical Aspects of Milieu Therapy.* Unpublished manuscript written as a Resident Physician in Psychiatry in The Menninger School of Psychiatry, Topeka, Kansas, June, 1959.

An Experiment in Training Volunteers. (pamphlet), The Advisory Committee on Service for the Aging, 1962.

Arnett, T.: Planning for the patient's discharge. *Mod. Hosp.,* 1956.

Azima, H.: Dynamic occupational therapy. *Dis. Nerv. Syst., 22, Suppl.,* April, 1961.

Baatz, Wilmer H.: Patient's library services and bibliotherapy. *Wilson Library Bulletin,* January 1961.

Baker, A., Davis, R. L., and Sivadon, P.: *Psychiatric Services and Architecture.* Geneva, Palais Des Nations, World Health Organization, 1959.

Balknap, Edward R.: Retrospect and prospect in educational therapy. *Amer. Arch. Rehabil. Ther., V,* December, 1957.

Bantz, Wilmer H.: Patients' library services and bibliotherapy. *Wilson Library Bulletin,* No. 35, 1961.

Barnard, Chester I.: *The Functions of the Executive.* Cambridge, Massachusetts, Harvard University Press, 1954.

Barton, Walter E.: *Administration in Psychiatry.* Springfield, Illinois, Chales C Thomas, 1962.

Bauer, Alfred: Hospital vocational rehabilitation. *Ment. Hosp.,* August, 1961.

Beers, Clifford: *A Mind That Found Itself.* An autobiography, Doubleday, 1953.

Bing, M.: Volunteers help head nurses at VA hospital. *RN, 18,* February, 1955.

Bengson, Evelyn: Nursing homes want activity programs. *AJOT, XV,* No. 4, 1961.

Bennett, A. E., Hargrove, Eugene A., and Engle, Bernice: *The Practice of Psychiatry in General Hospitals.* Berkeley, California, University of California Press, 1956.

Berne, Eric: *The Structure and Dynamics of Organization and Groups.* Philadelphia, Pennsylvania, J. B. Lippincott Company, 1963.

342

Bergman, Jr., Weston: An employee orientation program. *Ment. Hosp.,* October, 1957.

Black, James M.: *Developing Competent Subordinates.* New York, American Management Association, 1961.

Blackey, Eileen A.: *Group Leadership in Staff Training.* Washington, D. C., Department Of Health, Education, and Welfare, Children's Bureau and Bureau of Public Assistance, 1957.

Blakney, Preston C.: Educational therapy in a neuropsychiatric hospital. *Amer. Arch. Rehabil. Ther., V,* December, 1957.

Blumberg, A., and Aruenian, S.: A deeper look at volunteers. *Adult Leadership,* Vol. 2, June, 1960.

Broderick, Dorothy M.: Books aid the physically, mentally, and emotionally handicapped. *Library Journal,* No. *84,* December 15, 1959.

Brown, Esther L.: *Newer Dimensions of Patient Care.,* Part I, New York, Russell Sage Foundation, 1961.

Ibid, Part II, 1962.

Brown, Ray: The Milledgeville story. *Ment. Hosp.,* November, 1963.

Bullard, Dexter: The Chestnut Lodge community center. *Ment. Hosp.,* June, 1954.

Bursinger, Bess C.: Neuro-psychiatric hospital library. *Library Journal,* No. 79, November 15, 1954.

Bush, Charles K.: Hospital administration. *Ment. Hosp.,* September 1960.

Butler, George: *Playgrounds - Their Administration and Operations,* Rev. Ed., New York, A. S. Barnes and Company, 1951.

Caffey, Eugene: Writing up research, *Ment. Hosp.,* March 1963.

Changing Concepts and Practices in Psychiatric Occupational Therapy. Proceedings of the Alleyberry Conference, November 1956.

Chase, Mildred: How to keep personal relations personal. *Mod. Hosp.,* August 1961.

Copeland, Melvin T.: *The Executive at Work.* Cambridge, Massachusetts, Harvard University Press, 1952.

Correspondence study is useful tool to help re-orient mental patients. *The Alumni News,* a publication of the Kansas State Teachers College, Emporia, XXXIX, December 1960.

Cohen, Nathen E. (Ed.) : *The Citizen Volunteer.* Cleveland, Ohio, Western Reserve University, 1960.

Coleman, J. V.: Motivations of the volunteer in the health and welfare field. *Ment. Hyg., 41,* 1957.

Coville, Walter J.: Bibliotherapy. The Administrator and the Patients' Library, Paper read at a council meeting sponsored by the Committee on Patients' Libraries of the United Hospital Fund, New York, New York, March, 1959.

Crawshaw, Ralph: Present-Day adjunctive therapy in a hospital setting. *J. A. Phys. & Ment. Rehab., 12,* No. 1, January-February, 1958.

Dale, Ernest: *Planning and Developing the Company Organization Structure.* New York, American Management Association, 1952.

Dancik, Daniel: Administration of a medical rehabilitation service in a neuropsychiatric hospital. *Arch. Phys. Med.,* October, 1949.

Davis, John E.: *Clinical Application of Recreation Therapy.* Springfield, Illinois, Charles C Thomas, Publisher, 1952.

..........:*Rehabilitation, Its Principles and Practice.* Rev. Ed., New York, A. S. Barnes & Company, 1946.

Dimock, Marshall E.: *A Philosophy of Administration Toward Creative Growth.* New York, Harper & Bros., 1958.

The doctors and recreation in the hospital setting. North Carolina Recreation Commission, Raleigh, North Carolina, No. 30, January, 1962.

Doctors, hospitals, nurses, and children. *Child Study,* Vol. 34, Winter 1956-1957.

Dolch, E. T.: Books for the hospitalized child. *Amer. J. Nurs., 61:*66-68.

Dunton, Jr., William R., and Licht, Sidney: *Occupational Therapy - Principles and Practice.* 2nd Ed., Springfield, Illinois, Charles C Thomas, Publisher, 1956.

Dunton, Jr., William R.: *Prescribing Occupational Therapy.* Springfield, Illinois, Charles C Thomas, Publisher, 1947.

Duval, Addison M.: Management and the public mental hospital. *Ment. Hosp.,* October 1957.

Dyer, Gus W.: Educational therapy: objectives and values. *Ment. Hosp.,* January, 1964.

Dykens, James: Recruiting mental hospital workers. *Ment. Hosp.,* October, 1963.

Edgren, Gordon, Belyea, Robert, and Griffen, Ruth: A legacy of Education. *Ment. Health,* April, 1961.

Employment Interviewing. Washington, D. C., U. S. Government Printing Office, 1956.

Fidler, Gail S., and Fidler, Jr., Jan W.: *Introduction to Psychiatric Occupational Therapy.* New York, MacMillan, 1954.

Fink, Ludwig, and Dunning, Edward: Therapeutic utilization of mental hospitals industries. *Psychiat. Quart., 34,* 1960.

Fisher, S. H.: The recovered patient returns to the community. *Ment. Hyg.,* October, 1958.

Flandorf, Vera: Administration of the reading program in the pediatrics department of a hospital. *The Catholic Library World,* No. 30, December, 1958.

Fleck, S.: Recognition and utilization of the motivation of volunteers. *Ment. Hyg., 41,* 1957.

Full utilization of ancillary personnel. *Ment. Hosp.,* February 1959.

Gale, Mary, and Shatzky, Benjamin: P. S. 611 — Queens Annex: A school in a psychiatric hospital. *J. Hillside Hospital,* Adolescent Pavilion Number, IX, January-April, 1960.

Garber, Robert: Administration principles as adjuncts to therapy. *Ment. Hosp.,* July, 1964.

Gartenberg, Gerald: Developing procedural manuals for institutions. *Ment. Hosp.,* January, 1959.

Glover, John B., and Hower, Ralph H.: *The Administrator.* Homewood, Illinois, Richard D. Irwin, Inc., 1952.

Goodall, Frances Kessler: Interview information on volunteers in relation to placement and service experience with special reference to the volunteer service bureau. (Unpublished master's thesis. St. Louis, Missouri: George Warren Brown School of Social Work, Washington University, 1948.)

Guilfoile, Mabel S.: Short complete courses in educational therapy, *Amer. Arch. Rehabil., VI,* March, 1958.

Granger, Beverly J., and Doniger, Joan: A new perspective on training and practice in occupational therapy. *AJOT,* Vol. *XII,* No. 2 Part I, March-April, 1958.

Greenblatt, Milton and others (ed.): *The Patient and The Mental Hospital.* Glencoe, Illinois, Free Press, 1957.

Haddock, J. N., and Dunden, H. D.: Volunteer work in state hospital by college students. *Ment. Hyg.,* 35, October, 1951.

Haines, Robert A.: Taking a fix. *NAMT Book of Proceedings,* Lawrence, Kansas, Allen Press, 1958.

Hannah, Ruby: Navy bibliotherapy. *Library Journal,* No. 80, May, 1955.

Haring, Norris G., and Phillips, E. Lakin: *Educating Emotionally Disturbed Children.* New York: McGraw-Hill Book Company, Inc. 1962.

Hill, Beatrice: *Starting a Recreation Program in a Ciivlian Hospital,* New York, Nat. Rec. Assoc., 1955.

Huntting, Inez: Purpose and pathways in occupational therapy. *Ment. Health,* 1954.

Hyde, Robert J., Bockoven, Sanborune, Pfantz, Harold W., and York, Richard H.: *Milieu Rehabilitation,* Providence, R. I., Butler Health Center, 330 Grotto Avenue, April, 1962.

Indiana Mental Helath Volunteers Handbook and Guide. (pamphlet), State of Indiana, Department of Mental Health, December 1960.

Johnston, Ann: Help for the homebound. *Recreation,* No. *49,* 1956.

Kasprowicz, Alfred: Need of discharged patients. *Ment. Hosp.,* April 1960.

Kogan, Kate, and Jackson, Joan K.: Role perception in hospital interaction. *Nursing Research,* Vol. 10, No. 2, Spring, 1961.

Koller, Robert P.: Motivational technique in group classes of educational therapy patients. *Amer. Arch. Rehabil. Ther.,* V, September, 1957.

Kremens, Jack B.: Haverford - a new hospital for modern psychiatry. *Ment. Hosp.,* December, 1962.

Krygar, Clive, Jr.: We must re-evaluate our functions. *Ment. Hosp.,* March, 1964.

Langdon, Doris R.: Volunteer in crippled children program. *Community Health Bull.* 66, 1952.

Leadership and Supervision - A Management Report. U. S. Civil Service Commission, Personnel Management Series No. 9, Washington, D. C., U. S. Government Printing Office, December, 1955.

Lepawsky, Albert: *Administration - The Art and Science of Organization and Management.* New York, Alfred A. Knopf, Inc., 1949.

Licht, Sidney: *Occupational Therapy Source Book.* Baltimore, The Williams and Wilkins Company, 1948.

Linn, Louis: A philosophy of psychiatric research. *Ment. Hosp.,* January 1963.

Lozanoff, Paul: Educating disturbed children - a hospital community responsibility. *Ment. Hosp.,* July 1964.

Lundgren, Louis R.: A triple purpose activities building. *Ment. Hosp.,* January, 1959.

Mako, Alader, Crafis, Ewing, and Peer, Irwin: Defining and applying milieu therapy. *Ment. Hosp.,* October, 1962.

Manual For Supervisors of Student Affiliations: AOTA, Rev., April, 1962.

Manual on Organization of Women's Hospital Auxiliaries with Model Constitution and By-laws. (pamphlet) American Hospital Association, Chicago, 1950.

Manual for Volunteer Services Programs in California State Hospitals, Sacramento, California, Department of Mental Hygiene (undated pamphlet).

March, James G., and Simon, Herbert A.: *Organizations.* New York, John Wiley and Sons, 1958.

Martin, D. H.: Individual orientation for volunteers. *Ment. Hosp., 6,* September 1955.

Master control center for wired music system. *Ment. Hosp.,* September, 1956.

Mental health facilities: planning and construction issue. *Hospitals,* February 1, 1964.

McQuain, Clemmie L.: Proposed requirement for an acceptable school of educational therapy, undergraduate level. *Amer. Arch. Rehabil. Ther.,* V, March, 1957.

Miller, Norman P.: Christmas wishes for medical recreation. *Amer. Recreation J., 5,* No. 6, November-December, 1964.

Meyer, Harold D., and Brightbill, Charles K.: *Community Recreation.* Englewood Cliffs, New Jersey, Prentice-Hall, Inc., 1956.

Mullen, Francis A., and Blumenthal, Leroy H.: Principals of agency-school cooperation in a program for emotionally disturbed children. *Amer. J. Orthopsychiat., XXXII,* 1962.

Music Therapy as Taught. International Musicians, March, 1963.

New pathways from the mental hospital. J. Social Issues, 16:2, 1960.

Newman, William H.: *Administrative Action.* Englewood-Cliffs, New Jersey, Prentice-Hall, Inc., 1951.

Noroian, E. H.: *Research in Modern Concepts of Hospital Administration.* (ed.) Owen, J. K., Philadelphia, W. B. Saunders, 1962.

Occupational Therapy Reference Manual for Physicians. Dubuque, Iowa, William C. Brown Book Company, 1960.

Of recreation in the medical setting. North Carolina Recreation Commission, Raleigh, North Carolina, No. 27, November, 1959.

Orientation of Volunteers for Service in State Mental Hospitals. (pamphlet) Health and Welfare Federation of Allegheny County, 1956.

Osmond, Humphrey: Function as the basis of psychiatric ward design. *Ment. Hosp.,* April, 1957.

Owen, J. K.: *Modern Concepts of Hospital Administration.* Philadelphia, Pennsylvania. Saunders, 1962.

Palmer, M.: *Experiment in Use of Volunteers in Individual Relationships with Patients.* (Report submitted to the Rehabilitation Project at the Massachusetts Mental Health Center), November, 1956.

Parke, J. H.: Cost of free service. *Ment. Hosp. 4:*11, 1953.

Peszcynski, Mieczyslaw, and Tillock, Eugene E.: Clinical and administrative management of physical medicine and rehabilitation. *Hosp. Prog., 45,* March, 1964.

Pfiffner, John, and Sherwood, Frank P.: *Administrative Organization.* Englewood Cliffs, New Jersey, Prentice-Hall, 1960.

Phillips, Edwyn, and Draine, Catherine: Social Rehabilitation at a Mountain Resort. *Ment. Hosp.,* May, 1963.

Phillips, E. Lakin, Weiner, Daniel N., and Haring, Norris G.: *Discipline, Achievement, and Mental Health.* Englewood Cliffs, New Jersey, Prentice-Hall, Inc., 1960.

Planning for Long-term Patients. A Selected Bibliography, Washington, D. C.: U. S. Department of Health, Education, and Welfare, August, 1961.

Prentis, J., H. W.: Three c's of leadership. *Superv. Mgt. 7,* November, 1962.

Program outline for occupational therapy assistants in general practice. *AOTA, Rev.,* November, 1962.

Psychiatric Architecture. (ed.) Goshen, Charles E., American Psychiatric Association, 1700 Eighteenth Street, N. W., Washington, D. C., 1959.

Public relations: a responsibility of the mental hospital administrator. *Report #55,* New York, Group For The Advancement of Psychiatry, 1963.

Recreation contribution to the patient. North Carolina Recreation Commission, Raleigh, North Carolina, No. 32, September, 1963.

Recruitment and Retention of Volunteers for Service in Veterans Administration Hospitals. Report of a two year study by the Veterans Administration Voluntary Service Subcommittee on Recruitment and Retention of Volunteers, April, 1960.

Rehabilitation centers. *Architectural Rec.,* January, 1960.

Requirements of an acceptable training program for occupational therapy assistants. *AOTA, Rev.,* November, 1962.

Rosenfield, Isadore: A medical center for Puerto Rico. *Hospitals, 35,* June 1961.

Ross, Murray G., and Hendry, Charles E.: *New Understanding of Leadership.* New York, Association Press, 1957.

Rudy, Lester H., and Smith, Jackson A.: Modern concepts of hospital therapy. *Current Psychiatric Therapies, 1,* 1961.

Ruppenthal, Wayne W.: Objectivity in clinical practice. *NAMT Book of Proceedings,* 1957.

Rusk, H. A.: Philosophy of rehabilitation. *J. M. A. Alabama, 31,* May, 1962.

Ryan, J. T. Jr.: Responsibilities for leadership. *Hosp. Prog.,* 4, November, 1962.

Schlessinger, Lawrence: Patient motivation for rehabilitation. *AJOT,* XVII, 1, 1963.

Schultz, Walter J.: Educational therapy at the VA hospital, Downey, Illinois. *Amer. Arch. Rehabil. Ther., V,* September, 1957.

Scofield, John B.: Adolescent treatment in an adult hospital. *Amer. J. Orthopsychiat., XXXII,* 1962.

Selecting Supervisors. Washington, D. C., U. S. Government Printing Office, 1956.

Sewall, Lee G.: Methods of measuring hospital goals. *Ment. Hosp.,* February, 1964.

Sills, D. L.: *The Volunteers.* Bureau of Applied Social Research, Columbia University, 1957.

Simon, Herbert A.: *Administrative Behavior,* New York, MacMillan Company, 1947.

..........: The administrator as a decision-maker. *Hospital Administration,* Spring, 1958.

Smith, Harvey L.: Two lines of authority are one too many. *Mod. Hosp., 84,* March, 1955.

Snalldon, John L.: Architectural study. Architectural Supplement, *Ment. Hosp.,* June, 1961.

Sommers, Robert: Professionalization and occupational therapy. *Canad. J. O. T.,* No. 28, March, 1961.

Sorenson, Arthur A.: Research in educational therapy. *Amer. Arch. Rehabil. Ther.,* XI, March, 1963.

Statement of purpose and functions of a volunteer bureau. pamphlet approved by Advisory Committee on Citizen Participation of Community Chests and Councils of America, Inc., and the National Social Welfare Assembly, April 5, 1955.

Strandberg, B.: Educating and training of medical and non-medical personnel in physical medicine and rehabilitation. *Arch. Phys. Med. 43,* April, 1962.

Tead, Orway: *The Art of Administration.* New York, McGraw-Hill Book Company, 1951.

Tebow, Hilda: *Staff Development: an Integral Part of an Administration.* Report #35, Washington, D. C.: Department of Health, Education, and Welfare, 1959.

Traxler, Ralph Jr.: The qualities of an administrator. *Hosp. Adm., 6,* No. 4, 1961.

Triggs, Frances O.: *Personnel Work in Schools of Nursing.* Philadelphia, Pennsylvania, W. B. Saunders and Company, 1945.

Two recreational facilities. *Ment. Hosp.,* October, 1957.

Underwood, Mary B.: Experiment in group reading. *Library Journal,* No. 80, May, 1955.

Urwick, Lyndall: *Patterns of Organization.* Manchester, England, Manchester Press, 1946.

Volunteer gives and receives. *National Conference of Social Work Proceedings,* 1946.

Volunteer service guide for directors of state hospitals. Albany, New York, State Department of Mental Hygiene (undated pamphlet).

Volunteers in Minnesota's State Hospitals: St. Paul, Minnesota, State Department of Welfare (undated pamphlet).

Wade, Beatrice: Organizing an occupational therapy department. *Hospitals,* November, 1954.

Watson, Brantley: You and Management Development. *Hospital Management, 93,* March, 1962.

Weller, Evelyn G., and Kilborne, Elizabeth B.: *Citizen Participation in Public Welfare Programs.* Supplementary Services by Volunteers, U. S. Department of Health, Education and Welfare; Social Security Administration; Bureau of Public Assistance; Division of Technical Training; U. S. Government Printing Office; Washington, D. C. 1956.

West, Eilma, and Clark, Alonzo W.: Planning the complete occupational therapy service. *Hospitals, 25,* October, 1951.

Whisler, Thomas L.: Executives and their jobs: the changing organizational structure. *Hospital Administration, 9,* No. 3, Summer 1964.

White, H. F. Jr.: Strengths and weaknesses of volunteers and volunteer system. *Mod. Hosp. 80,* 1953.

Wilson, Gertrude, and Ryland, Gladys: *Social Group Work Practice.* Cambridge, Massachusetts, Houghton Mifflin Company, 1949.

Word is Hope. Austin, Texas: Hogg Foundation for Mental Health, 1961.

Worthy, James C.: Ethical and moral responsibilities of the executive. *Hospital Administration, 7:3,* 1962.

Writing job descriptions. (article) *Girl Scouts of the U. S. A.,* 1956.

Appendix A

SCHOOLS GRANTING DEGREES IN THE VARIOUS PROFESSIONS

LISTED BELOW ARE SCHOOLS who grant a degree in the various professions that usually make up the Activity Therapy Service. It should be noted that additional schools may have been added since the publication of this listing.

SCHOOLS GRANTING A DEGREE IN OCCUPATIONAL THERAPY*

Boston University, Sargeant College, Charles River Campus, University Road, Boston 15, Massachusetts.

Colorado State University, College of Home Economics, Fort Collins, Colorado.

Columbia University, College of Physicians and Surgeons, 630 West 168th Street, New York 32, New York.

Eastern Michigan University, Ypsilanti, Michigan.

Florida, University of, College of Health Related Services, Gainesville, Florida.

Illinois, University of, College of Medicine, 1853 West Polk Street, Chicago 12, Illinois.

Indiana University School of Medicine, 1200 West Michigan Street, Indianapolis 7, Indiana.

Iowa, State University of, College of Liberal Arts and College of Medicine, Iowa City, Iowa.

Kansas, University of, Lawrence, Kansas.

Loma Linda University, School of Medicine, Loma Linda, California.

Lawrence University, Appleton, Wisconsin (Milwaukee-Downer College).

Minnesota, University of, School of Medical Sciences, Minneapolis 14, Minnesota.

---

*AJOT, November, December, 1964 issue.

Mount Mary College, Milwaukee 10, Wisconsin.

New Hampshire, University of, College of Liberal Arts, Durham, New Hampshire.

New York University, School of Education, Washington Square, New York 3, New York.

New York, State University of, at Buffalo, School of Medicine 3435 Main Street, Buffalo 14, New York.

North Dakota, University of, Grand Forks, North Dakota.

Ohio State University, College of Education, Health Center, 410 West 10th Street, Columbus 10, Ohio.

Pennsylvania, University of, School of Allied Medical Professions, 3901 Pine Street, Philadelphia 4, Pennsylvania.

Puerto Rico, University of, School of Medicine, School of Physical and Occupational Therapy, Candelaria Esq. Mandry—Stop 22, Santurce, Puerto Rico.

Puget Sound, University of, Tacoma 6, Washington.

Richmond Professional Institute, Colleges of William and Mary, Richmond 20, Virginia.

Saint Catherine, College of, St. Paul 1, Minnesota.

San Jose State College, San Jose 14, California.

Southern California, University of, College of Letters, Arts, and Sciences, Box 274, Los Angeles 7, California.

Texas Woman's University, Denton, Texas.

Tufts University, Boston School of Occupational Therapy, College of Special Studies, 7 Harcourt Street, Boston 16, Massachusetts.

Washington University, School of Medicine, 4567 Scott Avenue, St. Louis 10, Missouri.

Washington, University of, School of Medicine, Department of Physical Medicine and Rehabilitation, CC-814 University Hospital, Seattle 5, Washington.

Wayne State University, College of Liberal Arts, Detroit 1, Michigan.

Western Michigan University, Kalamazoo 45, Michigan.

Wisconsin, University of, School of Medicine, 1300 University Avenue, Madison 6, Wisconsin.

SCHOOLS GRANTING A DEGREE IN RECREATION (HOSPITAL OR REHABILITATION MAJOR)

Teachers College, Columbia University, New York, New York.

New York University, New York, New York.

Sacramento State College, Sacramento, California.

San Francisco State College, San Francisco, California.

San Jose State College, San Jose, California.

Springfield College, Springfield, Massachusetts.

Texas Woman's University, Denton, Texas.

University of Minnesota, Minneapolis, Minnesota.

University of North Carolina, Chapel Hill, North Carolina.

University of Wisconsin, Madison, Wisconsin.

A listing of schools granting a degree in Recreation other than in the specialty of hospital or rehabilitation recreation may be secured from the National Recreation Association (Service Organization), 8 West Eighth Street, New York 11, New York, or American Recreation Society (Professional Organization), 1404 New York Avenue, N. W., Washington 5, D.C.*

SCHOOLS GRANTING A DEGREE IN MUSIC THERAPY

Alverno College, Milwaukee, Wisconsin.

Florida State University, Tallahasee, Florida.

Michigan State University, East Lansing, Michigan.

University of Kansas, Lawrence, Kansas.

Loyola University, New Orleans, Louisiana.

University of the Pacific, Stockton, California.

Indiana University, Bloomington, Indiana.

Ohio University, Athens, Ohio.

Texas Women's University, Denton, Texas.

Lincoln University, Jefferson City, Missouri.

SCHOOLS GRANTING A DEGREE IN LIBRARY SCIENCE (SPECIAL COURSES IN HOSPITAL AND MEDICAL LIBRARY SCIENCE)

University of Southern California, Los Angeles, California.

Catholic University of America, Washington, D.C.

---

*These two organizations have recently merged into the National Recreation and Park Association, 8 West Eight Street, New York 11, New York.

Emory University, Atlanta, Georgia.
University of Illinois, Urbana, Illinois.
University of Michigan, Ann Arbor, Michigan.
Columbia University, New York, New York.
University of North Carolina, Chapel Hill, North Carolina.
Western Reserve University, Cleveland, Ohio.
Drexel Institute of Technology, Philadelphia, Pennsylvania.

SCHOOLS GRANTING A DEGREE IN PHYSICAL THERAPY

Loma Linda University, Loma Linda, California.
Children's Hospital of Los Angeles, Los Angeles, California.
Stanford University Medical Center, Palo Alto, California.
University of California School of Medicine, San Francisco, California.
University of Colorado School of Medicine, Denver, Colorado.
University of Connecticut, Storrs, Connecticut.
University of Florida, College of Health Related Services, Gainesville, Florida.
Northwestern University Medical School, Chicago, Illinois.
Indiana University Medical Center, Indianapolis, Indiana.
State University of Iowa, Iowa City, Iowa.
University of Kansas Medical Center, Kansas City, Kansas.
University of Maryland School of Medicine, Baltimore, Maryland.
Boston University, Sargent College, Boston, Massachusetts.
Bouve-Boston School, Medford, Massachusetts.
Simons College, The Fenway, Boston, Massachusetts.
University of Michigan, Ann Arbor, Michigan.
University of Minnesota, Minneapolis, Minnesota.
Mayo Clinic, Rochester, Minnesota.
St. Louis University, St. Louis, Missouri.
Washington University, School of Medicine, St. Louis, Missouri.
Russel Sage College, Albany Medical College, Division of Physical Therapy, Albany, New York.
State University of New York at Buffalo, Buffalo, New York.
Ithaca College, Albert Einstein College of Medicine, New York, New York.

New York University School of Education, New York, New York.

University of North Carolina School of Medicine, Chapel Hill, North Carolina.

Duke University Medical Center, Durham, North Carolina.

Western Reserve University, Cleveland, Ohio.

Ohio State University, Columbus, Ohio.

University of Oklahoma, Oklahoma City, Oklahoma.

D. T. Watson School of Physiatrics, Division of Physical Therapy, Leetsdale, Pennsylvania.

University of Pennsylvania, Division of Physical Therapy, School of Allied Medical Professions, Philadelphia, Pennsylvania.

Baylor University, Medical Center, Dallas, Texas.

University of Puerto Rico, Street Number 2, Villa Nevarez, Rio Piedras.

University of Texas Medical Branch, Galveston, Texas.

Hermann Hospital, Houston, Texas.

Medical College of Virginia, Richmond, Virginia.

University of Washington, Seattle, Washington.

University of Wisconsin Medical School, Madison, Wisconsin.

Marquette University School of Medicine, Milwaukee, Wisconsin.

SCHOOLS GRANTING A DEGREE IN VOCATIONAL AND/OR INDUSTRIAL THERAPY

Degrees granted in the major area of vocational rehabilitation, manual arts, industrial arts, counseling and guidance, occupational therapy, sociology, psychology, and special education are usually applicable to this specialty.

SCHOOLS GRANTING A DEGREE IN EDUCATIONAL THERAPY

Degrees granted in the major area of special education applicable to this specialty. A state teaching certificate is also usually required.

SCHOOLS GRANTING A DEGREE IN VOLUNTEER SERVICES

Since no specific degree with a major in this field is provided at this time, consideration is given to those majoring in education, humancis, social science, health education, recreation, psychology, public health, and public administration.

PROFESSIONAL ORGANIZATIONS AND REGISTRATION (CERTIFICATION)

Occupational Therapy

Org. American Occupational Therapy Association
250 West 57th Street, New York 19, New York.

Reg. American Occupational Therapy Association
250 West 57th Street, New York 19, New York.

Org. Canadian Association of Occupational Therapy
331 Bloor Street, W., Toronto 5, Ontario.

Reg. Canadian Association of Occupational Therapy
331 Bloor Street, W., Toronto 5, Ontario.

Medical Recreation

Org. Hospital Recreation Section, American Park and Recreation Society.
1404 New York Avenue, N. W., Washington 5, D. C.
National Association of Recreation Therapist
Box 69
Vinita, Oklahoma.
Recreational Therapy Section, American Association of Health Physical Education and Recreation
1201 Sixteenth Street, N. W., Washington 6, D. C.

Reg. Council for the Advancement of Hospital Recreation
The Council is made up of representatives from the three organizations above. Application for registration at one of the three levels (director, leader, aide) is made through the respective professional organizations to which the individual belongs.
National Registration Board
National Recreation and Park Association
8 West Eight Street, New York 11, New York

Music Therapy

Org. National Association for Music Therapy, Inc.
  P. O. Box 610, Lawrence, Kansas.
Reg. National Association for Music Therapy, Inc.
  P. O. Box 610, Lawrence, Kansas.

Physical Therapy

Org. American Physical Therapy Association
  1790 Broadway, New York 19, New York.
Reg. American Registry of Physical Therapists
  30 W. Michigan, Avenue, Chicago 2, Illinois

Educational Therapy

Org. American Association of Rehabilitation Therapy, Inc.
  Box 4093, N. Little Rock, Arkansas 72116.
Reg. American Association of Rehabilitation Therapy, Inc.
  Box 17013, VA Hospital, Houston, Texas.

Library Science

Org. Association of Hospital and Institutional Libraries (a division of the American Library Association).
  50 East Huron Street, Chicago, Illinois.
Cert: Medical Library Association, 919 N. Michigan Avenue, Chicago, Illinois 60611.

Industrial and Manual Arts Therapy

Org. American Association of Rehabilitation Therapy, Inc.
  Box 4093, N. Little Rock, Arkansas 72116.
Reg. American Association of Rehabilitation Therapy, Inc.
  Box 17013, VA Hospital, Houston, Texas.

Directors and Coordinators

Org. American Academy of Physical Medicine and Rehabilitation
  30 N. Michigan Avenue, Chicago 2, Illinois (physicians only).

American Congress of Physical Medicine and Rehabilitation
30 N. Michigan Avenue, Chicago 2, Illinois (physicians only).

American Board of Physical Medicine and Rehabilitation
200 First Street, S. W., Rochester, Minnesota (physicians only).

American Medical Association
535 N. Dearborn Street, Chicago 10, Illinois (physicians only).

American Psychiatric Association
1700 - 18th Street, N. W., Washington 9, D. C. (physicians only).

Association for Medical Rehabilitation Directors and Co-ordinators
37 Clinton Avenue, Rockville Centre, New York (physicians and lay administrators).

Reg. Association for Medical Rehabilitation Directors and Co-ordinators
37 Clinton Avenue, Rockville Centre, New York (physicians and lay administrators).

American Board of Physical Medicine and Rehabilitation
30 N. Michigan Avenue, Chicago 2, Illinois (physicians only).

Volunteer Services

Org. American Association of Volunteer Service Coordinators
Mental Health Services, American Psychiatric Association
1700 - 18th Street, N. W., Washington, D. C.

Reg. None.

Corrective Therapy

Org. Association for Physical and Mental Rehabilitation
105 Lawrence Street, Rehoboth Beach, Delaware.

Reg. Association for Physical and Mental Rehabilitation
105 Lawrence Street, Rehoboth Beach, Delaware.

Appendix C

JOB SPECIFICATIONS FOR COORDINATOR

THE FOLLOWING PAGES provide a sampling of class specifications from federal, state, and private agencies employing a Coordinator or Administrator. Salary scales have been deleted.

COORDINATOR OF ACTIVITY THERAPY XIV[1]

Kind of Work

This is administrative work in coordinating various institutional activity therapy programs such as occupational therapy, recreation, music therapy, industrial therapy, vocational rehabilitation, and a patient library. Scope and emphasis of the program are determined by the Superintendent, but employee has wide latitude in the coordination of the activity therapies into the total treatment program.

Plans, develops and administers a comprehensive master integrated schedule of activity therapy to assure that each patient has an opportunity to receive treatment in the several localities included in this area.

Assists the clinical director in the selection of patients for assignment or prescription to one or more of the activity therapy programs.

Maintain close contact with the clinical director to develop and conduct medically approved plans and policies which will meet the needs, capabilities and interests of patients assigned to the activity therapy program.

Supervises the total program conducted by occupational therapy, recreation, music therapy, vocational rehabilitation, industrial therapy, and library.

Reviews budget estimates prepared by the directors of the activity therapy departments and makes changes when necessary.

Coordinates all records, statistics and reports, and reviews data prior to submission to clinical director or superintendent.

Performs related work as assigned.

Requirements for Work

Extensive knowledge of content of one activity therapy area, such as, occupational therapy or recreation and a knowledge and understanding of all other activity therapy areas.

Extensive knowledge of appropriate biological, physical, and social sciences, such as biology, physiology, psychology, and sociology.

Knowledge of the policies, principles, plans, practices, tools, and techniques of activity therapy administration.

Ability to adapt activity therapy policies, procedures, plans, practices, tools, and techniques to specific operational situations.

Minimum Experience and Educational Requirements

Two years of full-time paid experience as director of an institutional activity therapy program.

Eligibility for appointment as a Recreational Director XII, Occupational Director XII, Vocational and Industrial Therapy Director XII, or Music Therapist XII.

SUPERVISOR OF REHABILITATION SERVICES, MENTAL HOSPITALS[2]

Definition

Under medical direction, to plan, organize, and direct the rehabilitation services of a mental hospital; and to do other work as required.

Typical Tasks

Develops and supervises a program for the rehabilitation of patients through organized individual and group therapy activities, including creative and industrial arts, handicrafts, recreation, music and related therapies, the patients' library, and the volunteer services program; supervises a staff of occupational, recreation, music and industrial therapists and allied personnel; works with other staff members in coordinating the rehabilitation services program with medical, nursing, physical therapy, teaching, social work, and other therapeutic programs of the hospital; develops and directs a training program in the rehabilitation therapies for hospital employees and for students from educational institutions; recruits rehabilitation services personnel, evaluates their work, and takes or recommends appropriate action with respect to their work performance; establishes cooperative relationships with public and private agencies; addresses interested organizations on the rehabilitation program; orders equipment and supplies and prepares budgetary data for the rehabilitation services; keeps records and prepares reports.

Minimum Qualifications

Either I

One year of experience performing the duties of an Assistant Supervisor of Rehabilitation Services, Mental Hospitals, or performing the duties of a Coordinator of Volunteer Services or Senior Occupational Therapist in a California state mental hospital.

Or II

Experience: Two years of full-time paid experience in supervising an occupational therapy or a recreation or a music program and a staff of at least two professionally trained therapists, including or supplemented by one year of full-time paid experience as an occupational or as a recreation or a music therapist in a mental hospital: and

Education: Either

1. Registration with the National Registry of the American Occupational Therapy Association or eligibility for such registration; *or*
2. Equivalent to graduation from a recognized college with major work in recreation therapy, music therapy, vocational education or a closely related field,

and

Supervisor of Rehabilitation Services,
Mental Hospital

Knowledges and abilities:

Thorough knowledge of: theory and practice of mental and physical rehabilitation of mentally and physically handicapped persons.

Wide Knowledge of: principles and techniques of the rehabilitation services as practiced in occupational, recreation, music and industrial therapy and skill in their application; hospital organization and procedure; principles and techniques used in developing and conducting training courses for rehabilitation therapists; current trends in the rehabilitation therapy field; principles of effective supervision.

General knowledge of: basic pathology involved in diseases and injuries resulting in physical and mental handicaps and of the physical and psychological problems of the handicapped person; preventive mental health principles; accepted medical, nursing, physical therapy, teaching, and social work practices in mental institutions.

Ability to: direct the work of others; plan, organize, and direct a hospital rehabilitation services program; interpret rehabilitation programs to other staff members and to the public; analyze situations accurately and take effective action; speak and write effectively.

and

Special personal characteristics: Demonstrated supervisory ability; ability to establish and maintain cooperative interrelationships with individuals and groups; sympathetic and objective understanding of the problems of mentally and physically handicapped persons; tact; patience; emotional stability; pleasing personality and neat personal appearance.

PHYSICAL MEDICINE AND REHABILITATION COORDINATOR (AND REHABILITATION SPECIALIST— PHYSICAL MEDICINE)[3]

Duties

The duties of these positions require (medical) administrative supervision and coordination of a Physical Medicine and Rehabilitation Service at a V. A. hospital involving such functions as educational therapy, manual arts therapy, physical therapy, occupational therapy, corrective therapy, and blind rehabilitation, and the responsibility for coordinating such functions with other medical services and other rehabilitation functions within the V. A. At stations other than hospitals, these positions involve such functions as evaluation, appraisal and coordination of physical medicine and rehabilitation service programs within the area.

Experience Requirements

Applicants must show progressively responsible experience in work as described below, and in the total amount and amounts of specific types shown in the following table:

Type A. Medical administrative director, coordinator, or comparable official of a program of physical medicine and rehabilitation or reconditioning at the hospital or staff level in which the duties included medical administrative supervision and coordination of an organized group of therapeutic activities such as physical therapy, occupational therapy, corrective therapy, manual arts therapy, educational therapy, or similar medical rehabilitation activities characteristic of a physical medicine and rehabilitation program broad in scope.

Type B. Assistant to, or a trainee under, the medical administrative director or coordinator of a program of physical medicine and rehabilitation or reconditioning at the hospital level.

Type C. Chief or supervisor of a medical rehabilitation activity described in type A of a hospital program of physical medicine and rehabilitation or reconditioning.

Type D. Instructor, therapist, or instructor-therapist in a physical medicine and rehabilitation activity of a hospital program of medical rehabilitation or reconditioning such as described in Type A.

Type E. Experience in one or more of the following fields: Hospital management; medical administration involving such activities as registration, supply or personnel management; medical or psychiatric social work; vocational counseling, guidance, or placement for the physically disabled or handicapped;

clinical psychology; educational work as a teacher or supervisor of teachers of the handicapped in appropriate courses in a hospital, rehabilitation center, school for the handicapped, or homebound educational program.

Amount of Experience Required

Grade	Total	Specialized
GS-9	5 years	I year of type A, B, or C, or any combination of type A, B, or C.
GS-10	5½ years	1½ years of type A, B, or C, provided at least 3 months is shown in Type A or B.
GS-11	6 years	2 years type A, B, or C, provided at least 6 months is shown in type A.
GS-12	7 years	3 years type A, B, or C, provided at least one year is shown in type A.

Quality of Experience

For any grade the required amount of experience will not in itself be accepted as proof of qualification for any of these positions. The applicant's record of experience and training in coordinating medical rehabilitation activities must show that he has the ability to perform the duties of the position concerned. For all grades, applicants must show either six months of experience at a level of difficulty comparable to that of the next lower grade or one year of experience at a level of difficulty comparable to that of the second lower grade in the Federal service. Above GS-12: For any position at these grades, no additional amount of type of experience or education is required beyond that required for GS-12. However, there must have been a proportionate increase in the breadth and level of experience in the field in which outstanding professional stature was achieved and administrative acumen in program development, coordination, and implementation has been demonstrated.

Substitution of Education for Experience

1. Study in an accredited college or university may be substituted on the basis of one year of education for nine months of experience, up to a maximum of four years of education for three years of experience, provided that an average of at least six

semester hours per year was in one or any combination of the following subjects: Education (general, business, vocational, physical, or health), science, vocal studies, social work, personnel administration, hospital administration, vocational guidance and counseling, or psychology.

2. The successful completion of undergraduate college work in nonaccredited institutions will be accepted on the same basis as for accredited colleges provided that such institutions give instruction of definitely collegiate level and that the State University of the State in which the institution is located accepts the courses and gives advanced credit for them. (In those states where there is no State University, the evaluation and acceptance of college credit as made by the State Department of education will be accepted.

3. Graduation from an approved school of occupational therapy or physical therapy may be substituted for three years of experience.

4. No substitution may be made for the required specialized experience, nor for any experience required to be at a level of difficulty comparable to that of the next or second lower grade in the Federal service.

DIRECTOR, ADJUNCTIVE THERAPY[4]

Duties

To be responsible (1) for treatment planning and general administration of the Adjunctive Therapy section; (2) selection assignment, and professional development of personnel within the section; (3) interpretation of the function of the Adjunctive Therapies; (4) promotion and maintenance of working relationships with other departments, and (5) contribution to the development of the section and participation in total planning for the growth of the Foundation at professional meetings.

Educational Requirements

A masters degree in one of the Adjunctive Therapies (i.e., hospital recreation, music therapy, occupational therapy) A minimum of three years clinical experience in at least two of the adjunctive therapies. A minimum of two years supervisory experience directing a broad therapy program, in which executive and leadership ability have been demonstrated.

ACTIVITY THERAPY SUPERVISOR[5]

Duties

Plans and administers a coordinated master schedule of activity and rehabilitation therapies insuring that each patient receives prescribed treatment, including occupational, recreational, music, and industrial therapy. Directs in-service training programs in activity therapies for staff, college students, volunteer workers and employees. Reviews, revises if necessary, and coordinates budget estimates, reports and records prior to submission to clinical director or superintendent. Performs other related works as required.

Necessary Knowledge and Abilities

Knowledge of physiology, psychology and sociology; problems of mentally and physically ill; rehabilitative therapy; administration; educational methods.

Ability to supervise therapists, recreational personnel, volunteer workers; maintain effective patient therapy; establish effective working relationships with other departmental personnel; speak and write well.

Minimum Requirements

Master's degree from an accerdited college or university with a major in recreation, preferably hospital recreation, music therapy, social group work, vocational guidance and counseling, counseling psychology, manual arts, industrial arts, industrial arts or occupational therapy; *plus* three years of full time professional experience in an activity therapy program, two years of which must have been in an administrative capacity in directing a broad therapeutic program while supervising a staff of at least two professionally trained therapist

or

Graduation from an accredited school of occupational therapy;

plus five years of the experience as described above, two of which must have been at the administrative level as described above.

Special Requirements

The applicant must be registered with the National Registry of Occupational Therapy.

ADMINISTRATOR—EXECUTIVE DIRECTOR[6]

Minimum Requirements

Masters degree in public administration, post graduate study in psychology, guidance and counseling. Ten years successful administrative experience, ability to lead, develop and promote rehabilitation on local, state, and national levels.

Duties

1. Board of Directors—execute policies of, plan with and report to them on all phases of the Center and its operation.

2. Medical Advisory Committee—assist Medical Director in executing policies of, plan with, see that medical ethics are observed by the Staff.

3. Staff—employment of all staff, assignment of duties, and discharge for just cause.

4. Finance—prepare yearly budget, provide competent bookkeeping, account for all incomes and expenditures, control purchasing and see that annual audit is made.

5. National and State Organizations—serve as the representative of the Society and Crossroads, serve on committees and perform other functions.

MEDICAL DIRECTOR[7]

Minimum Requirements

A doctor of medicine in good standing with the State Medical Association. A Diplomate of the Board of Orthopedic Surgery, and a member in good standing with the American Medical Association.

Duties

1. To see that dictates of the Medical Advisory Committee are carried out. This includes matters on medical policies, ethics, and other factors which may be of a medical nature.

2. Directs the activities of the Medical Services. This includes Physical Therapy, Occupational Therapy, Speech Therapy, and Activities of Daily Living.

3. Confer with therapists as necessary to insure efficiency and harmony.

4. Serve as liaison between our Medical Department and Medical profession.

5. Supervision of professional staff in training program.

6. Show films, give talks, and make appearances before clubs, civic groups, and professional groups.

7. Handle medical problems that may need attention in the Vocational Workshop and other departments.

8. Serve as spokesman for the Medical Department in all matters which must be referred to outside sources.

9. Maintain high standards of medical and ethical treatment and conduct.

★   ★   ★

1. Indiana State Personnel Division, Indianapolis, Indiana, August, 1963.

2. California State Personnel Board, Sacramento, California, February, 1961.

3. Veterans Administration, Personnel Services, Washington, D. C., July, 1961.

4. The Meinninger Foundation, Topeka, Kansas, December, 1962.

5. Washington State Department of Personnel, Olympia, Washington, September, 1962.

6. Crossroads Rehabilitation Center, Indianapolis, Indiana, January, 1963.

7. Crossroads Rehabilitation Center, Indianapolis, Indiana, January, 1963.

SELECTED LIBRARY REFERENCES*

BOOKS SUITABLE FOR WORKING WITH VARIOUS TYPES OF PATIENTS

Dolch, Elaine T. A list of books which the author recommends for preschool children. Available from the *American Journal of Nursing,* 10 Columbus Circle, New York 19, New York.

Fenner, Phyllis, (Ed.): *Something Shared; Children and Books.* A personal treasury of articles and cartoons selected and with comments by the author editor. Day, 1959. The stories reveal the inner feelings of a child.

Illinois State Library: *Books For The Partially Sighted.* Titles suitable for young people and juveniles are indicated by "Y" and "J". All books in this list are in fourteen-point type.

Larrick Nancy: *A Parents' Guide to Children's Reading.* Garden City, New York. Doubleday and Company, 1958. A very fine guide for the volunteer in selecting suitable books, for children.

Massachusetts Library Association: Adult Education Committee, Comp. *Easy on your Eyes.* A listing of books printed in large clear type. 101 Tremont Street., Boston, Mass. The New England Council of Optometrists, 1962, 52p. (35¢) More than 600 books, printed in larger than normal type, for the patient who has difficulty in reading. Adult books for all ages, educational background and interest are listed.

New York Public Library: *For Tired Eyes, Books and Recordings.* New York Public Library, 5th Avenue and 42nd Street, New York 1961, 19 p. (25¢).

Rex, Jean: *Books About Parents and Their Children.* New York. Child Study Association of America, Inc. Many excellent reading suggestions. Useful for patients and institution libraries.

---

*This appendix prepared by Lucille K. Leuschner.

Wisconsin Free Library Commission: *Easy on the Eyes, Stimulating to the Mind, Adult Books in Clear Print.* Comp. by Work with Senior Citizens Committee, 1963. Available from Wis. Free Lib. Commission. Box 1437, Madison, Wisconsin 53701. (20¢) Books on many subjects offered. Books for reading aloud are indicated.

Books for Better Understanding of Self and Family. The books listed below, in various categories, have proved valuable. They will serve as a clue to the kinds of books that are useful. However, the titles listed represent only a few of the many books that could be used successfully.

Abrahamsen, David: *Road to Emotional Maturity,* Prentice-Hall, 1958. 399 pp. This book points out how we can learn to develop our hearts and minds to achieve and maintain emotional maturity and well-being.

Alvarez, Walter C.: *Live At Peace With Your Nerves.* Prentice-Hall, 1958. Dr. Alvarez, consultant emeritus for Mayo Clinic, explains that "Anxiety Neurosis" can be more dangerous to a person's health than the original ailment. He discusses causes of nervous tensions and their effect on work and daily living.

Bennett, Edward: *Search For Emotional Security.* Ronald, 1959. Discussion of conflicts to which the normal adult is exposed in daily business and personal life.

Bowman, Henry: *Marriage for Moderns,* 4th Ed., McGraw, 1960. Discusses problems which arise before and after marriage.

Bingham, June: *The Inside Story; Psychiatry and Everyday Life.* Knopf, 1953. Compiled under direction of Fritz Redlick; text written by June Bingham with the collaboration of Jacob Levine. Knopf, 1953. Cartoons aid in relating psychiatry's basic discoveries to everyday life.

Chafetz, Morris E.: *Alcoholism and Society.* Oxford, 1962, 319 p. This volume examines the causes of alcoholism, includes definition of alcoholism, psychological theories and other related scientific research. Final chapters are devoted to methods of alcoholism prevention.

Coleman, Lester: *Freedom from Fear.* Hawthorn Books, 1954. A doctor expresses concern over the increasing number of patients who are incapacitated more by fear and anxiety than by disease. He discusses the prevalence of fear, the reasons, and how it manifests itself.

Duvall, Evelyn M., and Hill, Reuben: *Being Married.* (with chapters in collaboration with Sylvanus Duvall) Association Press 1960, 44 pp. This book is a complete course on marriage and the preparation for marriage.

Egleson, Jim: *Parents without Partners.* A guide for divorced, widowed or separated parents by Jim Egleson and Frank Egleson. Dutton, 1961. An excellent guide for the single guide to parents' relationships with their children and development of sounder growth patterns for themselves.

Landis, Paul H.: *Making the Most of Marriage.* 2nd Ed., Appleton, 1960. (Sociology Ser.) A sound preparation for marriage and parenthood.

Magouen, F. Alexander: *Living a Happy Life,* Harper, 1960. To acquire happiness, man must find emotional maturity, self respect and self-fulfillment. The author shows how creative work gives significance to man's life.

May, Rollo: *Man's Search for Himself.* Norton, 1953. A famous American psychiatrist cites the causes of insecure feelings and describes values and goals to attain security.

Mann, Marty: *Marty Mann's New Primer on Alcoholism.* How people drink, how to recognize alcoholics, and what to do about them. Rinehart, 1958. A manual of practical knowledge to the alcoholic, his family, relatives and friends. Gives causes for alcoholism and defines an "alcoholic."

Overstreet, Harry Allen: *Mature Mind.* Norton, 1949. Defines maturity of the mind and examines emotions and social outlook in the light of psychological insights. Applies theories of maturity on conduct in home, education, politics and social relations.

Rogers, Carl R.: *On Becoming a Person.* Houghton-Mifflin, 1961. Explains the meaning of personal growth and how one person can help another.

Roosevelt, Eleanor: *You Learn By Living.* Harper, 1960, 211 pp. Mrs. Roosevelt has thought in practical terms about the questions we are all faced with in some way; How to conquer our fears; How to get the best out of ourselves and others; how to help other people; how to adjust to difficulties, etc.

Strecker, Edward, and Appel, Kenneth E.: *Discovering Ourselves*. 3rd Ed., MacMillan, 1958. A view of the human mind and how it works. An elementary book on psychology of motivation, behavior and human relations.

Schindler, John A.: *How to Live 365 Days a Year*. Prentice-Hall, 1955. Dr. Schindler discusses the six basic psychological needs and the problem of emotionally induced illness.

Weatherhead, Leslie: *Prescription for Anxiety*. Abingdon Press, 1956. A minister writes understandingly of patients' anxieties.

Young Adult Books

Breck, Vivian: *Maggie*. Doubleday, 1954.
Burnford, Sheila: *The Incredible Journey*. Little, 1961.
Coleman, Pauline: *The Different One*. Dodd, 1955.
Coolidge, Olivia: *Men of Athens,* Houghton, 1962.
Daly, Maureen: *Seventeenth Summer,* Dodd, 1948.
Forbes, Esther: *Johnny Tremain,* Houghton.
Keith, Harold: *Rifles for Watie,* Crowell, 1957.
Krumgold, Joseph: *Onion John,* Crowell, 1959.
Latham, Jean Lee: *Carry On, Mr. Bowditch*. Houghton Mifflin, 1955.
North, Sterling: *Rascal: A Memoir of a Better Era,* Dutton, 1963.
O'Dell, Scott: *Island of the Blue Dolphins,* Houghton, 1960.
Schaefer, Jack: *Old Roman,* Houghton, 1960.
Speare, Elizabeth: *The Bronz Bow,* Houghton, 1961.
Speare, Elizabeth: *Witch of Blackbird Pond,* Houghton, 1958.
Tunis, Edwin: *Frontier Living*. World Publishers, 1961.

Vocational Books

Angel, Juvenal L.: *Occupations For Men and Women After 45*. 3rd Ed., World Trade Academy, 1963.

Arco Publishing Company. Publishes study manuals for Civil Service Examinations in many fields of work.

Cohen, Nathan: *Vocational Training Directory of the United States.* 3rd Ed., Potomac Press, 1958.

Cunningham, Ed.: *Cunningham and Reed's Guide to Earning a Living.* Simon & Schuster, 1955. A complete survey of careers in business, the professions, trade, agriculture and government service.

Donahue, Wilma: *Earning Opportunities for Older Workers.* University of Michigan Press, 1955.

Feingold, S. Norman: *How to Get that Part-time Job.* Arco, 1958.

Gardiner, Glenn L.: *How You Can Get the Job You Want,* Harper, 1962.

Lovejoy, Clarence: *Lovejoy's Vocational School Guide, A Handbook of Job Training Opportunities.* Simon and Schuster, 1963.

Magoeun, F. Alexander: *Successfully Finding Yourself and Your Job.* Harper, 1959.

Marshall, Austin: *How To Get A Better Job.* Appleton, 1964. The new official book of the Job Finding Forum of the Advertising Club of New York.

Popham, Estelle. *Opportunities in Office Occupations.* Vocational Guidance Manuals, 1958.

Puchaski, B.: *What You Can Earn in Two Hundred and Fifty Different Careers.* Chilton, 1959.

United States Bureau of Labor Statistics: *Occupational Outlook Handbook.* U. S. Government Printing Office. Employment information on major occupations for use in guidance.

Material Suitable for Reading in Group Programs

Baker, Augusta, Comp.: *Stories to Tell and Read Aloud.* New York Public Library, 1959.

Beach, Steward (Ed.), *This Week Magazine: This Week's Short-Short Stories.*

Fadiman, Clifton: *Clifton Fadiman's Fireside Reader.* Simon and Schuster, 1961. An assortment of stories, non-fiction and verses chosen especially for reading aloud.

Gannett, Lewis: *The Family Book of Verse.,* Harper, 1961.

Gilberth, Frank: *Cheaper By The Dozen.* Crowell, 1948.

Giniger, K. S.: *A Treasury of Golden Memories.* Hansen House, 1958.

Hodnett, Edwards: *Poems to be Read Aloud.* Norton, 1957.

Kerr, Jean: *Please Don't Eat the Daisies.* Doubleday, 1957.

Laughton, Charles: *Tell Me a Story.* An Anthology, McGraw, 1957.

McGinley, Phyllis: *The Province of the Heart.* Viking, 1959.

Ross, David: *Poet's Gold: Poems for Reading Aloud.* 2nd Rev. Ed., Devin Adair, 1956.

Woods, Ralph: *Famous Poems and the Little Known Stories Behind Them.* Hawthorn, 1961.

Woods, Ralph: *Second Treasury of the Familiar.* McMillan, 1959.

Suggested Sources for Obtaining Material for Discussion Program

Center for Study of Democratic Institutions. (Main activity of the Fund for the Republic, Inc. Robert M. Hutchins, Chairman). You may write for list of pamphlet titles. Box 4068, Santa Barbara, California or 133 East 54 Street, New York 22, New York.

Intercom: An information Service for Citizen Education and Activity in World Affairs, a magazine published by Foreign Policy Association—World Affairs Center, 345 East 46th Street, New York 17. It reports on new programs, books, techniques, visual aids, pamphlets, speakers, public opinion and sources of information.

The Great Books: A reading-discussion program on great books of the world. For information on the program and for help in getting started, write to the Great Books Foundation, 37 South Wabash, Chicago 3.

The Great Ideas Program is based on Great Books of the Western World. There are lists of readings, study guides, and self testing questions.

Reading for an Age of Change, published by the American Library Association in cooperation with the Public Affairs Committee, Inc. The series is available from the Public Affairs Pamphlets, 22 East 38th Street, New York 16, New York. Single copies 60 cents each. Subscription to the Series (one copy of all five titles) $2.50.

Books and Pamphlets helpful in organizing groups and developing techniques for good discussions:

Auer, John: *Handbook for Discussion Leaders*. Harper, 1959.

Cheavers, Frank: *Leading Group Discussions*. Hogg Foundation for Mental Health, 1958. University of Texas, Austin 12, Texas. 25¢.

Utterback, William: *Decision Through Discussion*. 3rd Ed. Rinehart, 1958. A manual for Group Leaders.

Lee, Robert: *The Library Sponsored Discussion Group*. A.L.A. 1959, $1.25. (May be purchased from American Library Association, 50 East Huron Street, Chicago 11, Illinois.) Methods by which an effective adult education program based on group discussion can be planned and organized in the library and how to evaluate one program. Included also are sources for locating materials suitable for discussion and a list of packaged programs.

Lee, Robert: *Getting the Most Out of Discussion—A guide for Participants*. Library Community Project, A. L. A., 1956.

How To Use The Reading For An Age of Change Series: *A Handbook for Librarians*, by Mrs. Helen Lyman, may be purchased from Adult Services Division, American Library Association, 50 East Huron Street, Chicago 11, Illinois. 50¢ each. Very helpful aid for using each guide in serving the individual or group. Suggestions are made for in-service training and the use of the guide in program planning.

Our American Heritage—A Program Sponsored by the American Library Association, based on readings from Gerald W. Johnson, "This American People," and Henry S. Commager, "Living Ideas in American."

Many Excellent Documentary and Educational Films are Available from Various Sources

Sources of Free Films:

Association Films, Incorporated, 1108 Jackson Street, Dallas, Texas. 561 Hillgrove Avenue, Las Grange, Illinois. Broad at Elm,

Ridgefield, New Jersey. 799 Stevenson Street, San Francisco 3, California.

Canadian Travel Film Library, 111 North Wabash Avenue, Suite 1412, Chicago, Illinois, serves Ohio, Indiana, Illinois, Missouri, Arkansas, Louisiana and all states west, 680 Fifth Avenue, New York 19, New York.

Ford Motor Company, American Road, Dearborn, Michigan. 16 East 52nd Street, New York 22, New York. 4303 Telegraph Avenue, Oakland, California.

General Motors Corporation, Public Relations Staff, 1775 Broadway, New York 19, New York.

Ideal Pictures, Incorporated, 58 East South Water Street, Chicago, Illinois.

Modern Talking Picture Service, 3 East Fifty-Fourth Street, New York, New York (Borrower pays transportation charge both ways).

Vocational Films "American at Work" series provided by A. F. L.-C. I. O. Unions and may be available through State Education Department.

Educators Guide To Free Films, Educators Progress Service, Randolph, Wisconsin. $6.00.

Educators Guide to Free Slide Films, Educators Progressive Service, Randolph, Wisconsin $6.00.

Catalogue Cards may be Purchased from:

1. H. W. Wilson Co., 950 University Avenue, New York 52, New York.
2. Library of Congress Cards—to be ordered from Card Division Library of Congress, Building 159, Navy Yard Annex, Washington, D. C. 20541.

At additional cost, these companies will provide processing and cataloging service for books purchased from them.

1. Alanar Book Processing Center (a subsidiary of Bro-Dart industries) Box 921, Williamsport, Pennsylvania.
2. Alesco, Harristown Road, Glen Rock, New Jersey.

Appnedix E

BIBLIOGRAPHY OF INDUSTRIAL
THERAPY*

LEIGHTON A. PRICE, M.S.

T HE FOLLOWING BIBLIOGRAPHY was assembled to facilitate tracing the history of an area of rehabilitation variously referred to as industrial therapy, work therapy, therapeutic hospital industries, and ergotherapy. The use of the techniques that characterize industrial therapy has a long history, and the status of this kind of therapeutic program has varied widely from one decade, country, and type of rehabilitation to another.

During the past ten years, interest in applying the techniques of industrial therapy to treat mental illness has surged. Although there are several bibliographic sources for the field of rehabilitation in general and some sources that deal with more specific aspects, there is no comprehensive bibliography for industrial therapy. Moreover, people writing on industrial therapy often cite few references, most of which are only tangetially related. A comprehensive bibliography of the appropriate literature would, therefore, seem most useful.

The general state of the industrial therapy literature gives the impression that many persons currently concerned with the application of these techniques to the problems of mental illness have lost sight of the extensive body of literature in the area. This can perhaps best be explained by the fact that there have been such wide variations in the popularity of industrial therapy techniques and in the rehabilitation purposes for which they have been applied. After each period of decline in the popularity of industrial therapy, it appears to have been rediscovered in a new rehabilitation context, with little awareness of its earlier use.

---

*The first draft of the bibliography was prepared by Leighton A. Price. Later editorial revision was done by Ruth B. Ekstrom and Norman Wexler with the final copy being prepared by Kathryn Neil, all of the Educational Testing Service, Princeton, New Jersey.

Since industrial therapy has such a varied history, the bibliography includes publications on work therapy techniques in halfway houses, curative workshops, and sanatoria, as well as in hospitals. In order to demonstrate how much attention has been paid to work therapy in different countries at various times, the bibliography has been subdivided. The major division is between English and foreign language sources. Both of these sections have been divided into five time periods.

Many of the references in this bibliography were read in order to check the appropriateness of their inclusion. For others, selection was based on only a brief abstract or on the content of their titles. There are relatively few references for which the appropriateness of inclusion is uncertain.

This bibliography does not pretend to be exhaustive. The outer limits of the subject matter are vague, and there are many publications at the heart of the subject that have been cited in few or in obscure sources. That so few references are cited by current writers in the area not only constituted a principal obstacle to the exhaustiveness of this bibliography but also demonstarted the importance of assembling it.

ENGLISH LANGUAGE REFERENCES

Before 1920

Bickmore, A.: *Industries for the Feeble-minded and Imbecile.* London, Adlard & Son, 1913.

Brigham, A.: The moral treatment of insanity. *Amer. J. Insanity, 4:*1-15, 1847.

Browne, W. A. F.: *What Asylums Were, Are, and Ought to Be.* Edinburgh, Scotland, A & C. Black, 1837.

Butler, J. S.: *The Curability of Insanity and the Individualized Treatment of the Insane.* New York, G. P. Putnam's Sons, 1887.

Dickens, C.: *American Notes for General Circulation.* 3rd Ed., London, Chapman & Hall, 1842.

Earle, P.: *The Curability of Insanity.* Philadelphia, J. B. Lippincott, 1887.

Earle, P.: *History, Description and Statistics of the Bloomingdale Asylum for the Insane.* New York, Egberg, Hovey & King, 1848.

Eddy, T.: Hints for introducing an improved mode of treating the insane in the asylum. Paper read before the governors of the New York Hospital, 1815.

Ellis, W. C.: *A Treatise on the Nature, Symptoms, Causes, and Treatment of Insanity.* London, Holdsworth, 1838.

Hallaran, W. S.: *The Cure of Insanity.* Cork, Ireland, Edwards & Savage, 1810. (Reprinted in *Occupational Therapy and Rehabilitation, 26:*3-7, 1947.)

Hammond, W. A.: The non-asylum treatment of the insane. *Trans. Med. Soc. New York,* Syracuse, 1879.

Haslam, J.: *Considerations on the Moral Management of Insane Persons.* London, Hunter, 1817.

Kirkman, J.: *Annual report of the Suffolk Lunatic Asylum.* 1848.

Page, C. W., and Butler, John S.: The man and his hospital methods. *Amer. J. Insanity, 57*:477-499, 1901.

Pinel, P.: *A Treatise on Insanity.* Translated by D. D. Davis, M.D., Sheffield, England, Cadell & Davis, 1806. (Facsimile ed., New York, Hafner, 1962.)

Reid, E. C.: Ergotherapy in the treatment of mental disorders. *Boston Med. Surg. J., 171*:300, 1914. (Reprinted in *Occupational Therapy and Rehabilitation, 26:* 461-467, 1947.)

Tuke, S.: A letter on pauper lunatic asylum, 1815. (Reprinted in *A Psychiatric Milestone: Bloomingdale Hospital Centenary.* New York, Privately printed by the Society of the New York Hospital, 1921, pp. 195-199.)

Withers, T.: *Observations on Chronic Weakness.* York, England, Cadell & Nicoll, 1777.

Woodward, S. B.: *Annual report of the Worcester Lunatic Hospital.* 1842.

Woodward, S. B.: *12th annual report of the Worcester State Lunatic Hospital.* Boston, Dutton & Wentworth, 1844.

Woodward, S. B.: The medical treatment of the insane. Address to the Association of Medical Superintendents of American Institutions for the Insane, 1846.

1920-1929

Baker, A. F.: Organizing occupational therapy in a small hospital. *Occup. Ther. & Rehabil., 6*:315-319, 1927.

Bond, E. D.: A mental hospital in the 'fabulous forties." *Amer. J. Psychiat., 4*:527-536, 1925.

Bowen, A. L.: How to improve the care and treatment of the mentally ill. *Mod. Hosp., 18*:506-508, 1922.

Brainerd, W.: Workshops in a general hospital. *Arch. Occup. Ther., 2*:109-114, 1923.

Brown, P. K.: Vocational training vs. occupational therapy. *Nation's Health, 3:* 536, 1921.

Bryant, L. C.: Manual work with the mentally defective child patient. *Mod. Hosp., 27*:61-63, 1926.

Crain, R. B.: Industrial workshops and their importance in relation to placing the handicapped. *J. Indust. Hyg., 11*:257-265, 1929.

Dean, T. N.: The value of curative work in workmen's compensation cases. *Occup. Ther. & Rehabil., 7*:11-19, 1928.

Evans, A. E.: Tour of Dutch mental hospitals and clinics. *J. Ment. Sci., 75*:192-208, 1929.

Evans, E. V.: The organization of a curative workshop. *Occup. Ther. & Rehabil., 8:* 49-62, 1929.

Foley, E. A.: Pre-industrial value of occupational therapy in mental hospitals. *Arch. Occup. Ther., 3*:109-112, 1924.

Goodfriend, J.: Occupational therapy in a hospital for chronic diseases. *Occup. Ther. & Rehabil., 6*:265-275, 1927.

Harman, B. M.: The hospital or sanatorium magazine as an occupational therapy activity. *Occup. Ther. & Rehabil.,* 6:213-219, 1927.

Henderson, D. K.: Occupational therapy. *Occup. Ther. & Rehabil.,* 4:7-16, 1925.

Kefauver, H. J.: Agriculture as occupational therapy in the neuropsychiatric hospitals. *U. S. Veterans Bureau Med. Bull.,* 2:592-600, 1926.

Kefauver, H. J.: Occupational therapy and agriculture in the United States Veteran's Hospitals for the calendar year 1927. *U. S. Veterans Bureau Med. Bull.,* 4: 721-724, 1928.

Kefauver, H. J.: Occupational therapy in relation to agriculture. *Occup. Ther. & Rehabil.,* 7:189-197, 1928.

Kenna, W. M.: Occupational therapy and hospital industries. *Occup. Ther. & Rehabil.,* 6:453-461, 1927.

Kidner, T. B.: Occupational therapy in 1922. *Mod. Hosp.,* 20:43-46, 1923.

Kidner, T. B.: The hospital pre-industrial shop. *Occup. Ther. & Rehabil.,* 4:187-194, 1925.

Leavitt, M. A.: *Handicapped Wage Earners.* New York, The Jewish Social Service Association, Inc., 1928.

Livingston, W. H.: Useful occupational therapy vs. useless occupational therapy. *Mod. Hosp.,* 21:210-212, 1923.

MacLeisch, I. M.: Half-way House, curative workshop. *Occup. Ther. & Rehabil.,* 8:173-176, 1929.

Mattison, J. A.: Occupational therapy in general hospitals. *Occup. Ther. & Rehabil.,* 6:105-111, 1927.

Morrow, J. R.: The new program of the National Tuberculosis Association for the after-care of sanatorium patients, and its bearing on curative work in the sanatorium. *Occup. Ther. & Rehabil.,* 8:159-169, 1929.

Robeson, H. A.: The pre-industrial shop: Problems, organization and methods. *Occup. Ther. & Rehabil.,* 7:401-406, 1928.

Rollier, A.: The work-cure in surgical tuberculosis. *Brit. J. Tuberc.,* 22:101-112, 1928.

Ruhl, M. E.: Wood-shop work for convalescents. *Mod. Hosp.,* 18:298, 1922.

Sample, G.: Combining curative work with vocational training in tuberculosis sanatoria. *Occup. Ther. & Rehabil.,* 6:143-148, 1927.

Sands, I. F.: When is occupation curative? *Occup. Ther. & Rehabil.,* 7:115-122, 1928.

Skottowe, I.: On the methods in vogue at the Boston Psychopathic Hospital. *J. Ment. Sci.,* 74:474-487, 1928.

Sullivan, O. M.: The inter-relation between occupational therapy and subsequent vocational or industrial rehabilitation. *Occup. Ther. & Rehabil.,* 6:175-185, 1927.

Tower, L. F.: Occupational therapy for mental defectives at Syracuse State School. *Occup. Ther. & Rehabil.,* 11:353-359, 1932.

Treatment of disease by employment at St. Elizabeth's hospital. *Mod. Hosp.,* 20: 198-200, 1923.

Young, J.: Curative work in the Mercer Sanatorium. *Mod. Hosp.,* 25:170-172, 1925.

1930-1939

Atwood, S. M.: The pine tree cure for delinquency. *The Survey,* 68:603, 1932.

Brody, M. W.: The value of "free association" in state hospital practice for placement of patients into industrial therapy. *Occup. Ther. & Rehabil.,* 16:319-326, 1937.

Bryan, W. A.: *Administrative Psychiatry*. New York, W. W. Norton, 1936.

Collier, G. K.: Directed industrial therapy as an aid to the general practitioner and the specialist. *Occup. Ther. & Rehabil., 11:*425-432, 1932.

Cooke, D. W.: Industrial therapy as applied in an occupational therapy department. *Occup. Ther. & Rehabil., 16:*39-45, 1937.

Evans, A. E.: A tour of some mental hospitals of western Germany. *J. Ment. Sci., 79:*150-166, 1933.

Gratiot, L.: Occupational therapy and a sheltered workshop sponsored by the Junior League of St. Louis. *Occup. Ther. & Rehabil., 10:*151-159, 1931.

Harrison, E.: A curative workshop. *Rehabil. Rev., 8:*25-31, 1934.

Inch, G. F.: Therapeutic placement of mental patients in state hospital industries. *Occup. Ther. & Rehabil., 15:*241-248, 1936.

Kessler, H. H.: The curative workshop and the rehabilitation of the disabled. *Rehabil. Rev., 9:*12-16, 1935.

Marsh, L. C.: An experiment in the group treatment of patients at the Worcester State Hospital. *Ment. Hyg., 17:*396-416, 1933.

Noble, M. O.: Aims and objectives of the Toronto curative workshop. *Occup. Ther. & Rehabil., 16:*223-236, 1937.

Patterson, W. J.: The field of occupational therapy in central workshops in large cities. *Occup. Ther. & Rehabil., 18:*365-371, 1939.

Rosell, R. R.: Occupational therapy and vocational training in a sanatorium and their relation to after-care: An outsider's viewpoint. *Occup. Ther. & Rehabil., 10:*169-173, 1931.

Rowe, M. L.: Occupational therapy and vocational training in a sanatorium and their relation to after-care: An outsider's viewpoint. *Occup. Ther. & Rehabil., 10:*175-177, 1931.

Russell, J. I.: *The Occupational Treatment of Mental Illness*. Baltimore, William Wood, 1938.

Stevenson, G. H.: The healing influence of work and play in a mental hospital. *Occup. Ther. & Rehabil., 11:*85-89, 1932.

Thornton, S. H.: Gardening and the feebleminded. *Ment. Welfare, 16:*8-11, 1935.

Tower, L. F.: Occupational therapy for mental defectives at Syracuse State School. *Occup. Ther. & Rehabil., 11:*353-359, 1932.

Wertham, F.: Progress in psychiatry: The active work therapy of Dr. Simon. *Arch. Neurol. & Psychiat., 24:*150-160, 1930.

Worchel, P.: Program for industrial therapy. *Occup. Ther. & Rehabil., 17:*117-122, 1938.

Young, E. S.: Setting up an industrial program for the tuberculous. *Occup. Ther. & Rehabil., 18:*155-164, 1939.

1940-1949

American Psychiatric Association: *One Hundred Years of American Psychiatry*. New York, Columbia University Press, 1944.

Bennett, A. E., and Engle, B.: Psychiatric nursing and occupational therapy. In E. A. Spiegel (Ed.): *Progress in Neurology and Psychotherapy*. New York, Grune & Stratton, 1947, Vol. 2, p. 491-499.

Casson, E.: Forty cases treated at the Allendale Curative Workshop. *Lancet, 241* (2): 516-517, 1941.

Close, O. H.: California camps for delinquents. In *Social Correctives for Delinquency: National Probation Association Yearbook 1945.* New York, National Probation Association, 1946, p. 136-147.

Davis, J. E.: Employment is nature's best physician. *Hygeia, 20:*268, 1942.

Deutsch, A.: *Mentally Ill in America: A History of Their Care and Treatment from Colonial Times.* 2nd Ed., New York, Columbia University Press, 1949.

Fetterman, J. L.: A note on rehabilitation: Work as therapy. *Ohio State Med. J., 40:* 117-122, 1944.

Fore, M. O.: An experiment in parole and hospital employment for the mentally ill in Iowa. *Ment. Hyg., 29:*423-428, 1945.

Grant, I.: Occupation is participation. *Amer. J. Occup. Ther., 2:*237-239, 1948.

Greve, B.: Curative workshop. *Virginia Med. Month., 71:*180-182, 1944.

Harrison, H. M.: If you work—you win. *Hygeia, 23:*916, 1945.

Hart, H. H.: Work as integration. *Med. Rec., 160:*735-739, 1947.

Hochauser, E.: Objectives of sheltered workshops. *Jewish Soc. Serv. Quart., 25:* 533-545, 1949.

Hurley, C. F.: Overall occupational therapy program of a mental hospital. *Amer. J. Occup. Ther., 2:*191-195, 1948.

Hurt, S. P.: Occupational therapy in the rehabilitation of the poliomyelitis patient. *Amer. J. Occup. Ther., 2:*83-87, 1948.

Hyde, R. W., and Atwell, C. R.: Evaluating the effectiveness of a psychiatric occupational therapy program. *Amer. J. Occup. Ther., 2:*232-339, 1948.

Jones, H. M.: Adaptation of industrial operations to occupational therapy in a naval hospital. *Occup. Ther. & Rehabil., 24:*179-182, 1945.

Licht, S. (Ed.) : *Occupational Therapy Source Book.* Baltimore, Williams & Wilkins, 1948.

Menninger, K.: Work as a sublimation. *Bull. Menninger Clin., 6:*170-182, 1942.

Merritt, M. E.: Organization of a workshop in a general hospital. *Occup. Ther. & Rehabil., 21:*289-291, 1942.

Moeller, H. G.: The Natural Bridge Camp. In *Bulwarks Against Crime: National Probation and Parole Association Yearbook, 1948.* New York, National Probation and Parole Association, 1949, p. 162-173.

Nickels, M. M.: A state hospital as a source of man power in the present emergency. *Ment. Hyg., 27:*390-393, 1943.

Preston, G. H.: Relating occupational therapy to reality. *Occup. Ther. & Rehabil., 21:*17-24, 1942.

Price, H. G., and Corcoran, L.: Work therapy in a private neuropsychiatric hospital. *Occup. Ther. & Rehabil., 24:*155-159, 1945.

Psychiatric Rehabilitation Symposium. *Occupational Therapy and Rehabilitation, 28:*267-285, 1949.

Reggio, A. W.: Some thoughts on occupational therapy, work shops, and rehabilitation. *Amer. J. Occup. Ther., 2:*164-165, 1948.

Rudolph, H. L.: Work therapy in an Army general hospital. *Arch. Phys. Med. & Rehabil., 26:*741-747, 1945.

Sallak, V. J.: Today's rule is no more busy work; job fitness is goal of occupational therapy. *Hospitals, 17* (9) *:*97-102, 1943.

Scholten, W.: Occupational therapy as a preliminary to industrial therapy. *Occup. Ther. & Rehabil., 21:*86-89, 1942.

Stover, E. M.: Industry brings jobs to veterans in hospitals. *Occupations, 22:*474-476, 1944.

Valliant, N.: Practical application in curative workshops. *Occup. Ther. & Rehabil., 21:*292-293, 1942.

Valliant, N.: End results obtained in Baltimore Junior League curative workshops. *Bull. School Med. Univ. Maryland, 27* (3) :96-102, 1942.

Verzi, M. A.: Job cart for hospitalized G. I.'s. *Occupations, 24:*413, 1946.

Veterans Administration. Increased employment opportunities within VA installations for domiciliary members, *VA Technical Bulletin TB 5-80,* Washington, D. C., May 21, 1948.

Wade, B.: A survey of occupational and industrial therapy in the Illinois state hospitals. *Illinois Psychiat. J., 2* (1) :23-31, 1942.

Walkiewicz, S. T.: Convalescent patients as mental hospital employees. *Smith College Studies in Social Work, 16:*282-284, 1946.

Willard, H. S., and Spackman, C. S. (Eds.) : *Principles of Occupational Therapy.* Philadelphia, Lippincott, 1947.

Woodman, R.: *What state hospitals can do to prevent unnecessary decline in the quality of state care and treatment for the mentally ill.* National Committee for Mental Hygiene, 1945.

1950-1959

Anderson, A. S., Hard, M. E., and Betlach, R.: Industrial therapy at Roseburg VA Hospital. In *Program guide, physical medicine and rehabilitation: G-2, M-2, Part VIII.* Washington, D. C.: Office of the Chief Medical Director Veterans Administration, Department of Medicine and Surgery, August 1955, p. 30-32.

Appleby, L., and Bliss, B.: For mental patients physically impaired—a hospital program of service. *J. Rehabil., 24* (2) :16-17; 47-49, 1958.

Appleby, L., and Page, C. W.: Member-employee program: Rehabilitation for chronic mental patients—an evaluation. Unpublished manuscript, Osawatomie (Kan.) State Hospital, 1959.

Ayres, A. J.: A pilot study on the relationship between work habits and workshop production. *Amer. J. Occup. Ther., 9:*264-267, 1955.

Baganz, C. N., Namen, J. M., Hall, R., and Swickle, J. A.: The industrial therapy program at Lyons. In *Program guide, physical medicine and rehabilitation: G-2, M-2 Part VIII.* Washington, D. C.: Office of the Chief Medical Director Veterans Administration, Department of Medicine and Surgery, August 1955, p. 3-7.

Bailey, J. D.: The work trial method of vocational evaluation. *J. Rehabil., 24* (1) : 12-14, 1958.

Baker, A. A.: Factory in a hospital. *Lancet, 270* (1) :278-279, 1956.

Ball, M., and Dotte, P.: Artisan therapy: A new focus on therapeutic activities. *Amer. J. Occup. Ther., 13:*257-263, 1959.

Banks, O. M., and Watkins, A. L.: The Bay State Medical Rehabilitation Center. *J. Rehabil., 25* (4) :12-14, 1959.

Bay, A. P., and Schlotter, B.: *Working and playing to health.* 16 mm. motion picture, b and w, sound, 35 min., 1954.

Baxt, R., Lurie, A., and Miller, J. S. A.: Vocational adjustment for the emotionally disturbed, *J. Hillside Hospital, 3:*25-31, 1954.

Beck, B. M.: *Youth Within Walls.* New York, Community Service Society of New York, 1950.

Belknap, I.: *Human Problems of a State Mental Hospital.* New York, McGraw Hill, 1956.

Bellak, L., Black, B. J., Lurie, A., and Miller, J. S. A.: Rehabilitation of the mentally ill through controlled transitional employment. *Amer. J. Orthopsychiat., 26:* 285-296, 1956.

Bennett, A. E., and Engle, B.: Psychiatric nursing and occupational therapy. In E. A. Spiegel (Ed.) : *Progress in Neurology and Psychiatry.* New York, Grune & Stratton, 1957, Vol. 12, p. 625-633.

Bettag, O. L.: *Industrial therapy assignments.* Mental Health Regulation No. 70. (Rev. ed.) Springfield, Ill.: Department of Public Welfare, 1956.

Bockhoven, J. S.: Moral treatment in American psychiatry. *J. Nerv. Ment. Dis., 124:* 167-194; 292-321, 1956.

Bolin, B. J., and Scott, D.: Patient industry and the workers' attitudes toward their jobs. *Amer. J. Psychiat.,* 115:246-247, 1958.

Boorstein, S.: Ego autonomy in psychiatric practice. *Bull. Menninger Clin., 23:*148-156, 1959.

Boyle, R. W., Schwartz, L., and Prosser, E. L.: A sheltered workshop program in a geriatric hospital. *Geriatrics,* 10:436-439, 1955.

Breed, A. F.: California youth authority forestry camp program. In S. Glueck (Ed.) : *The Problem of Delinquency.* Boston, Houghton Mifflin, 1959, p. 705-711.

Burr, J.: Group work therapy in Holland. *Lancet, 269* (2) :1083, 1955.

Carstairs, G. M.: Industrial work as a means of rehabilitation for chronic schizophrenics. In *Second International Congress of Psychiatry Report I.* Zurich: Orell Fussli Arts Graphiques S. A., 1959, pp. 99-102.

Carstairs, G. M., Clark, D. H., and O'Connor, N.: Occupational treatment of chronic psychotics: Observations in Holland, Belgium, and France. *Lancet, 269* (2) :1025-1030, 1955.

Carstairs, G. M., O'Connor, N., and Rawnsley, K.: Organization of a hospital workshop for chronic psychotic patients. *Brit. J. Prevent. & Soc. Med.,* 10:136-140, 1956.

Charlton, E. P. H.: The place of work in the treatment of mental disorder. In *Proceedings of a Conference of the National Association for Mental Health (Great Britain).* London, 1959, p. 29.

Christrup, H. H.: The new look in industrial therapy. *Amer. J. Occup. Ther., 11:* 276-277, 1957.

Clarke, A. D. B., and Clarke, A. M.: A rehabilitation program for certified mental defectives. *Ment. Health, 14:*4-10, 1954.

Cohen, L.: Vocational planning and mental illness. *Personnel and Guidance J., 34:* 28-32, 1955.

Collins, S. D., Flynn, S. J., Manners, F., and Morgan, R.: Factory in a ward. *Lancet,* 2:609-611, 1959.

Combs, M. H.: An activities program in a custodial care group. *Amer. J. Occup. Ther., 13:*5-8, 1959.

Conners, J. E.: A new step in the rehabilitation of the chronic mental patient. *J. Counsel. Psychol., 5:*115-119, 1958.

Conners, J. E., and Margolin, R. J.: Member-employee follow-up and implications for rehabilitation of the psychiatric patient. *Personnel and Guidance J., 37:* 369-374, 1959.

Cross, K. W., Harrington, J. A., and Mayer-Gross, W.: A survey of chronic patients in a mental hospital. *J. Ment. Sci., 103:*146-171, 1957.

Curry, A. E.: Developing a training program for industrial personnel. *Ment. Hosp.,* *10* (4) :40-41, 1959.

Dancik, D.: Industrial therapy. In *Program guide, physical medicine and rehabilitation: G-2, M-2, Part VIII.* Washington, D. C.: Office of the Chief Medical Director Veterans Administration, Department of Medicine and Surgery, August 1955, pp. 1-2.

Davies, J. B. M.: The handicapped adult in the community. *Lancet, 268* (1) : 1212-1213, 1955.

Dax, E. C.: Industrial occupations in Dutch and English mental hospitals. *Ment. Hosp., 9* (9) :14-18, 1958.

Diethelm, O.: *Treatment in Psychiatry.* 2nd Ed., Springfield, Thomas, 1950.

Dodd, D. D., and Allison, D. D.: Growth of a hospital industry unit. In *Program guide, physical medicine and rehabilitation: G-2, M-2, Part VIII.* Washington, D. C.: Office of the Chief Medical Director Veterans Administration, Department of Medicine and Surgery, August 1955. Pp. 33-36.

DuBois, F. S.: Occupational therapy. *Amer. J. Psychiat., 112:*550-553, 1956.

DuBois, F. S.: Rehabilitation and occupational therapy. *Amer. J. Psychiat., 113:* 637-641, 1957.

DuBois, F. S.: Rehabilitation and occupational therapy. *Amer. J. Psychiat., 114:* 632-636, 1958.

DuBois, F. S.: Rehabilitation and occupational therapy. *Amer. J. Psychiat., 115:* 635-640, 1959.

Dunton, W. R., Jr., and Licht, S. (Eds.) : *Occupational Therapy: Principles and Practice.* Springfield, Thomas, 1950.

Edwards, J. E.: The value of the mental hospital farm. *Ment. Hosp., 10* (6) :43-44, 1959.

Elkins, H. K., Hively, C. H., and Dietrich, R. W.: Hospital industry program at VA hospital, Palo Alto, California. In *Program guide, physical medicine and rehabilitation: G-2, M-2, Part VIII.* Washington, D. C.: Office of the Chief Medical Director Veterans Administration, Department of Medicine and Surgery, August 1955, pp. 16-18.

Elton, F. C.: Vocational activity: A therapy. *Bull. Amer. Rehabil. Comm., 1:*1, July 1952.

Feintuch, A.: Classification of sheltered workshops. *Occupations, 29:*515-517, 1951.

Feintuch, A.: Sheltered workshops—a conceptual framework. *J. Rehabil., 24* (1) :9-10, 1958.

Feuss, C. D., and Maltby, J. W.: Occupational therapy in the therapeutic community. *Amer. J. Occup. Ther., 13:*9-12, 1959.

Fidler, G. S.: The role of occupational therapy in a multi-discipline approach to psychiatric illness. *Amer. J. Occup. Ther., 11:*8-12, 1957.

Forrer, G. R.: Work therapy program at Northville State Hospital. *Amer. J. Occup. Ther., 9:*154-155, 1955.

Gardner, J., and Morgan, N. C.: Industrial therapy. *Amer. J. Occup. Ther., 7:* 250-252, 1953.

Gilmore, H.: Some observations on treatment in the terminal phases of hospitalization. *Amer. J. Psychiat., 108:*749-754, 1952.

Ginsberg, S. T., and Saunders, R.: Advances in psychosocial treatment of the neuropsychiatric patient. *Information Bull.* Washington, D. C., 1957, pp. 10-90.

Gold, J. G.: Occupational therapy and physical therapy leading to rehabilitation. *Amer. J. Occup. Ther., 6:*20-23, 1952.

Goldberg, I. I.: A survey of the present status of vocational rehabilitation of the mentally retarded residents in state-supported institutions. *Amer. J. Ment. Def., 61:*698-705, 1957.

Goldstein, H. K.: Social service participation in member-employee program. *Information Bull.* Veterans Administration Department of Medicine and Surgery, August 1954, pp. 22-24.

Goril, R. B., and Erickson, P. O.: Industrial therapy: Planning and activation. In *Program guide, physical medicine and rehabilitation: G-2, M-2, Part VIII.* Washington, D. C.: Office of the Chief Medical Director Veterans Administration, Department of Medicine and Surgery, August 1955, pp. 8-11.

Gregory, C. C., and Jacobs, D. F.: The member-employee program as a therapeutic agent. *J. Counsel. Psychol., 6:*121-126, 1959.

Griffiths, H.: The bridge between treatment and employment. *Rehabilitation, 4:* 2-5, 1952.

Grobman, M. E., McMillen, M. L., and Turner, E. M.: Industrial therapy at VA center, Waco, Texas. In *Program guide, physical medicine and rehabilitation: G-2, M-2, Part VIII.* Washington, D. C.: Office of the Chief Medical Director Veterans Administration, Department of Medicine and Surgery, August 1955, pp. 40-41.

Heninger, O. P.: Should occupational therapy pay for itself? *Amer. J. Occup. Ther., 8:*1-2, 1954.

Hirsch, D. K.: A work trial program for the severely handicapped. *J. Rehabil., 16* (6) :3-6, 1950.

Hockhauser, E.: The sheltered workshop in a program for the rehabilitation of the chronically ill. New York, Author, 1951. 16pp. (Mimeo.)

Hoffman, J. L.: Rehabilitation concepts in mental hospital practice. *J. Rehabil., 22* (4) :4-6; 16-19, 1956.

Hooper, W. H.: The industrial therapy program at Topeka State Hospital. *Kansas Acad. Sci., 55:*87-91, 1952.

Houston, F.: A project for a mental-health village settlement. *Lancet, 269* (2) :1133-1134, 1955.

Hunt, R. C.: Summary of observations. *Mental health programs in Britain and Holland.* Albany, N. Y., Hunt-WHO, 1958.

Huseth, B.: Halfway houses: A new rehabilitation measure. *Ment. Hosp., 9* (8) :5-9, 1958.

Infield, H. F.: Community and psychotherapy: A study of Gould Farm. *J. Human Relations, 5* (1) :50-78, 1956 *(Psychol. Abstr. 32:*532) .

Ivany, E., and Rothschild, D.: Relationship of the occupational therapy department to hospital industries. *Amer. J. Occup. Ther., 5:*16-22, 1951.

Isaacson, J.: From sitter to citizen: A project of vocational and social rehabilitation. *Ment. Hyg., 42:*538-543, 1958.

Izutsu, S.: A sheltered workshop in a hospital setting. *Canad. J. Occup. Ther., 26:* 11-21, 1959.

Jones, M.: *The therapeutic community: A new treatment method in psychiatry.* New York, Basic Books, 1953.

Jones, M.: Industrial rehabilitation of mental patients still in hospital. *Lancet, 271* (2) :985, 1956.

Jones, M.: The treatment of personality disorders in a therapeutic community. *Psychiatry, 20:*211-220, 1957.

Jones, M., Pomryn, B. A., and Skellern, E.: Work therapy. *Lancet, 270* (1) :343-344, 1956.

Kaplan, J. A., and Soden, W. H.: Therapeutic hospital industries. In *Program guide, physical medicine and rehabilitation: G-2, M-2, Part VIII.* Washington, D. C.: Office of the Chief Medical Director Veterans Administration. Department of Medicine and Surgery, August 1955, pp. 44-45.

Kaufmann, P., and Sewall, L. G.: Hospital industries: Honest therapy or slave labor? In *Program guide, physical medicine and rehabilitation: G-2, M-2, Part VIII.* Washington, D. C.: Office of the Chief Medical Director Veterans Administration, Department of Medicine and Surgery, August 1955, pp. 21-23.

Klapper, M.: *A Program of Vocational Rehabilitation.* New York, National Association for Mental Health, 1958.

Knudson, A. B. C.: Rehabilitation of the mentally ill in the Veterans Administration. In M. Greenblatt, and B. Simon (Eds.) : *Rehabilitation of the Mentally Ill: Social and Economic Aspects.* Washington, D. C., American Association for the Advancement of Science, 1959, pp. 141-146.

Koven, B., and Shuff, F.: Group therapy with the chronically ill. *Amer. J. Occup. Ther., 7:*208-209, 1953.

Kratter, F. E.: An English hospital for the mentally defective. *Ment. Hosp., 10* (3) : 14-16, 1959.

Kratz, J. A.: Vocational rehabilitation, past, present, and future in the United States. *Bull. Amer. Rehabil. Comm., 2:*1-6, May, 1954.

Krusen, F. H.: Relationships between occupational therapy and physical medicine and rehabilitation. *Canad. J. Occup. Ther., 21:*3-9, 1954.

Laing, J. K. C.: Occupational therapy. *Amer. J. Ment. Def., 56:*125-131, 1951.

Landy, D.: *The work supervisors group: Some factors in the hospital work program.* Annual Report of Rehabilitation Project, Massachusetts Mental Health Center, to Office of Vocational Rehabilitation, 1956-1957, pp. 72-85.

Landy, D., and Raulet, H.: The hospital work program. In M. Greenblatt and B. Simon (Eds.) : *Rehabilitation of the Mentally Ill: Social and Economic Aspects.* Washington, D. C., American Association for the Advancement of Science, 1959, pp. 71-87.

Lavine, L. A., and Sandeen, E. W.: Industrial therapy: Seven years of progress. *Ment. Hosp., 10* (7) :17-18, 1959.

Leavitt, C. M.: Activating the aged: Geriatric patients develop their own O. T. area. *Ment. Hosp., 10* (8) :16-17, 1959.

Levine, D., Marks, H. K., and Hall, R.: Differential effect of factors in an activity therapy program. *Amer. J. Psychiat., 114:*532-535, 1957.

Lewis, A.: Resettlement of the chronic schizophrenic. In *Second International Congress of Psychiatry—Report I.* Zurich: Orell Fussli Arts Graphiques S. A., 1959, pp. 223-228. (Also in *Journal of the All India Institute of Mental Health, 1:* 22-28, 1958.

Linder, M. P., and Landy, D.: Post-discharge experience and vocational rehabilitation needs of psychiatric patients. *Ment. Hyg., 42:*29, 1958.

Loos, F. M., and Tizard, J.: The employment of adult imbeciles in a hospital workshop. *Amer. J. Ment. Def., 59:*395-403, 1955.

Margolin, R. J.: Member-employee program: New hope for the mentally ill. *Amer. Arch. Rehabil. Ther., 3* (3) :69-81, 1955.

Margolin, R. J., and Haefner, D. P.: Questions for research study of rehabilitation programs with special reference to the member-employee programs. *Amer. Arch. Rehabil. Ther., 7:*41-44, 1959.

Marks, M., and Greene, L. B.: Rehabilitation. In E. A. Spiegel (Ed.) : *Progress in Neurology and Psychiatry.* New York, Grune & Stratton, 1955, Vol. 10, pp. 619-629.

Martin, G. J., Reisman, M. J., and Noyes, A. P.: Vocational rehabilitation in a psychiatric hospital: An initial report. *Ment. Hyg., 38:*107-112, 1954.

Martin, H., *et al.*: Vocational rehabilitation in the mental hospital. *Ment. Hosp., 10* (2) :27-29, 1959.

Merker, F. F., Vehlow, E. L., and Nelson, A. V.: Patient treatment possibilities of industrial therapy at Winter VA Hospital. In *Program guide, physical medicine and rehabilitation: G-2, M-2, Part VIII.* Washington, D. C.: Office of the Chief Medical Director Veterans Administration, Department of Medicine and Surgery, August 1955, pp. 12-15.

Moss, F. B.: A program for geriatric patients from hospital to community *Amer. J. Occup. Ther., 13:*268-271, 1959.

Newcombe, J. A., Charlton, E. R., and Farrier, R. F.: The industrial therapy program, Roanoke, Virginia. In *Program guide, physical medicine and rehabilitation: G-2, M-2, Part VIII.* Washington, D. C.: Office of the Chief Medical Director Veterans Administration, Department of Medicine and Surgery, August 1955, pp. 42-44.

Oberndorf, C. P.: Psychopathology of work. *Bull. Menninger Clin., 15:*77-84, 1951.

O'Connor, N.: Defectives working in the community. *Amer. J. Ment. Def., 59:*173-180, 1954.

O'Connor, N., and Rawnsley, K.: Incentives with paranoid and nonparanoid schizophrenics in a workshop. *Brit. J. Med. Psychol., 32:*133-143, 1959.

O'Connor, W., and Tizard, J.: *The Social Problem of Mental Deficiency.* New York, Pergamon, 1956.

O'Neill, F. J., and Agnew, H. B.: Pilot industrial program productive. *Ment. Hosp. 10* (4) :38-39, 1959.

O'Reilly, D. E.: Rehabilitation in the general hospital. *Amer. J. Occup. Ther., 6:* 4-8, 1952.

Osmund, H.: Rehabilitation services within the hospital. *Ment. Hosp., 9* (5) :45-47, 1958.

Osterheld, R. G.: Work therapy for epileptics. *Ment. Hosp., 10* (9) :33, 1959.

Padula, H.: Long-term patients receive job training. *Ment. Hosp., 9* (3) :20, 1958.

Peffer, P. A.: Money: A rehabilitation incentive for mental patients. *Amer. J. Psychiat., 110:*84-92, 1953.

Peffer, P. A.: Motivation of the chronic mental patient. *Amer. J. Psychiat., 113:* 55-59, 1956.

Peffer, P. A., Margolin, R. J., Stotsky, B. A., and Mason, A. S. (Eds.) : *Member-employee program: A new approach to the rehabilitation of the chronic mental patient.* (Rev. ed.) Brockton, Mass., Veterans Administration Hospital, 1957.

Peffer, P. A., Margolin, R. J., and Conners, J. E.: Integrative forces in the development and follow-up of a member-employee program. *Amer. Arch. Rehabil., 6:* 8-14, 1958.

Progress Report, 1957-58, Project on rehabilitation of the mentally ill. Boston, Mental Health Center, 1958.

Rabinowitz, H. S.: Morale and productivity in a sheltered workshop for the severely disabled. *Arch. Phys. Med. & Rehabil., 39:*152-157, 1958.

Querido, A.: *Mental Health in the Netherlands.* Netherlands National Federation for Mental Health, 1954.

Ranno, F. S., and Satre, R. P. O.: Some considerations in the operation of industrial therapy. In *Program guide, physical medicine and rehabilitation: G-2, M-2, Part VIII.* Washington, D. C.: Office of the Chief Medical Director Veterans Administration, Department of Medicine and Surgery, August 1955, pp. 19-21.

Rapp, V. W., Fishbune, L., and Awtry, H. N.: Industrial therapy in a neuropsychiatric hospital. In *Program guide, physical medicine and rehabilitation: G-2, M-2, Part VIII.* Washington, D. C.: Office of the Chief Medical Director Veterans Administration, Department of Medicine and Surgery, August 1955, pp. 45-56.

Rees, T. P., and Whitley, J. S.: Occupational therapy in mental disease. *World Mental Health, 9:*109-118, 1957.

Rennie, T. A. C., Burling, T., and Woodward, L. C.: *Vocational Rehabilitation of Psychiatric Patients.* Cambridge, Mass., Commonwealth Fund, 1950.

Reik, L. E.: The half-way house: The role of laymen's organizations in the rehabilitation of the mentally ill. *Ment. Hyg., 37:*615-618, 1953.

Riemer, D., Kilmartin, H. E., Feri, O. W., Slater, R. W., Brewer, L. R., and Lynch, P. H.: Hospital industries at Bedford Veterans Administration Hospital. *Psychiat. Quart. Suppl., 30:*74-82, 1956.

Rothschild, B. F., and Weiss, B. A.: A vocational placement and training program in a state psychiatric institution. *Personnel and Guidance J., 37:*226-229, 1958.

Rudd, J. L., and Margolin, R. J.: Industrial therapy in a member-employee hospital. *Amer. Arch. Rehabil. Ther., 4* (4) :225-230, 1956.

Schillinger, A. A., and Fridovich, D.: Monetary patient-hospital relationships in the Veterans Administration: The member-employee. *Psychiat. Quart. Suppl., 32:*82-98, 1958.

Schnadt, F.: A plan for rehabilitating improved psychotic patients. *Amer. J. Psychiat., 110:*253-260, 1953.

Schossberger, J.: Therapeutic atmosphere in a work village for mental patients in Israel. In J. H. Masserman and J. L. Moreno (Eds.) : *Progress in Psychotherapy.* New York, Grune & Stratton, 1959, Vol. 4, pp. 279-288.

Schwartz, C.: *Rehabilitation of mental hospital patients: Review of the literature.* Public Health Monogr. No. 17. Washington, D. C.: U. S. Department of Health, Education, and Welfare, 1953.

Schwartz, L.: Occupational rehabilitation at a state residential center for retarded youth. *Amer. J. Ment. Def., 63:*408-414, 1958.

Shires, E. B.: A vocational work adjustment unit: Eight months' experience. *Arch. Phys. Med. & Rehabil., 40:*113-117, 1959.

Smith, H. W.: A sheltered employment project in an institution for mental defectives. *Amer. J. Ment. Def., 61:*665-671, 1957.

Soforenko, A. Z.: Farm training program for emotionally disturbed and mentally retarded children. *Agricultural Education Magazine, 32:*61-62, 1959.

Spiegel, E. A. (Ed.) : *Progress in Neurology and Psychiatry.* New York, Grune & Stratton, 1957, Vol. 10.

Stanley, R.: The place of work in the treatment of mental disorder. In *Proc. Nat. A. Ment. Health (Great Britain)*, London, 1959, p. 39.

Stathakis, J., and Pritchard, D. C.: Community retraining—a member of the rehabilitation team. In *Program guide, physical medicine and rehabilitation: G-2, M-2, Part VIII.* Washington, D. C.: Office of the Chief Medical Director Veterans Administration, Department of Medicine and Surgery, August 1955, pp. 24-29.

Stern, E. S.: Operation Rip Van Winkle. *Lancet, 2:*62-63, 1959.

Stotsky, B. A.: A new look at rehabilitation. *Amer. Arch. Rehabil. Ther., 3* (1) : 22-27, 1955.

Stotsky, B. A.: Predicting success on the member-employee rehabilitation program. *J. Consult. Psychol., 19:*274, 1955.

Stotsky, B. A., and Weinberg, H.: The prediction of the psychiatric patient's work adjustment. *J. Counsel. Psychol., 3:*3-7, 1956.

Stringham, J. A.: Rehabilitating chronic neuropsychiatric patients. *Amer. J. Psychiat., 108:*924-928, 1952.

Strader, S. E., and Gibb, J.: Lexington VA Hospital—hospital industry program. In *Program guide, physical medicine and rehabilitation: G-2, M-2, Part VIII.* Washington, D. C.: Office of the Chief Medical Director Veterans Administration, Department of Medicine and Surgery, August 1955, pp. 37-39.

Stubbins, J., and Napoli, P. J.: Vocational goals for the psychiatric patient. *Personnel and Guidance J., 33:*471-475, 1955.

A Survey of Sheltered Workshops Operated by Jewish Vocational Service Agencies. New York, Jewish Occupational Council, 1954.

Switzer, M. E.: Progress and future plans of the federal vocational rehabilitation program. *J. Chron. Dis., 3:*318-322, 1956.

Taggert, D. L.: The role of occupational therapy in the rehabilitation therapies program of the California state hospitals. *Amer. J. Occup. Ther., 7:*128-130, 1953.

Tizard, J.: Institutional defectives. *Amer. J. Ment. Def., 59:*158-165, 1954.

Tizard, J., and O'Connor, N.: The occupational adaptation of high-grade mental defectives. *Lancet, 263* (2) :620-623, 1952.

Toppen, J. T., and Wolfe, H. E.: Vocational rehabilitation as a therapeutic tool. *Dis. Nerv. Sys., 20:*425-426, 1959.

Veterans Administration. *Department of Medicine and Surgery Manual,* M-1, Part III, and M-2, Part X. (undated)

Veterans Administration. Member-employee programs in psychiatric hospitals. *VA Technical Bulletin,* No. IV, TV 10-355, December 15, 1953.

Viscardi, H., Jr.: *Give us the tools.* New York, Eriksson-Taplinger, 1959.

Wadsworth, W. V., Scott, R. F., and Tonge, W. L.: A hospital workshop. *Lancet, 2:* 896-897, 1958.

Walk, A.: Some aspects of the "moral treatment" of the insane up to 1854. *J. Ment. Sci., 100:*807-837, 1954.

Wayne, G. J.: Work as therapy, with special reference to the elderly. *Ment. Hyg., 39:* 79-88, 1955.

White, A. A.: Industrial rehabilitation of psychiatric cases in England. *Amer. J. Psys. Med., 32:*207-212, 1953.

Whitehouse, F. A.: Vocational training in a rehabilitation center. *J. Rehabil., 17* (2) : 19-23, 1951.

Wing, J. K., and Giddens, R. G. T.: Industrial rehabilitation of male chronic schizophrenic patients. *Lancet, 2:*505-507, 1959.

Wittkower, E. D., and Azima, H.: Dynamic aspects of occupational therapy. *AMA Arch. Neurol. & Psychiat., 79:*706-710. Also in M. Greenblatt and B. Simon (Eds.) : *Rehabilitation of the Mentally Ill: Social and Economic Aspects.* Washington, D. C., American Association for the Advancement of Science, 1959, pp. 103-111.

Wright, F. H.: An evaluation of the candidate employee program in the rehabilitation of psychiatric patients. *Diss. Abst., 17:*1604, 1957.

Wright, F. H.: Rehabilitation in twenty-five European NP hospitals. *J. Counsel. Psychol., 6:*275-279, 1959.

Wright, F. H.: The exit unit program for psychotic patients. *J. Counsel. Psychol., 6:* 116-120, 1959.

Yost, O. R.: Therapeutic value of gardening. *South. Med. Surg., 113:*33-35, 1951.

1960-1963

Agnew, P. C.: An experiment in replacing gift distribution with work therapy on a psychiatric ward. *Psychiat. Quart. Suppl., 35:*270-280, 1961.

Alberts, D., Hudec, M., Lever, P. G., and West, F. R.: Farm project proves successful for Florida mental patients. *J. Rehabil., 28* (2) :15, 1962.

Ananian, M., and Biddle, W. E.: The Prep Shop: Work for willing hands. *Ment. Hosp., 13:*436-439, 1962.

Annesley, P. T.: A rehabilitation unit on group therapy lines for long-stay patients. *Psychiat. Quart., 35:*231-237, 1961.

Appleby, L., and Ray, E. L.: Selective job placements for patients. *Ment. Hosp., 11* (9) :37-40, 1960.

Arbegast, A. W.: Homemaking for mentally ill patients as rehabilitative training. *J. Home Economics, 55:*640-642, 1963.

Arnholter, E. G.: A sheltered workshop approach to rehabilitation of the "unemployables." In H. Gerjuoy (Ed.) : *Rehabilitation: Pathways in a Changing World.* Toledo, Ohio, The University of Toledo Research Foundation, 1962, pp. 35-39.

Bartlett, F. L.: Institutional peonage: Our exploitation of mental patients. *Atlantic Monthly, 214:*116-119, 1964.

Basham, J.: A rehabilitation challenge. *Ment. Hosp., 11* (3) :14-16, 1960.

Baur, A. K.: Hospital vocational rehabilitation. *Ment. Hosp., 12* (8) :9-10, 1961.

Bayne, R.: The remedial workshop at Ste. Anne's Veterans Hospital, Ste. Anne de Bellevue, Province of Quebec, Canada. *Amer. Arch. Rehabil. Ther., 11:*51-54, 1963.

Bennett, A. E., and Engle, B.: Psychiatric nursing and occupational therapy. In E. A. Spiegel (Ed.) : *Progress in Neurology and Psychiatry.* New York, Grune & Stratton, 1961, Vol. 16, pp. 575-584.

Bennett, A. E., and Engle, B.: Psychiatric nursing and occupational therapy. In E. A. Spiegel (Ed.) : *Progress in Neurology and Psychiatry.* New York, Grune & Stratton, 1962, Vol. 17, pp. 572-582.

Bennett, A. E., and Engle, B.: Psychiatric nursing and occupational therapy. In E. A. Spiegel (Ed.) : *Progress in Neurology and Psychiatry.* New York, Grune & Stratton, 1963, Vol. 18, pp. 659-669.

Bockoven, J. S.: *Moral Treatment in American Psychiatry.* New York, Springer, 1963.

Bond, R. J.: Work as a therapeutic medium in the treatment of delinquents. In K. I. Wollan (Ed.) : The work camp as a resource for the treatment of delinquents—Workshop 1961. *Amer. J. Orthopsychiat., 32:*846-850, 1962.

Bradshaw, F. J., Jr.: Member-employee program as means of rehabilitation. *Ment. Hyg., 46:*573-579, 1962.

Brooks, G. W.: Rehabilitation of hospitalized patients. In Appleby, L., *et al.: Chronic Schizophrenia.* Glencoe, Free Press, 1960.

Brooks, G. W.: Motivation for work in psychiatric rehabilitation. *Dis. Nerv. Syst., 22* (4) :129-132, 1961.

Burke, J., and Lafave, H. G.: Attitudes of chronic mental patients to a program of rehabilitation. *Ment. Hyg., 47:*123-128, 1963.

Cary, L. J.: History of the work camp as a method of treating delinquents. In K. I. Wollan (Ed.) : The work camp as a resource for the treatment of delinquents—Workshop 1961. *Amer. J. Orthopsychiat., 32:*818-823, 1962.

Casey, J. F., Rackow, L. L., and Sperry, A. W.: *Observations on the treatment of the mentally ill in Europe.* Washington, D. C., Veterans Administration, July 1960.

Chittick, R. A., Brooks, G. W., Irons, F. S., and Deane, W. N.: *The Vermont story: Rehabilitation of chronic schizophrenic patients.* Burlington, Queen City Printers, 1961.

Clark, D. H.: Background and present day status of industrial and occupational therapy programs in English hospitals. *Amer. Arch. Rehabil. Ther., 11:*35-47, 1963.

Clark, D. H., Hooper, D. F., and Oram, E. G.: Creating a therapeutic community in a psychiatric ward. *Human Relations, 15:*123-127, 1962.

Cohen, J. S.: A workshop operation within the framework of a state institution. *Amer. J. Ment. Def., 66:*51-56, 1962.

Cohen, J. S.: Community day work in an institutional vocational training program. *Amer. J. Ment. Def., 66:*574-579, 1962.

Cohen, J. S., and Williams, C. E.: A five phase vocational training program in a residential school. *Amer. J. Ment. Def., 66:*230-237, 1961.

Conners, J. E., Wolkon, G. H., Haefner, D. P., and Stotsky, B. A.: Outcome of post-hospital rehabilitative treatment of mental patients as a function of ego strength. *J. Counsel. Psychol., 7:*278-282, 1960.

Cooper, A. B., and Early, D. F.: Evolution in the mental hospital: Review of a hospital population. *Brit. Med. J., 2:*1600-1603, 1961.

Cumming, J., and Cumming, E.: *Ego and Milieu: Theory and Practice of Environment Therapy.* New York, Atherton, 1962.

Dain, N., and Carlson, E. T.: Milieu therapy in the nineteenth century: Patient care at the Friends' Asylum, Frankford, Pennsylvania, 1817-1861. *J. Nerv. Ment. Dis., 131:*277-290, 1960.

Deane, W. N., and Dodd, M. L.: Educational techniques for the rehabilitation of chronic schizophrenic patients. *Amer. J. Occup. Ther., 14:*7-12, 1960.

Denber, H. C. B.: Industrial workshop for psychiatric patients. *Ment. Hosp., 11* (6) : 16-18, 1960.

Denber, H. C. B.: A therapeutic community: Analysis of its operation after two years. In H. C. B. Denber (Ed.) : *Research Conference on Therapeutic Community.* Springfield, Thomas, 1960, pp. 57-77.

Denber, H. C. B.: Work therapy for psychiatric patients. *Comp. Psychiat., 1:*49-54, 1960.

Denber, H. C. B., and Rajotte, P.: Problems and theoretical considerations of work therapy for psychiatric patients. *Canad. Psychiat. A. J., 7:*25-33, 1962.

Desroches, H. F., and Walter, C. L.: Daily preferences and institutionalization. *J. Psychol., 55:*397-400, 1963.

Dorgan, J.: Obeservations on industrial therapy in United Kingdom mental hospitals. *Canad. Ment. Health, Suppl.,* 9, 1961.

DuBois, F. S.: Rehabilitation and occupational therapy. *Amer. J. Psychiat., 116:* 657-662, 1960.

DuBois, F. S.: Rehabilitation and occupational therapy. *Amer. J. Psychiat., 117:* 657-663, 1961.

Durling, D.: State hospitals make a new start in vocational rehabilitation. *Ment. Hyg., 44:*105-110, 1960.

Early, D. F.: The industrial therapy organization (Bristol): A development of work in hospital. *Lancet, 2:*754-757, 1960.

Edgerton, R. B., Tarjan, G., and Dingman, H. F.: Free enterprise in a captive society. *Amer. J. Ment. Def., 66:*35-41, 1961.

Fairweather, G. W., Simon, R., Gebhard, M. E., Weingarten, E., Holland, J. L., Sanders, R., Stone, G. B., and Reahl, J. E.: Relative effectiveness of psychotherapeutic programs: A multicriteria comparison of four programs for three different patient groups. *Psychol. Monog.: General and Applied, 74* (5, Whole No. 492), 1960.

Filer, R. N., and O'Connell, D. D.: A useful contribution climate for the aging. *J. Gerontol., 17:*51-57, 1962.

Fink, L., and Dunning, E.: Therapeutic utilization of mental hospital industries. *Psychiat. Quart. Suppl., 34:*76-87, 1960.

Fisher, S. H.: Psychiatric rehabilitation in Israel. *Ment. Hyg., 47:*239-248, 1963.

Folkard, S.: Aggressive behavior in relation to open wards in a mental hospital. *Ment. Hyg., 44:*155-161, 1960.

Gage, R. M., and Wolfson, I. N.: Four years of experience with day work program at Letchworth Village. *Amer. J. Ment. Def., 67:*563-568, 1963.

George, I. W.: O. T. adapted to rehabilitation. *Ment. Hosp., 11* (1):22-24, 1960.

Gerjuoy, H.: The industrial therapy curriculum. *Amer. Arch. Rehabil., 10:*12-23, 1962.

Gerjuoy, H. (Ed.): *Rehabilitation: Pathways in a Changing World.* Toledo, Ohio, The University of Toledo Research Foundation, 1962.

Goldman, E., and Soloff, A.: Issues in rehabilitation workshops. *Personnel and Guidance J., 40:*169-173, 1961.

Gordon, H. L., and Allen, G. D.: A member-employee program as a rehabilitation technique. *Amer. J. Phys. Med., 39:*114-119, 1960.

Gordon, H. L.: *Member-employee programs in VA NP hospitals: An interpretive review of the literature.* Washington, D. C.: Psychiatric Evaluation Project, Veterans Administration Hospital, 1961.

Gordon, H. L., and Groth, C.: Mental patients wanting to stay in the hospital. *Arch. Gen. Psychiat., 4:*124-130, 1961.

Gratke, B. E., and Lux, P. A.: Psychiatric occupational therapy in a milieu setting. *Amer. J. Occup. Ther., 14:*13-16, 1960.

Greenland, C.: Work as therapy in the treatment of chronic mental illness. *Canad. Psychiat. A. J., 7*:11-15, 1962.

Green thumb therapy. *Amer. Arch. Rehabil. Ther., 9* (3) :16-19, 1961.

Griffith, W. D.: Laboratory for practical rehabilitation. *Ment. Hosp., 12* (4) :25-27, 1961.

Grold, L. J.: Resistance to changing a psychiatric ward. *Ment. Hosp., 11* (4) :16-18, 1960.

Guthrie, D I.: An experiment in industrial rehabilitation. *South African Med., 35* (1) :306-310, 1961.

Guyette, H., and Deane, W. N.: Industrial therapy: Vermont State Hospital OVR Project. *J. Rehabil., 27* (5) :32, 1961.

Hadly, J. M.: Work as therapy. *Amer. Arch. Rehabil. Ther., 8* (1) :11-16, 1960.

Hallenbeck, C. E. (Ed.) : *An investigation into the vocational potentials of hospitalized patients with chronic disabilities.* Special project grant 41-56. Final report of the Highland Shop, Inc. Washington, D. C., Office of Vocational Rehabilitation, Department of Health, Education, and Welfare, 1960.

Hamilton, V., and Salmon, P.: Psychological changes in chronic schizophrenics following differential activity programmes. *J. Ment. Sci., 108*:505-520, 1962.

Havens, L. L., and Harding, F. A.: Rehabilitating the mentally disabled: A report of the Massachusetts Commission's methods and experience. *J. Rehabil., 27* (6) :22-23, 1961.

Hooper, D. F.: Changing the milieu in a psychiatric ward. *Human Relations, 15:* 111-122, 1962.

Hubbs, R. S.: Rehabilitation means restoration: The sheltered workship. *Ment. Hosp., 11* (4) :7-9, 1960.

Huseth, B.: England's halfway houses. *Ment. Hosp., 13*:422-424, 1962.

Hutton, G.: Management in a changing mental hospital. *Human Relations, 15:* 283-310, 1962.

Hyde, R. W., Bockoven, J. S., Pfautz, H. W., and York, R. H.: *Milieu Rehabilitation: For Physical and Mental Handicaps.* Providence, R. I., Butler Health Center, 1962.

Jacobs, D. F.: Vocational rehabilitation of the psychiatric patient: A hospital-community problem. *Personnel and Guidance J., 38*:642-647, 1960.

Jensen, M. B., and Yanagi, G. H.: Directive treatment of long-term closed ward schizophrenics. *J. Clin. Psychol., 17*:139-141, 1961.

Johnson, W.: Rehabilitation as it seems to be and as it might be. *Etc, 10* (2) :203-223, 1963.

Jones, M.: Social rehabilitation with emphasis on work therapy as a form of group therapy. *Brit. J. Med. Psychol., 33*:67-71, 1960.

Kaplan, S.: The growing importance of the trainable in an institutional setting. *Amer. J. Ment. Def., 66*:393-398, 1961.

Kissin, G., and Carmichael, D. M.: Rehabilitation of psychiatric patients. *J. Rehabil., 26* (5) :24-28, 1960.

Kraepelin, E.: One Hundred Years of Psychiatry. (Trans. by W. Baskin) , New York, Citadel, 1962.

Krygar, C., Jr.: Clerical work in psychiatric occupational therapy. *Amer. J. Occup. Ther., 14*:64, 1960.

Leavitt, L. A.: Industrial therapy: Its role in a complete rehabilitation program. *Amer. Arch. Rehabil. Ther., 8* (4) :4-8, 1960.

Lerner, M. J.: Responsiveness of chronic schizophrenic to the social behavior of others in a meaningful task situation. *J. Abnorm. Soc. Psychol., 67*:295-299, 1963.

Lerner, M. J., and Fairweather, G. W.: Social behavior of chronic schizophrenics in supervised and unsupervised work groups. *J. Abnorm. Soc. Psychol., 67*:219-225, 1963.

Luger, M. J.: Extending the work camp concept. In K. I. Wollan (Ed.) : The work camp as a resource for the treatment of delinquents—Workshop, 1961. *Amer. J. Orthopsychiat., 32*:850-853, 1962.

Mann, W. A., and Terhune, W. B.: Rehabilitation and occupational therapy. *Amer. J. Psychiat., 118*:650-654, 1962.

Mann, W. A., and Terhune, W. B.: Rehabilitation and occupational therapy. *Amer. J. Psychiat., 119*:686-690, 1963.

Martin, H. R., and Schaefer, I. J.: Mental illness and vocational handicap. *Ment. Hosp., 12* (8) :6-7, 1961.

Martinson, M. C.: General considerations basic to a work experience program. *Ed. Rep., 2,* 1961.

McCourt, J. F., and Goldstein, G.: The pharmacy: Unique setting for rehabilitation of mental patients. *Ment. Hyg., 47*:602-606, 1963.

McGowan, J. F. (Ed.) : *An introduction to the vocational rehabilitation process: A manual for orientation of in-service training.* Washington, D. C., U. S. Department of Health, Education, and Welfare, Office of Vocational Rehabilitation, 1960.

McGrath, V., and Burke, B. B.: Compensated work therapy programs in the New York State Department of Mental Hygiene. *Amer. Arch. Rehabil. Ther., 11*: 48-50, 1963.

McPheeters, H. L.: A treatment unit for alcoholics. *Ment. Hosp., 11* (3) :41-42, 1960

Mills, D. F.: *Recidivism patterns for selected veterans in a neuropsychiatric hospital* Paper read at American Personnel and Guidance Association, Boston, Mass., April 1963.

Mindlin, D. F.: Evaluation of therapy for alcoholics in a workhouse setting. *Quart. J. Studies on Alcohol, 21*:90-112, 1960.

Morehouse, R. E.: The Brockton ceramics project: A semi-industrial workshop. *Amer. J. Occup. Ther., 15*:256-257, 1961.

Moseley, L.: Returning the ex-patient to employment. *J. Rehabil., 27* (5) :22-34, 1961.

Nagler, B., and Kirkland, M.: Institutional work programs—boon or bane? *Amer. J. Ment. Def., 66*:375-380, 1961.

Norton, Y., and Gaster, B.: Progressive activities for rehabilitation. *Ment. Hosp., 13*: 418, 1962.

Oliver, B. M.: A laundry evolves into a therapy center. *Ment. Hosp., 12* (8) :34-35, 1961.

Olshansky, S., and Unterberger, H.: The meaning of work and its implications for the ex-mental hospital patient. *Ment. Hyg., 47*:139-149, 1963.

Oseas, L.: Therapeutic potentials in work. *Arch. Gen. Psychiat., 4*:622-631, 1961.

Oseas, L.: A model for establishing therapeutic work conditions. *J. Counsel. Psychol., 10*:368-372, 1963.

Pavorsky, B.: Volunteering for step-by-step rehabilitation. *Ment. Hosp., 11* (3) :21-25, 1960.

Peffer, P. A.: Cadre-Employee Program. *Ment. Hosp., 12* (10) :33-34, 1961.

Peters,, J. S., Payne, R. A., and Bole, A. E.: Socio-egocentrism of patients in a half-way hospital. *Vocational Guid. Quart., 11:*110-115, 1963.

Pinner, J. I.: Job placement of ex-mental patients. *Dis. Nerv. Syst., 22* (4) :122-124, 1961.

Planansky, K., and Dillman, E.: An experience with work therapy in the management of disturbed patients. *Nursing Res., 11:*101-104, 1962.

Reiser, M., and Waldman, M.: *The Work Adjustment Center—A Bridge to Employability*. Philadelphia, Work Adjustment Center, 1961.

Richman, S., and Zinn, S.: Work as a central focus in therapy. *Ment. Hosp., 13:* 603-609, 1962.

Risk, J. W.: The hospital farm—boon or bane to patients? *Ment. Hosp., 16* (6) : 22-23, 1961.

Roberts, S.: Occupational therapy and sheltered workshop program in a home for the aged. *J. Amer. Geriat. Soc., 10* (1) :532-534, 1962.

Rusalem, H., and Spciser, A.: The meaningfulness of work. *Vocational Guid. Quart., 12:*119-122, 1963.

Sacks, J. M.: Transitional programs for psychiatric patients. *Ment. Hyg., 44:* 577-581, 1960.

Seagar, C. P.: An interim report on open hospitals in Great Britain. *Ment. Hosp., 11* (4) :21-25, 1960.

Smith-e-Incas, J.: The mentally retarded psychotic. *Ment. Hosp., 11* (4) :30, 1960.

Soloff, A.: The work therapy research center. *J. Jewish Communal Serv., 38:*171-177, 1961.

St. Pierre, R. G.: Therapeutic incentive program. *Amer. Arch. Rehabil. Ther., 11* (2) :33-34, 1963.

Thompson, J. R.: The effects of industrial therapy upon personality and behavior. *Diss. Abst., 21:*3170, 1961.

Wadsworth, W. V.: Industrial therapy in a mental hospital. *Nursing Times, 57:* 446, 1961.

Wadsworth, W. V., Scott, R. F., and Wells, B. W. P.: Employability of long-stay schizophrenic patients. *Lancet, 2:*593-595, 1961.

Wadsworth, W. V., Scott, R. F., and Wells, B. W. P.: The employability of chronic schizophrenics. *J. Ment. Sci., 108:*300-303, 1962.

Wadsworth, W. V., Wells, B. W. P., and Scott, R. F.: A comparative study of the fatigability of a group of chronic schizophrenics and a group of hospitalized non-psychotic depressives. *J. Ment. Sci., 108:*304-308, 1962.

Wadsworth, W. V., Wells, B. W. P., and Scott, R. F.: Quantity and quality of industrial therapy. *Lancet, 2:*1375-1376, 1962.

Wadsworth, W. V., Wells, B. W. P., and Scott, R. F.: The organization of a sheltered workshop. *J. Ment. Sci., 108:*780-785, 1962.

Wayne, G. J.: Work therapy in the Soviet Union. *Ment. Hosp., 12* (8) :20-23, 1961.

Weber, G. H.: The organization of camps for delinquent boys. In K. I. Wollan (Ed.) : The work camp as a resource for the treatment of delinquents—Workshop, 1961. *Amer. J. Orthopsychiat., 32:*824-836, 1962.

Weschler, H. W.: Transitional residences for former mental patients: A survey of halfway houses and related rehabilitation facilities. *Ment. Hyg., 45:*65-76, 1961.

White, J. S.: Patients cook their way back to health. *Mod. Hosp., 97* (2) :112-117, 1961.

Wolfe, H. E.: A survey of vocational rehabilitation at Longview State Hospital for 1959. *Ment. Hyg.*, *45*:167-170, 1961.

Wolfe, H. E.: The role of vocational rehabilitation in today's state mental hospital. *Ment. Hyg.*, *46*:192-198, 1962.

Wolfe, H. E.: A two year analysis of an in-hospital vocational rehabilitation program. *Dis. Nerv. Syst.*, *23*:640-641, 1962.

FOREIGN LANGUAGE REFERENCES

Before 1920

Jaspers, K. (1913) : Quoted in *Allgemeine Psychopathologie*. 14th Ed. Berlin, 1948, p. 700.

Leuret, F.: *Du traitement moral de la folie*. [On the moral treatment of insanity.] Paris, France: Baillière, 1840. (A translated passage is in *Occup. Ther. & Rehabil.*, *27*:27-33, 1948.)

1920-1929

Calmels: [Treatment of mental disease by work.] *Annales Médico-psychologiques*, *85* (1) :277-283, 1927.

Courbon, P.: Un voyage d'études dans les asiles de Hollande. *Annales Médico-Psychologiques*, *86* (2) :289-306, 1928.

Garmendia, F. S., and Darder, V. C.: [Work in treatment of mental disease.] *Anales de la Facultad de Medicina*. Universidad de Montevideo. *10*:783-791, 1925.

Gilabert, F. Z.: [Value of work in mental diseases.] *Archivos de Médicina, Cirugia y Especialidades, 31*:36-43, 1929.

Goetz, Nobbe and Powells: Erfahrungen mit der Beschäftigungstherapie nach Simon in den ostpreussisschen Provinzialanstalten. *Allgemeine Zeitschrift für Psychiatrica, 86*:102-111, 1927.

Gross, A.: Der Umbau einer Zellenabteilung. *Allgemeine Zeitschrift für Psychiatrica, 84*:183-204, 1926.

Gross, A.: Graeplin's Bedeutung für die Anstaltspsychiatrie. *Archic für Psychiatrie und Nervenkrankheiten, 87*:50-67, 1929.

Gründler, W.: Bericht über die Dienstreise nach Gütersloh. *Psychiatrisch-neurologische Wochenschrift, 29*:347-351, 1927.

Halberstadt, G.: A propos de "l'Ergothérapie." *Annales Médico-Psychologiques, 87* (1) :193-198, 1929.

Herting: [Exhibit of industrial employment of insane at the Gesolei, Stuttgart.] *Psychiatrisch-neurologische Wochenschrift, 28*:539-541, 1926.

Hinrichs and Grabow: Erfolge der Dauerschlafbehandlung und Arbeitsherapie in der Landesheil-und Pflegeanstalt Neustadt in Holst. *Psychiatrisch-neurologische Wochenschrift, 29*:410-413, 1927.

Ilberg, G.: Neber den Umfang der Arbeitstherapie. *Psychiatrisch-neurologische Wochenschrift, 28*:433-435, 1926.

Ilberg, G.: Anregungen zur Verbesserung der Irrenpflege. *Viener Medizinische Wochenschrift, 77*:1232-1235, 1927.

Ilberg, G.: Erfahrungen mit erweiterter Beschäftigungstherapie. *Allgemeine Zeitschrift für Psychiatrica, 88*:108-113, 1928.

Kahlbaum: Aktivere Arbeitstherapie bei Psychisch-Kranken. *Klinische Wochenschrift, 6:*1294-1296, 1927.

Köhler, F.: [Sanatoriums for occupational treatment.] *Tuberkulose, 9:*5, 1929.

Löwenstein, O.: Ueber einige experimentelle und klinische Grundlagen für die Anwendung der Psychotherapie bei Psychosen mit besonderem Hinblick auf die Arbeitstherapie. *Zeitschrift für die gesamte Neurologie und Psychiatrie, 110:* 50-59, 1927.

Maier, H., and Römer: Die Frühentlassung der Schizophrenen. *Zentralblatt für die gesamte Neurologie und Psychiatrie, 53:*662-663, 1929.

Meltzer, E.: Die neuen Ziele der Psychotherapie. *Psychiatrisch-neurologische Wochenschrift, 29:*108-113; 117-121, 1927.

Meltzer, E.: Muss der Anstaltsarzt wissenschaftlich arbeiten? *Psychiatrisch-neurologische Wochenschrift, 31:*405-410, 1929.

Müller, G.: Die Beschäftigungsbehandlung in der Lippeschen Heil—und Pflegeanstalt Lindenhaus bei Brake in Lippe. *Psychiatrisch-neurologische Wochenschrift, 27:*491-494, 1925.

Neisser, C.: Bettbehandlung, Arbeit, aktivere Therapie. *Archiv für Psychiatrie und Nervenkrankheiten, 77:*663-664, 1926.

Neisser, C.: Die Weiterentwicklung der praktischen Psychiatrie, insbesondere der Anstaltstherapie im Sinne Griesinger's. *Monatsschrift für Psychiatrie und Neurologie, 63:*314-335, 1927.

Reinelt, E.: [Active employment for insane; statistical records.] *Psychiatrisch-neurologische Wochenschrift, 29:*83-86, 1927.

Reiss: Die aktivere Beschäftigungbehandlung der Heil-und Pflegeanstalten. *Psychiatrisch-neurologische Wochenschrift, 31:*105-111, 1929.

Sanz, E. F.: [Sanatoriums laying particular emphasis on the therapeutic value of work in benign psychoses.] *Archivos de Medicina, Cirugia y Especialidades, 28:* 725-727, 1928.

Sicco, A.: [Simon's use of manual labor adapted to the individual.] *Revista de Criminologiá, Psiquiatriá y Medicina Legal, 15:*539-549, 1928.

Sicco, A.: *Sobre laborterapia, el metodo del Dr. Hermann Simon.* Buenos Aires: Talleres Graficos de la Penitenciaria Nacional, 1928.

Simon, H.: Aktivere Therapie in der Irrenanstalt. *Allgemeine Zeitschrift für Psychiatrica, 81:*425-428, 1925.

Simon, H.: Psychotherapie in der Irrenanstalt, Bericht über den II. Allg. ärztl. Kongr. f. Psychotherapie. Leipzig, S. Hirzel, 1927.

Simon, H.: [More active treatment of patients in the psychiatric institution.] *Allgemeine Zeitschrift für Psychiatrica, 87:*97-145, 1927.

Simon, H.: Arbeitstherapie in der Irrenanstalt und ihre moderne Ausgestaltung. *Allgemeine Zeitschrift für Psycvhiatrica, 86:*446-451, 1927.

Simon, H.: Aktivere Krankenbehandlung in der Irrenanstalt. II. Erfahrungen und Gedanken eines praktischen Psychiaters zur Psychotherapie der Geisteskrankheiten. [More active treatment of mental patients in hospital.] *Allgemeine Zeitschrift für Psychiatrica, 90:*69-73; 245-309, 1929.

Thumm, M.: [experiences with "active" therapy in psychoses.] *Zeitschrift für die gesamte Neurologie und Psychiatrie, 103:*225-236, 1926.

Thumm, M.: Beschaftigungsgrad und aktive Therapie. *Psychiatrisch-neurologische Wochenschrift, 29:*242-244, 1927.

Thumm, M.: Literaturbericht zur aktiveren (Beschäftigungs-) Therapie nach Simon. *Allgemeine Zeitschrift für Psychiatrica, 89:*154-166, 1928.

Tramer, M.: [Work and suggestion as therapeutic agents in neuroses.] *Schweizer Archiv für Neurologie und Psychiatrie, 21:*187-213, 1927.

Tramer, M.: [Work and suggestion as therapeutic agents in neuroses.] *Schweizer Archiv für Neurologie und Psychiatrie, 22:*122-144, 1928.

Trapet: Die Simonsche Beschäftigungstherapie. *Psychiatrisch-neurologische Wochenschrift, 28:*94-95, 1926.

Van der Scheer, W. M.: Ueber einige wichtige Behändlungsmethoden in unserer Anstalt. *Psychiatrisch-neurologische Wochenschrift, 28:*73-74, 1926.

Van der Scheer, W. M.: Rückblick über zwanzig Jahre Irrenpflege und Betrachtungen über die aktivere Therapie in der Provinzial Heilanstalt bei Santpoort (früher Meerenberg, Holland). *Zeitschrift für Psychische Hygiene, 1:*161-177, 1928.

Van der Scheer, W. M.: [Value of work and working skill of insane.] *Neurotherapie, 11:*1-31, 1929. (Supplement in *Psychiatrische en Neurologische, 33:*1-35, 1929.)

Wickel: Fortschritte in der Erkenntnis und Behandlung der Geisteskrankheiten. *Münchener Medizinische Wochenschrift, 73* (2) :1463-1464, 1926.

Wiest, A.: [Various occupations for patients and convalescents.] *Deutsche Medizinische Wochenschrift, 55* (2) :1559, 1929.

1930-1939

Aiginger, J.: [Effect of work on the human psyche, with notes on present status of occupational therapy in Austria.] *Wiener Klinische Wochenschrift, 49* (2) :1256-1258, 1936.

Alexander, H.: [Comparative value of sanatorium at high altitude and of work sanatorium.] *Müchener Medizinische Wochenschrift, 79* (1) :801-802, 1932.

Anton, W.: [Comparative value of sanatorium at high altitude and of work sanatorium.] *Münchener Medizinische Wochenschrift, 79* (1) :554-556, 1932.

Anton, W.: Zauberberg und Arbeitssanatorium. (Zu den Erwiderungen von Alexander und Kattendidt auf meinen Aufsatz.) *Münchener Medizinische Wochenschrift, 79* (1) :841-842, 1932.

Bozhovsky, V. G.: [Physical work as treatment in sanatoriums.] *Vrachebnaya Gezeta, 35:*820-823, 1931.

Brieger, E.: [Workshop settlements in sanatoriums as unlimited treatment for patients with chronic tuberculosis.] *Zeitschrift für Tuberkulose, 60:*353-365, 1931.

Bronkhorst, W.: [Work cure as last phase in therapy.] *Zeitschrift für Tuberkulose, 74:*321-333, 1936.

Bugaisky, J. P.: ["Active" (work) therapy in psychiatric hospitals.] *Jurnal Nevropatologii i Psikhiatrii, 23:*111-122, 1930.

Bugaisky, J. P.: [Importance of work and collective activity.] *Zeitschrift für die gesamte Neurologie und Psychiatrie, 129:*299-312, 1930.

Cabitto, L.: [Value of work associated with sulfur fever therapy in mental disease.] *Note e Rivista di Psichiatria, 62:*285-295, 1933.

d'Ambrosio, R.: [Sanatorial and postsanatorial work: trends and results in Ramazzini Sanatorium.] *Difesa Sociale, 17:*39-69, 1938.

Damiani, F.: [Behavior of therapeutic pneumothorax in patients during work therapy.] *Lotta contra la Tubercolosi, 9* (2) :1144-1162, 1938.

del Greco, F.: [Psychologic and therapeutic value of work in mental diseases.] *Archivo Generale di Neuralogia, Psichiatria, e Psicoanalisi, 13*:35-40, 1932.

del Rosso, L. M.: [Occupational colonies for patients before and after sanatorium treatment.] *Medicina Italiana* [Milan], *11*:697-707, 1930.

di Aichelburg, U.: [Importance of recreation and work as therapeutic factors in hospital patients.] *Giornale di Batteriologia, Virologia et Immunologia, 22:* 499-513, 1939.

Dorn, E.: Arbeitstherapie und Lungentuberkulose. Bemerkungen zu der Arbeit von Dr. Schnurrer: Neue Wege Ausnutzung eines der wichigsten Heilfaktoren bei der Behandlung der Lungentuberkulose, namlich die "Arbeitstherapie," durch engste Verbindung der Heilanstalt mit einem landwirtschaftlichen Gutsbetriebe und Siedlung. *Münchener Medizinische Wochenschrift, 78*:1439-1440, 1931.

Dorn, E.: [Provision of suitable work for patients.] *Deutsches Tuberkulose-Blatt, 13*:230-235, 1939.

Ferrari, G. C.: [Original method of applying restless insane to methodical, but active work.] *Rassegna di Studi Psichiatrici, 19*:834-846, 1930.

Gaudier, H.: [International workshop clinic at Leysin for surgical tuberculosis.] *Echo Médicine du Nord, 36*:313-317, 1932.

Genkina, M. N., and Zelenin, N. V.: [Collective work as therapeutic factor.] *Sovietskaya Nevropatologiya, Psikhiatriya i Psikhogigiena, 1*:837-841, 1932.

Gorriz, M.: [Work as therapeutic means in mental diseases.] *Medicana, 3*:363-373, 1932.

Ichok, G.: [Influence of work on mental and physical conditions of patients; problems related to choice of occupation after recovery.] *Progresos de la Clínica, 41:* 27-35, 1933.

Kattentidt, B.: [Comparative value of a sanatorium at high altitude and of a work sanatorium.] *Münchener Medizinische Wochenschrift, 79* (1) :802-803, 1932.

Kirchmann, H.: [Comparative value of a sanatorium at high altitude and of a work sanatorium.] *Münchener Medizinische Wochenschrift, 79* (2) :1125-1126, 1932.

Marabotti, P. M.: [Curative effects of work.] *Difesa Sociale, 11*:344-350, 1932.

Oldenburg, F., and Seisoff, C.: [Statistics regarding recovery of railway employees who have been treated in industrial sanatoriums; proposals for establishing workshop clinics for those with open tuberculosis.] *Zeitschrift für Tuberkulose, 61*:334-349, 1931.

Paasch, G.: [Course of treatment during graded work in workshop settlements.] *Zeitschrift für Tuberkulose, 60*:365-370, 1931.

Parry, B. E.: European and American practice in hospital and workshop. *Nosokomeion, 6*:136-141, 1935.

Pecker, A.: [Work of patients.] *Progrès Médical*, p. 738-743, 1932.

Pernambucano, U.: [Work of insane in Colony for Assistance for Psychopaths of Pernambuco.] *Revista Medica de Pernambuco, 5*:263-272, 1935.

Poerzgen, H.: [Comparative value of sanatorium at high altitude and of a work sanatorium.] *Munchener Medizinische Wochenschrift, 79* (2) :1125, 1932.

Roederer, C.: [Value of work for patients; results of Hague Conference.] *Journal de Médecine de Paris, 52*:640-642, 1932.

Rollier, A.: [International factory clinic at Leysin, for Leliotherapy and occupational cure of indigent patients with surgical tuberculosis.] *Revue Scientifique, 68:*641-650, 1930.

Roussel, P.: [Sunlight, climate and work in treatment.] *Revue d'Actinologie et de Physiothérapie, 7:*142-158, 1931.

Sarno, A.: [Workshop of occupational reeducation and readaptation in Fermin Ferreyra Hospital.] *Revista de Tuberculosis del Uruguay, 7:*475-477, 1938.

Schnurrer: [New ideas of occupational therapy of pulmonary tuberculosis (combining sanatorium with agricultural enterprise and settlement).] *Münchener Medizinische Wochenschrift, 78* (2) :1185-1187, 1931.

Shershen, M. M.: [Experiences with educational work in a ward for restless patients at a psychiatric hospital.] *Sovietskaya Nevropatologiya, Psikhiatriya i Psikhogigiena, 2:*98-110, 1933.

Waldvogel, W.: [Hop-picking as therapy for mental patients.] *Psychiatrisch-neurologische Wochenschrift, 40:*65-66, 1938.

1940-1949

Alvarez, R. P.: [Work therapy and its place in the total scheme of an anti-tuberculosis campaign.] *Medicinia Colonial Madrid, 3:*42-56, 1944.

d'Arcangelo, D.: [Clinical observations on sanatorial work therapy practiced in Addis Ababa, and consideration on particular suitability of Ethiopian plains for organization of sanatorial work colonies.] *Bolletino delia Societa Italiana di Medicina e Igiene Tropicale, 4:*389-403; 405-418, 1944.

Kogan, M. S.: Diferentsirovaniia sistema organizatsii trudovoi terapii i trudoustroistva pri psikhonevrologicheskom dispaansere. [A differential system of organization of work therapy and work training in the psycho-neurological dispensary.] *Nevropatalogiia i Psikhiatriia, 17* (5) :67-71, 1948.

Nebias, O.: [Work in treatment and rehabilitation.] *Revista Paulista de Tisiologia, 11:*191-196, 1945.

Neidhard, E.: [Twenty-five years activity of a workshop in the Oskar-Helene Home for cripples.] *Zeitschrift für Kruppelfürsorge, 35:*17-20, 1942.

Snell, W. E.: Some thoughts on outdoor employment of sanatorium patients. *Tubercle, 23:*101-103, 1942.

1950-1959

Beeck, M.: [Psychological aspects in work therapy and occupational therapy.] *Acta Psychotherapeutica, Psychosomatica et Orthopaedagogica, 7:*172-173, 1959.

Berglin, C. G.: [Convalescence and readjustment to work.] *Svencka Läkartidningen, 56* (6) :3157-3166, 1959.

Birzele, K.: Training der Arbeitswilligkeit. [Training of Willingness to work.] *Wiener Medizinische Wochenschrift, 107* (1) :443, 1957.

Eriksson, G.: [Convalescence—readjustment to work.] *Svenska Läkartidningen, 56* (6) :3166-3196, 1959.

Fernandez-Zoila, A., and Lebreton, M.: Aspects psychopathologiques due travail thérepeutique. [Psychopathological aspects of work therapy: Its temperal and rhythmic components.] *Evolution Psychiatrique, 4:*739-756, 1958.

Fries, P. E.: Om industriell arbetsterapi. [Industrial work therapy.] *Social-medizinsk Tidskrift, 33:*17-19, 1956.

Ianushevskii, I. K.: Opyt trudovi terapii v ncvropsikhiatricheskikh uchrezhdeniiakh. [Work therapy in mental institutions.] *Zhurnal Nevropatologii i Psikhiatrii, 57:* 249-252, 1957.

Koechlin, P.: Schema de l'utilisation du travail en fonction des niveaux de sociabilite. [A scheme for the utilization of occupational therapy at different levels of social interaction.] *Hygiène Mentale, 41* (1) :12-22, 1952.

Leistner, R., and Branton, H.: Die Grenzen der Methodik; Betrachtungen uber den Wert der Schematik in der Arbeitstherapie. [The Frontiers of the methodic approach; comments on the worth of the schematic approach in work therapy.] *Internationale Zeitschrift für Individual-Psychologie, 19:*174-177, 1950.

Neumann, R., and Prohaska, L.: [Work as part of therapy.] *Wiener Klinische Wochenschrift, 63* (2) :588-590, 1951.

Schunk, J. G.: Uber Erfahrungen in der Organisation der Arbeitstherapie. [On experiences in the organization of work therapy.] *Psychiatrie, Neurologie und Medizinische Psychologie,* Leipzig, *8:*82-85, 1956.

Shternberg, E. IA., and Luninskaia, I. R.: O vluanii trudovoi terapii na razvitie mikrotsefalov. [Effect of work therapy on the development in mocrocephaly.] *Zhurnal Nevropathologii i Psikhiatrii, 57:*897-903, 1957.

Sivadon, P. D.: Principes généraux de thérapeutique par le travail. [General principles of work therapy.] *Hygiène Mentale, 44:*54-65, 1955.

Torok, I., and Lesch, G.: [Role of payment of wages in the occupational therapy of mental disorders.] *Ideggyogy Szemle, 12:*306-307, 1959.

Wagner, W., and Schlepckow, D.: [Working establishment connected with sanatorium; experiences during fourteen years.] *Beitraege zur Klinik der Tuberkulose und Spezifischen Tuberkulose-Forschung, 108:*259-264, 1953.

Župic, S.: Pitanje rehabilitacije dŭsevnih bolesnika i dŭsevno difektnih lica. [Problem of rehabilitation of mental deficiency and mental disorders.] *Neuropsihijatrija, 2:*240-247, 1954.

1960-1963

Adachi, T.: [The work treatment transition of the pulmonary consumption patients. The transition of the work treatment.] *Niigata Medical Journal, 75:* 1140-1143, 1961.

Bimbad, Sla.: [Organization and effectiveness of work therapy in the P. P. Kashchenko Hospital.] *Voprosy Psikhiatrii i Nevropatologii, 7:*305-311, 1961.

Caccuri, S.: [Clinical aspects of the use of the disabled.] *Rivista degli Infortuni e delle Mallattie Professionali, 48:*996-1038, 1961.

Faurbye, A.: [Principles of work and occupational therapy in a mental hospital.] *Nordisk Medicin, 64* (2) :1327-1329, 1960.

Filion, N.: [Attempt at group work in rehabilitation.] *Canad. J. Occup. Ther., 28:* 97-103, 1961.

Filion, N.: [Attempt at group work in rehabilitation. (3)] *Canad. J. Occup. Ther., 28:*129-134, 1961.

Filion, N.: [Essay on group work in rehabilitation. (4)] *Canad. J. Occup. Ther., 29:* 21-26, 1962.

Gad, P. G.: [Work assignment and rehabilitation.] *Nordisk Medicin, 63* (1) :113-120, 1960.

Gálfi, Béla.: [Labor therapy in the Institute for Labor Therapy at Pomaz.] *Magyar Pszichologiai Szemle, 18:*173-183, 1961.

Gogstad, A. C.: [Work training—a form of treatment in rehabilitation medicine.] *Nordisk Medicin, 68* (2) :1381-1386, 1962.

Leroy: [From the bed to the workshop.] *Techniques Hospitalières, Medico-Sociales et Sanitaires, 17:*69-73, 1961.

Mirskaia, M. M., Povorinskii, Iu. A., and Rubinova, R. S.: [On the problem of the differentiation of work therapy and biological therapy in psychiatric wards for acute conditions.] *Voprosy Psikhiatrii i Nevropatologii, 7:*312-318, 1961.

Tsvetanov, B., Khinov, V., and Atanasova, Ts.: [Work therapy and work capacity of patients in osteoarticular therapy.] *Khirugiia, 15:*310-312, 1962.

INDEX

Vocational and industrial therapy *(see also* industrial therapy) , 17, 18
director, 111
facilities, 295, 299, 309
place of, 17
Vocational counseling, 17, 110
Vocational placement, 17, 18
Vocational Rehabilitation Administration, xii, 337
Vocational Rehabilitation Division, 17
Vocational training, 110
Vocational rehabilitation, 17
vocational therapy in, 44-46
Vocational therapy *(see also* industrial and/or work therapy) , 17
Volunteer and the Psychiatric Patient, 205
Volunteer services, 18, 203-226, 233
administration of, 214-225
administrative functions of, 222
assignment guide for, 216
budget, 207
classified, 214
community relations, 224-225
concept of, 203
coordinator of, 207, 209, 216, 217, 218, 220, 224
evaluating need for, 210
facilities, 299
historical development of, 203-205
hospital-community council, 212, 218
interviewing for, 218, 219
material donations for, 216, 217
organization of program for, 204-214, 221, 222
orientation for, 207, 215, 216, 218, 220
professional organization, 357
recruiting for, 207, 217, 218
screening for, 207, 218, 219

selection of coordinator for, 207
job description, 208
staff advisory committee for, 210
supervision of volunteers for, 207
trends in, 225-226
volunteers
assignment of, 218, 221
occasional, 214, 215
recognition of, 218, 222
regular, 214, 215
training of, 218, 220, 327
Volunteer Services in Mental Hospitals, 205

W

Warren, John C., 137
Washburn Project *(see also Project 52)* , 7, 13
Wasteland, 164
Weekly Patients Activity Schedule, 287
West, Wilma, 298
Western Reserve University, 148
Willard, Helen S., 32, 120
Wilson Co., H. W., 153
catalogue cards, 155
fiction catalogue, 156
Wilson Library Bulletin, 170
Wittkower, Ed., 113
Wolberg, Lewis, 143
Wolfe, Corinne, 316, 317
Worchester Royal Infirmary, 138
Works Progress Administration, 78
Work therapy *(see also* industrial and vocational therapy) , 17

Y

YMCA-YWCA, 68, 283

Z

Zubaithes, Christina, 178, 180

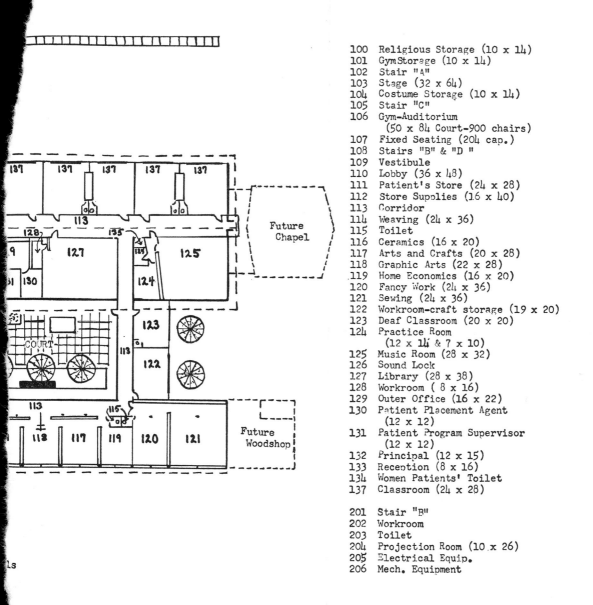

100 Religious Storage (10 x 14)
101 Gym Storage (10 x 14)
102 Stair "A"
103 Stage (32 x 64)
104 Costume Storage (10 x 14)
105 Stair "C"
106 Gym-Auditorium
    (50 x 84 Court-900 chairs)
107 Fixed Seating (204 cap.)
108 Stairs "B" & "D "
109 Vestibule
110 Lobby (36 x 48)
111 Patient's Store (24 x 28)
112 Store Supplies (16 x 40)
113 Corridor
114 Weaving (24 x 36)
115 Toilet
116 Ceramics (16 x 20)
117 Arts and Crafts (20 x 28)
118 Graphic Arts (22 x 28)
119 Home Economics (16 x 20)
120 Fancy Work (24 x 36)
121 Sewing (24 x 36)
122 Workroom-craft storage (19 x 20)
123 Deaf Classroom (20 x 20)
124 Practice Room
    (12 x 14 & 7 x 10)
125 Music Room (28 x 32)
126 Sound Lock
127 Library (28 x 38)
128 Workroom (8 x 16)
129 Outer Office (16 x 22)
130 Patient Placement Agent
    (12 x 12)
131 Patient Program Supervisor
    (12 x 12)
132 Principal (12 x 15)
133 Reception (8 x 16)
134 Women Patients' Toilet
137 Classroom (24 x 28)

201 Stair "B"
202 Workroom
203 Toilet
204 Projection Room (10 x 26)
205 Electrical Equip.
206 Mech. Equipment

ate School and Hospital (permission to reprint courtesy of *Mental Hospitals*).

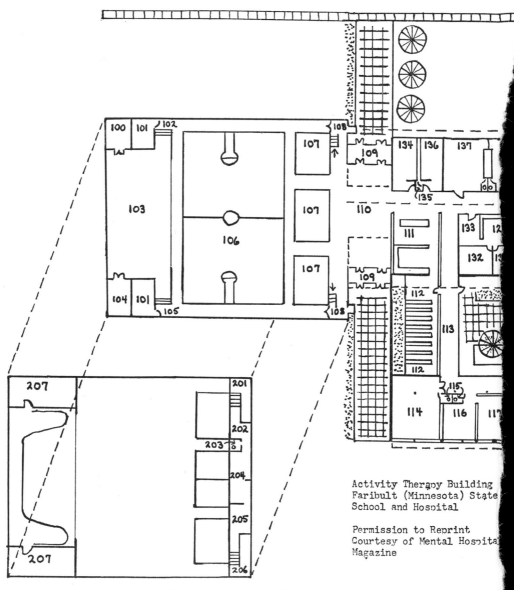

Activity Therapy Building
Faribult (Minnesota) State
School and Hospital

Permission to Reprint
Courtesy of Mental Hospital
Magazine

Figure 14. Activity Therapy Building, Faribult (Minnesota) S